Biological Monitoring Methods for Industrial Chemicals

Biological Monitoring Methods for Industrial Chemicals

RANDALL C. BASELT, Ph.D.
Associate Professor, Department of Pathology
Director, Toxicology and Drug Analysis Laboratory
University of California Medical Center, Sacramento

Biomedical Publications

Library of Congress Cataloging in Publication Data

Baselt, Randall C.
Biological monitoring methods for industrial chemicals.

Includes bibliographies and index.
1. Industrial toxicology. 2. Poisons — Analysis.
3. Body fluids — Analysis. 4. Indicators (Biology)
5. Environmental monitoring. I. Title.
[DNLM: 1. Environmental pollutants — Analysis.
2. Monitoring, Physiologic — Methods.
3. Poisons — Analysis. WA671 B299b]
RA1229.B37 615.9'02 79-56927
ISBN 0-931890-04-7

PREFACE

Much concern has been expressed during the last decade regarding the numerous toxic substances to which man is exposed at home and at work. In a few short years, we have seen the creation of large federal agencies, such as OSHA, NIOSH, EPA and NIEHS, each devoted wholly or partially to a particular aspect of the control of chemicals in our environment. One of the most promising areas of activity in our war on environmental and industrial poisons is the field of biological monitoring, the routine analysis of human tissues or excreta for direct or indirect evidence of exposure to chemical substances. It has been predicted that within a few more years the use of biological monitoring data, in conjunction with prudently established biological threshold limit values, will be a common, if not mandatory, practice in the management of chemical exposures in the workplace.

Before that is possible, a great deal of research must be done and much data collected and sifted. The purpose of this book is to compile into manageable form the existing data on the human disposition of chemicals which are amenable to biological monitoring, and to provide practical analytical methods for these chemicals or their metabolites in the appropriate specimens. Some of the methods included are currently employed in industry as routine tools, and their application to biological monitoring problems and the interpretive use of their quantitative data are well understood. Other substances, and methods for their determination, have been included to illustrate the potential for understanding their behavior in humans and to inspire further investigation on these and other important chemicals. It is hoped that this collection will act in some small way as a catalyst for the adoption of biological monitoring as a standard preventive measure in the practice of industrial hygiene and environmental safety.

RCB

CONTENTS

Biological Monitoring Methods for Industrial Chemicals

INTRODUCTION

PURPOSES OF BIOLOGICAL MONITORING

Biological monitoring is one element of a total environmental program for control of industrial chemical exposure, which also includes aspects such as employee physical examinations, environmental controls, protective clothing and equipment, and the monitoring of contaminants in workroom air. Due to ethical considerations in performing research on humans and obvious limitations in analytical methodology, it has been one of the least invoked and understood elements of a control program. Yet, as a highly sensitive index of an individual employee's exposure to chemicals, biological monitoring can be an effective and powerful tool for the industrial hygienist.

The methods used in routine biological monitoring are also often applicable to instances of chemical intoxication, in which it is necessary to confirm or to rule out the possibility that a particular substance has caused a toxic response. This type of laboratory examination is helpful not only in the treatment of an intoxicated individual, but in the prevention of further similar occurrences as well as in the establishment of liability for a chemical exposure.

SCOPE OF BIOLOGICAL MONITORING

Elkins (1954) is considered to be among the first to advocate the adoption of biological monitoring as an essential element of an industrial hygiene program, and has done pioneering work on correlations between exposure concentrations of industrial chemicals and their concentrations in body fluids. More recently, he has proposed the establishment of biological threshold limit values for chemicals in biological specimens, comparable to the threshold limit values for substances in the industrial atmosphere which have been used for many years (Elkins, 1967). Several excellent monographs or review articles have since appeared which deal with the general aspects of biological monitoring programs (Linch, 1974; Waritz, 1979), choice of specimens (Berlin et al., 1979), application of analytical methodology to specific chemicals (Piotrowski, 1971) or interpretation of analytical results in relation to the severity of exposure (Lauwerys, 1975). While biological monitoring is a young and rapidly developing science, it is apparent that it has many proponents and numerous advantages to offer to chemical exposure control programs.

CHOICE OF SPECIMENS

The many concerns over the type of specimen to use for biological monitoring have been addressed in recent reviews (Linch, 1974; Waritz, 1979). The primary variables to be considered in choosing a specimen include its routine availability, the metabolic profile of the specific chemical, availability of published reference limits, route of exposure, time of sampling, and characteristics of the analytical method to be employed.

Urine is one of the most frequently analyzed biological specimens, due to the ease of collection and the presence of nearly all exogenous chemicals or their metabolites in amounts which are often proportional to the absorbed dose. Urine may be collected as a spot sample, a timed specimen over a several hour period, or a 24 hour specimen. The latter type of collection, although desirable for purposes of accuracy in estimating exposure, has been found to be impractical in routine applications (Turner and Merlis, 1971). In most cases, urine should be stored refrigerated or frozen until the analysis is accomplished, rather than adding chemical preservatives (although some analytes require pH adjustment for stability). An allowance for urine dilution, when made, is usually based on specific gravity or creatinine content. The customary procedure in the United States involves correction to a specific gravity of 1.024 (Elkins et al., 1974), although other investigators have claimed average values of 1.016 for residents of England (Buchwald, 1965) and 1.018 for U.S. workers (Fishbeck et al., 1975). Due to these inconsistencies, it is probably preferable to express urine data in terms of creatinine content or on the basis of excretory rate of a substance.

Breath is also a specimen which is easily obtained without discomfort to the donor, but its use is limited to analysis of those substances of sufficiently high volatility to appear in breath in measurable amounts. The marked influence of atmospheric substance concentrations on breath concentrations and the rapid excretion of most volatile substances further limit the collection of expired breath specimens to a time point just after the end of exposure. One of the most serious considerations in breath sampling is the collection device which is used. It is highly recommended that a standardized device, of known integrity and compatability with the analyte, be used and that it be stored at a constant (preferably elevated) temperature until analysis (Pasquini, 1978).

Theoretically, blood is the body fluid which should show the best correlation with the atmospheric concentration of a substance, the amount absorbed (regardless of the route of administration), the degree of retention and the severity of effect. Due to practical considerations, however, such as the difficulty of obtaining frequent specimens, the low concentrations produced and its general unsuitability as an analytical matrix, blood is often avoided in favor of urine or breath. Blood containers and collection devices must usually be selected carefully for a specific application. For instance, whole blood is required for lead, erythrocyte cholinesterase or carbon monoxide analysis, necessitating the presence of an anticoagulant which does not interfere with the determination of the analyte. Fluoride and oxalate are good anticoagulants, but may be analytes themselves on occasion, and fluoride is known to inhibit enzymes such as cholinesterase. EDTA may interfere with lead analysis by some procedures, and heparin has been found to interfere in certain colorimetric methods. Furthermore, most commercial vacuum blood tubes are unsuitable for trace metal analyses due to contamination.

Other specimens which have been investigated for biological monitoring purposes include biopsy fat, saliva, breast milk, hair, nails and feces. Each of these specimens offers an advantage for specific monitoring situations, but each is fraught with its own difficulties in collection, storage and analysis. These difficulties must be recognized and solved prior to institution of a successful monitoring program.

LABORATORY QUALITY CONTROL

The requirements for a quality control program in a biological monitoring laboratory have been thoroughly discussed elsewhere (Linch, 1974; Berlin et al., 1979), and will not be repeated here. However, several items of special importance in the analysis of biological specimens bear stressing. The first is that the standards used to calibrate a method should resemble as closely as possible the specimen to be analyzed, in order to duplicate the effects of the biological materials on recovery and on background readings. When the analyte is a natural component of the specimen, which occurs frequently, it may be necessary to use aqueous standards or to invoke the method of standard additions. Second, the use of bulk quality control materials, an aliquot of which is analyzed together with each batch of specimens, contributes greatly to the reliability of each day's results. This material does not necessarily have to be of the same matrix as the specimen (although it is preferable) but it should be of a stable, homogenous nature; unfortunately, not all analytes are stable in solution for prolonged periods of time and therefore not all analytical procedures are subject to control by this method. Needless to say, both standards and quality control materials must be treated in a manner identical to that of the specimens during the analysis procedure.

References

A. Berlin, A. H. Wolff and Y. Hasegawa (eds.). *The Use of Biological Specimens for the Assessment of Human Exposure to Environment Pollutants,* Martinus Nyhoff, The Hague, 1979.

H. Buchwald. The specific gravity of urine specimens. Ann. Occ. Hyg. 8: 265, 1965.

H. B. Elkins. Analyses of biological materials as indices of exposure to organic solvents. Arch. Ind. Hyg. Occ. Med. 9: 212 - 222, 1954.

H. B. Elkins. Excretory and biological threshold limits. Am. Ind. Hyg. Asso. J. 28: 305 - 314, 1967.

H. B. Elkins, L. D. Pagnotto and H. L. Smith. Concentration adjustments in urinalysis. Am. Ind. Hyg. Asso. J. 35: 559 - 565, 1974.

W. A. Fishbeck, R. R. Langer and R. J. Kociba. Elevated urinary phenol levels not related to benzene exposure. Am. Ind. Hyg. Asso. J. 36: 820 - 824, 1975.

R. Lauwerys. Biological criteria for selected industrial toxic chemicals: a review. Scand. J. Work Env. Health 1: 139 - 172, 1975.

A. L. Linch. *Biological Monitoring for Industrial Chemical Exposure Control,* CRC Press, W. Palm Beach, Florida, 1974.

D. A. Pasquini. Evaluation of glass sampling tubes for industrial breath analysis. Am. Ind. Hyg. Asso. J. 39: 55 - 62, 1978.

J. K. Piotrowski. *The Application of Metabolic and Excretion Kinetics to Problems of Industrial Toxicology,* U.S. Government Printing Office, Washington, D.C., 1971.

J. K. Piotrowski. *Exposure Tests for Organic Compounds in Industrial Toxicology,* U.S. Government Printing Office, Washington, D.C., 1977.

W. J. Turner and S. Merlis. Vicissitudes in research: the twenty-four hour urine collection. Clin. Pharm. Ther. 12: 163 - 166, 1971.

R. S. Waritz. Biological indicators of chemical dosage and burden. In *Patty's Industrial Hygiene and Toxicology,* Vol. 3 (L. V. Cralley and L. J. Cralley, eds.), John Wiley and Sons, New York, 1979, pp. 257 - 318.

ACETALDEHYDE

Occurrence and Usage. Acetaldehyde is a volatile liquid used in the manufacture of a number of synthetic chemical products, including certain plastics, dyes and resins. It is also present in fairly high concentrations in cigarette smoke. The current threshold limit value is 100 ppm (180 mg/m^3) in the industrial atmosphere.

Blood Concentrations. Acetaldehyde has not been determined in the blood of persons exposed to the vapor. The substance is a metabolite of ethanol and paraldehyde, however, and has been measured following the administration of these drugs. Endogenous blood acetaldehyde levels probably do not exceed 0.2 mg/L. An acute oral dose of ethanol to volunteers produces blood acetaldehyde concentrations of 0.9 - 1.3 mg/L, whereas in chronic alcoholics, these levels may range from 1.7 - 2.5 mg/L (Korsten et al., 1975). Following co-administration of ethanol and an inhibitor of acetaldehyde metabolism, such as disulfiram or calcium carbamide, acetaldehyde blood concentrations may increase five to tenfold over normal levels (Truitt and Walsh, 1971).

Metabolism and Excretion. The major portion of a dose of acetaldehyde is metabolized to acetic acid and then to carbon dioxide. Urinary excretion of acetaldehyde during periods of elevated blood levels has been suggested, but not documented (Truitt and Walsh, 1971). A certain portion is also excreted unchanged in the expired breath. A single acute dose of ethanol (78 mL/70 kg) produces maximal breath acetaldehyde concentrations of 0.007 - 0.010 mg/L (Freund and O'Hollaren, 1965).

Toxicity. Low to moderate air concentrations of acetaldehyde (50 - 200 ppm) cause eye irritation and upper respiratory discomfort. Higher concentrations may cause dyspnea and central nervous system depression.

Biological Monitoring. Acetaldehyde concentrations in breath, blood or urine have not been correlated with occupational exposure to acetaldehyde. It is likely that breath and blood acetaldehyde concentrations correlate best with the degree of exposure, and that breath concentrations exceeding 0.01 mg/L and blood concentrations exceeding 0.5 mg/L represent significant exposure to acetaldehyde in subjects who have not recently ingested ethanol.

Analysis. A procedure is presented for the analysis of blood or urine acetaldehyde by direct-injection gas chromatography (Brien and Loomis, 1978). The technique is also applicable to the determination of breath samples.

References

J. F. Brien and C. W. Loomis. Gas-liquid chromatographic determination of ethanol and acetaldehyde in blood. Clin. Chim. Acta 87: 175 - 180, 1978.

G. Freund and P. O'Hollaren. Acetaldehyde concentrations in alveolar air following a standard dose of ethanol in man. J. Lipid Res. 6: 471 - 477, 1965.

M. A. Korsten, S. Matsuzaki, L. Feinman and C. S. Lieber. High blood acetaldehyde levels after ethanol administration. New Eng. J. Med. 292: 386 - 389, 1975.

E. B. Truitt, Jr. and M. J. Walsh. In *The Biology of Alcoholism*, Vol. 1 (B. Kissin and H. Begleiter, eds.), Plenum Press, New York, 1971, pp. 161 - 195.

Blood and Urine Acetaldehyde by Gas Chromatography

Principle:

An internal standard is added to the specimen. The solution is deproteinized with perchloric acid and the supernatant is subjected to headspace analysis using flame-ionization gas chromatography.

Reagents:

Stock solution — 1 mg/mL acetaldehyde in water
Blood or urine standards — 1, 2, 5, 10 and 20 mg/L
7.6% Thiourea in water
Internal standard — 3.0 g/L 1-propanol in water
34 g/L Perchloric acid

Solutions are to be cooled to 4° C. prior to analysis.

Instrumental Conditions:

Gas chromatograph with flame-ionization detector
1.8 m x 2 mm i.d. glass column containing 5% Carbowax 20M on Haloport F
Injector, 100° C.; column, 90° C.; detector, 150° C.
Helium flow rate, 30 mL/min

Procedure:

1. Transfer 1 mL blood or urine to a 30 mL polycarbonate tube. Add 100 μL 7.6% thiourea and 250 μL internal standard and vortex.
2. Add 8.65 mL dilute perchloric acid and vortex for 15 sec. Centrifuge for 10 min at 4° C.
3. Transfer 2 mL of the supernatant to a 30 mL vial and seal with a rubber septum. Heat the vial at 60° C. for 30 min and inject 1 mL of the headspace into the chromatograph.

	Retention time (min)
acetaldehyde	0.7
internal standard	2.2

Calculation:

Calculation is based on a standard curve prepared each time an analysis is performed. This procedure cannot be controlled by the usual methods due to the instability of acetaldehyde-containing solutions.

Evaluation:

Sensitivity: 0.25 mg/L
Linearity: 0.25 - 20 mg/L
C.V.: 6% at 10 mg/L
Relative Recovery: 105%

Interferences:

Ethanol is known to separate from acetaldehyde, but other volatiles have not been studied for potential interference. The addition of thiourea to blood inhibits the non-enzymatic formation of acetaldehyde.

ACETONE

Occurrence and Usage. Acetone is frequently employed as a solvent for paints, plastics and adhesives and as a chemical intermediate. The current threshold limit value for industry is 1000 ppm (2400 mg/m^3) of the vapor in the air, although this will likely be lowered to 750 ppm in the near future.

Blood Concentrations. In healthy adults, endogenous acetone blood levels (up to 10 mg/L) are unmeasurable by routine gas chromatographic techniques. Acetone concentrations are markedly elevated during diabetic or fasting ketoacidosis and may range from 100-700 mg/L (Ramu et al., 1978). Blood acetone levels in 8 volunteers peaked at 20 and 100 mg/L at the end of a 2 hour exposure to 100 and 500 ppm, respectively, of acetone vapor. The levels declined with a half-life of 3 hours (DiVincenzo et al., 1973).

Some accumulation occurs when acetone is breathed on a daily basis; in a subject exposed to air containing 2100 ppm for 8 hours daily, accumulation occurred for 3 days until steady-state was attained. The peak blood level (at the end of the 8-hour day) was 182 mg/L and the trough level measured 16 hours later was 91 mg/L. Intoxication was not observed in subjects with blood concentrations as high as 330 mg/L (Haggard et al., 1944).

Metabolism and Excretion. Acetone is metabolized by oxidation at a relatively slow rate, 1 - 3 mg/kg/hr in most subjects tested. At higher blood concentrations, the majority of the chemical is removed by excretion, primarily in the breath and to a lesser extent in the urine. The average blood/breath acetone concentration ratio is 330 (range 322 - 339), whereas the average ratio between urine and blood is 1.34 (Haggard et al., 1944). In 4 subjects who were exposed to 500 ppm of acetone for 2 hours, the 24-hour urine specimens contained an average of 3.5 mg of acetone (DiVincenzo et al., 1973).

Toxicity. Acetone is considered to be relatively nontoxic, causing eye irritation at air concentrations of 1000 - 6000 ppm and central nervous system depression at concentrations exceeding 10,000 ppm. Several workers who developed symptoms of acute intoxication (dizziness and muscular weakness) on exposure to air concentrations of at least 12,000 ppm exhibited urine acetone concentrations of 46-72 mg/L (Ross, 1973). Hyperglycemia has been noted as a frequent finding during acetone intoxication resulting from either ingestion or inhalation of the chemical (Gitelson et al., 1966). An individual who ingested acetone and became lethargic was noted to have a blood acetone level of 2500 mg/L which declined with a half-life of 31 hours (Ramu et al., 1978).

Biological Monitoring. Specimens of breath, blood or urine taken at the end of a work shift which contain more than 0.6, 200 or 270 mg/L of acetone, respectively, are indicative of excessive exposure to acetone. Pre-exposure specimens should be analyzed to insure the absence of significant levels of acetone resulting from metabolism of endogenous substances.

Analysis. The following gas chromatographic method is applicable to the determination of acetone and other volatiles in blood, breath and urine (Baselt and Barrett, 1975).

References

R. Baselt and C. Barrett. Unpublished results, 1975.

G. D. DiVincenzo, F. J. Yanno and B. D. Astill. Exposure of man and dog to low concentrations of acetone vapor. Am. Ind. Hyg. Asso. J. 34: 329 - 336, 1973.

S. Gitelson, A. Werczberger and J.B. Herman. Coma and hyperglycemia following drinking of acetone. Diabetes 15: 810 - 811, 1966.

H. W. Haggard, L. A. Greenberg and J. M. Turner. The physiological principles governing the action of acetone together with determination of toxicity. J. Ind. Hyg. Tox. 5: 133 - 151, 1944.

A. Ramu, J. Rosenbaum and T. F. Blaschke. Disposition of acetone following acute acetone intoxication. West. J. Med. 129: 429-432, 1978.

D. S. Ross. Acute acetone intoxication involving eight male workers. Ann. Occ. Hyg. 16: 73-75, 1973.

Blood and Urine Volatiles by Gas Chromatography

Principle:

The specimen is diluted with an equal volume of the internal standard, an aqueous solution of methyl ethyl ketone. The mixture is injected directly into a gas chromatograph equipped with a flame-ionization detector.

Reagents:

Stock solutions — 100 mg/mL aqueous solutions of acetaldehyde, acetone, ethanol, isopropanol and methanol

Blood or urine standards — 50, 100, 200, 500 and 1000 mg/L for each chemical

Internal standard solution — 1 mL methyl ethyl ketone per L of water

Instrumental Conditions:

Gas chromatograph with replaceable glass injector sleeve and flame-ionization detector

6′ x 1/8″ stainless-steel column containing 0.2% Carbowax on 60/80 mesh Carbopack C (Supelco)

Injector, 200° C.; column, 125° C.; detector, 200° C.

Nitrogen flow rate, 17 mL/min

Procedure:

1. Transfer 100 μL blood or urine to a plastic micro-centrifuge tube. Add 100 μL internal standard and vortex.
2. Inject 0.5 μL of the solution into the gas chromatograph using a 5 μL direct-injection syringe (Hamilton #7105 N) which has been pre-loaded with 0.5 μL of water. Withdraw the needle and immediately rinse the syringe with water.

	Retention time (min)
acetaldehyde	0.6
methanol	0.6
ethanol	0.9
acetone	1.1
isopropanol	1.3
internal standard	2.3

Calculation:

Calculation is based on a response factor derived from a standard curve. A quality control specimen containing 200 mg/L of each of the appropriate chemicals is analyzed daily.

Evaluation:

Sensitivity: 25 mg/L
Linearity: 50 - 1000 mg/L
C.V.: 2 - 4%
Relative recovery: not established

Interferences:

The injection technique must be standardized in order to obtain reproducible results. The glass insert for the injector should be replaced after every 10 - 20 injections, replacing the septum at the same time. Acetaldehyde co-elutes with methanol in this procedure; if this presents a problem, a column containing Porapak Q will resolve these two substances. Breath samples may be analyzed by direct injection of 1 - 2 mL, using as standards suitably prepared dilutions of the appropriate chemical in air.

ACETONITRILE

Occurrence and Usage. Acetonitrile, or methyl cyanide, is a clear liquid used as a laboratory and industrial solvent and as a synthetic intermediate. The current threshold limit value is 40 ppm (70 mg/m^3) in the industrial atmosphere, which is approximately the odor threshold of the vapor.

Blood Concentrations. Acetonitrile has not been measured in blood or plasma. However, the metabolites of acetonitrile, cyanide and thiocyanate, may be determined in blood as an index of exposure. In normal persons, blood cyanide is usually less than 0.04 mg/L and plasma thiocyanate levels less than 12 mg/L. Cyanide was not detected in the blood of volunteers exposed to a concentration of 160 ppm acetonitrile vapor for four hours (Pozzani, 1959).

Metabolism and Excretion. Acetonitrile is known to produce cyanide *in vivo,* which is further metabolized to thiocyanate. It has been estimated that at least 12% of an inhaled dose of the chemical is metabolized in this manner, and undoubtedly a substantial portion is exhaled unchanged in the breath. In normal subjects thiocyanate urine levels may range from 1 - 17 mg/L. Urine thiocyanate concentrations were not significantly elevated in volunteers exposed to a concentration of 160 ppm acetonitrile vapor for four hours (Pozzani, 1959).

Toxicity. Acetonitrile vapor concentrations of up to 500 ppm cause irritation of mucous membranes, whereas higher concentrations may produce weakness, nausea, convulsions and death. Blood cyanide concentrations of 3 - 11 mg/L and serum thiocyanate levels of 160 - 230 mg/L were observed in two workers suffering severe toxicity due to exposure to high concentrations of acetonitrile. Serum thiocyanate concentrations of less than 120 mg/L were associated with less severe symptoms such as weakness, nausea and abdominal pain in other subjects. An individual who died about 2 hours after a 12 hour exposure to acetonitrile had the following cyanide concentrations detected in his tissues at autopsy (Amdur, 1959):

Cyanide Concentrations in an Acetonitrile Fatality (mg/L or mg/kg)

Blood	Lung	Liver	Spleen	Kidney	Urine
8.0	1.3	0	3.2	2.0	2.2

Biological Monitoring. Blood cyanide concentrations exceeding 0.1 mg/L or plasma or urine thiocyanate concentrations exceeding 20 mg/L in workers exposed to acetonitrile are indicative of excessive exposure. Pre-exposure specimens should be analyzed to establish each individual's background levels, which are often elevated in smokers.

Analysis. Procedures are presented for the analysis of blood cyanide and plasma and urine thiocyanate in the section on cyanide (p. 94).

References

M. L. Amdur. Accidental group exposure to acetonitrile. J. Occ. Med. 1: 627 - 633, 1959.

U. C. Pozzani, C. P. Carpenter, P. E. Palm et al. Mammalian toxicity of acetonitrile. J. Occ. Med. 1: 634 - 642, 1959.

ACRYLONITRILE

Occurrence and Usage. Acrylonitrile (vinyl cyanide) is used extensively in the manufacture of plastics, synthetic fibers and adhesives. It is also employed as a chemical intermediate and as a fumigant. The current threshold limit value for the vapor is 20 ppm (45 mg/m^3). Acrylonitrile has been proposed for classification as a carcinogen, with no assigned exposure limit.

Blood Concentrations. The compound is readily absorbed following inhalation of the vapor or during dermal contact with the liquid. Acrylonitrile has not been detected in the blood of animals exposed to lethal concentrations of the vapor. The metabolites of acrylonitrile, cyanide and thiocyanate, may be measured in blood as an index of exposure (Brieger et al., 1952). In normal unexposed subjects, blood cyanide is usually less than 0.04 mg/L and plasma thiocyanate levels less than 12 mg/L. Plasma thiocyanate achieves a maximum at the end of an exposure to acrylonitrile; Lawton et al. (1943) stated that levels exceeding 20 mg/L in non-smokers and 30 mg/L in smokers were indicative of overexposure to the chemical.

Metabolism and Excretion. Acrylonitrile is known to produce cyanide *in vivo,* which is further metabolized to thiocyanate. The extent of this biotransformation is unknown, and it is likely that a portion of an absorbed dose of the chemical is exhaled unchanged in the breath. Attempts to relate urine thiocyanate concentrations to the level of exposure to acrylonitrile vapor were unsuccessful due to the wide normal range of thiocyanate in urine (Brieger et al., 1952). However, Lawton et al. (1943) found that urinary thiocyanate levels reached a maximum 24 to 48 hours after an exposure, and that levels exceeding 2 mg/24 hours in non-smokers and 16 mg/24 hours in smokers were indicative of overexposure to the chemical.

Toxicity. Mild cases of intoxication due to acrylonitrile usually involve eye irritation, headache, nausea and weakness. Severe toxicity results in asphyxia and death due to cyanide poisoning. Exposure to concentrations exceeding 150 ppm for four hours has caused serious toxicity in monkeys (Dudley et al., 1942).

Biological Monitoring. Blood cyanide concentrations exceeding 0.1 mg/L or plasma or urine thiocyanate concentrations exceeding 20 mg/L in workers exposed to acrylonitrile are indicative of excessive exposure. Pre-exposure specimens should be analyzed to establish each individual's background levels, which are often elevated in smokers. The pending reclassification of acrylonitrile as a carcinogen will require that no exposure be detectable using the most sensitive method available.

Analysis. Procedures are presented for the analysis of blood cyanide and plasma and urine thiocyanate in the section on cyanide (p. 94).

References

H. Brieger, F. Rieders and W. A. Hodes. Acrylonitrile: spectrophotometric determination, acute toxicity, and mechanism of action. Arch. Ind. Hyg. Occ. Med. 6: 128 - 140, 1952.

H. C. Dudley, T. R. Sweeney and J. W. Miller. Toxicology of acrylonitrile (vinyl cyanide). J. Ind. Hyg. Tox. 24: 255 - 258, 1942.

A. H. Lawton, T. R. Sweeney and H. C. Dudley. Toxicology of acrylonitrile (vinyl cyanide). J. Ind. Hyg. Tox. 25: 13 - 19, 1943.

ALDRIN

Occurrence and Usage. Aldrin (octalene) is a chlorinated naphthalene derivative which has been used as an insecticide since 1950. It is closely related to two other members of the cyclodiene class, dieldrin and endrin. Aldrin has been banned from use in some countries due to its persistence in the environment and its potential for chronic toxicity. The current threshold limit value for industrial exposure is 0.25 mg/m^3.

Blood Concentrations. Blood concentrations of dieldrin, an aldrin metabolite, averaged 0.0014 mg/L in 10 persons with no occupational exposure to insecticides. About 80% of whole blood dieldrin was restricted to the plasma. Serum concentrations in persons with low to high occupational exposure to aldrin and dieldrin averaged 0.0007 - 0.0023 mg/L for aldrin and 0.0094 - 0.0270 mg/L for dieldrin (Dale et al., 1966). The average half-life of dieldrin in blood is 97 days, with a range of 50 - 167 days (Brown et al., 1964).

Metabolism and Excretion. Aldrin is metabolized in man by epoxide formation, converting it to dieldrin. Aldrin and dieldrin are approximately equitoxic, but it is as dieldrin that the compound accumulates in the body fat of man and other animals. Concentrations of dieldrin in fat from 131 autopsies in England averaged 0.21 mg/kg (range 0 - 1.29), with no significant correlation to sex, age, place of abode or cause of death (Hunter et al., 1963). In industrially exposed workers, dieldrin concentrations in fat averaged 6.12 mg/kg (range 0.60 - 32). Aldrin is slowly eliminated from the body, primarily as unknown hydrophilic metabolites, in feces and to a slight extent in urine. Unchanged aldrin is not found in the urine of workers exposed to the chemical, although dieldrin concentrations may range up to 0.07 mg/L (Hayes and Curley, 1968).

Toxicity. Aldrin produces central nervous system excitation after both acute and chronic overexposure; poisoning is manifested by nausea, dizziness, headache, involuntary movements, convulsions and loss of consciousness. Blood dieldrin concentrations of 4 aldrin workers who displayed moderate to severe symptoms of chronic intoxication ranged from 0.04 - 0.53 mg/L; fat concentrations in 2 of these subjects 2 - 3 weeks after the last exposure were 60 and 149 mg/kg (Kazantzis et al., 1964). Brown et al. (1964) have established a threshold blood dieldrin concentration of 0.16 - 0.25 mg/L for the expression of signs of intoxication due to aldrin or dieldrin. An individual who ingested aldrin was found to have characteristic signs of poisoning and aldrin and dieldrin plasma concentrations of 0.036 and 0.279 mg/L, respectively, 18 hours after ingestion; after 20 days, when recovering, these concentrations had fallen to 0.002 and 0.090 mg/L, respectively (Dale et al., 1966). The acute lethal dose of aldrin in man is believed to range from 3 - 7 g of the compound (Spiotta, 1951).

Biological Monitoring. Plasma dieldrin concentrations in excess of 0.005 mg/L are indicative of significant exposure in workers occupationally exposed to aldrin.

Analysis. Aldrin and dieldrin may be determined in biological specimens by electron-capture gas chromatography, using a scheme which includes many other organochlorine insecticides (Dale et al., 1966).

References

V. K. H. Brown, C. G. Hunter and A. Richardson. A blood test diagnostic of exposure to aldrin and dieldrin. Brit. J. Ind. Med. 21: 283 - 286, 1964.

W. E. Dale, A. Curley and C. Cueto, Jr. Hexane extractable chlorinated insecticides in human blood. Life Sci. 5: 47 - 54, 1966.

W. J. Hayes and A. Curley. Storage and excretion of dieldrin and related compounds. Arch. Env. Health 16: 155 - 162, 1968.

C. G. Hunter, J. Robinson and A. Richardson. Chlorinated insecticide content of human body fat in southern England. Brit. Med. J. 1: 221 - 224, 1963.

G. Kazantzis, A. I. G. McLaughlin and P. F. Prior. Poisoning in industrial workers by the insecticide aldrin. Brit. J. Ind. Med. 21: 46 - 51, 1964.

E. J. Spiotta. Aldrin poisoning in man. Arch. Ind. Hyg. Occ. Med. 4: 560 - 566, 1951.

Plasma Organochlorine Pesticides by Electron-Capture Gas Chromatography

Principle:

The chlorinated hydrocarbon insecticides and their metabolites are extracted from plasma with hexane. The concentrated extract is analyzed by electron-capture gas chromatography on 10% DEGS, using a second column for confirmation of positive results.

Reagents:

Stock solutions — 1 mg/L hexane solutions of the appropriate agents
Plasma standards — 0.001, 0.005, 0.010, 0.050 and 0.100 mg/L of the appropriate agent
Hexane (nanograde)
Sodium sulfate — anhydrous Na_2SO_4

Instrumental Conditions:

Gas chromatograph with electron-capture detector
2 m x 2 mm i.d. aluminum column containing 10% diethylene glycol succinate on 60/80 mesh Chromosorb G

1.2 m x 2 mm i.d. aluminum column containing 5% Dow 200 on 60/80 mesh Chromosorb G
Injector, 224° C.; column, 180° C.; detector, 224° C.
Nitrogen flow rate, 80 mL/min

Procedure:

1. Transfer 2 mL plasma to a 15 mL glass-stoppered centrifuge tube. Add 5 mL hexane and shake to extract.
2. Centrifuge and discard the lower aqueous phase with the aid of a disposable pipet. Add a small amount of solid Na_2SO_4 and vortex.
3. Transfer 4 mL of the hexane to a 15 mL centrifuge tube and evaporate to dryness under a stream of nitrogen at 40° C.
4. Dissolve the residue in 50 μL hexane and inject 10 μL into the gas chromatograph, using either column.

	Retention time (min)	
	10% DEGS	5% Dow 200
aldrin	3.1	11.3
α - BHC	4.4	4.2
γ - BHC (lindane)	7.0	5.2
o,p′ - DDE	8.4	17.8
heptachlor epoxide	9.6	14.4
p,p′ - DDE	11.3	22.0
dieldrin	14.4	22.0
o,p′ - DDT	16.0	28.7
δ - BHC	21.0	5.2
β - BHC	23.8	4.6
p,p′ - DDT	30.3	38.2
p,p′ - DDD	38.3	28.7

Calculation:

Calculation is based on a response factor derived from a standard curve. A quality control specimen containing the appropriate agent at a mid-range concentration is analyzed daily.

Evaluation:

Sensitivity: 0.0001 mg/L
Linearity: 0.001 - 0.100 mg/L
C.V.: not established
Relative recovery: not established

Interferences:

In order to prevent contamination from reagents and glassware, reagent blanks must be frequently analyzed. The use of two chromatographic columns to confirm positive results increases the specificity of the method.

ANILINE

Occurrence and Usage. Aniline is a colorless aromatic liquid which tends to darken on exposure to light. The compound is widely used as a chemical intermediate and solvent and in the manufacture of synthetic dyes. The threshold limit value in the industrial atmosphere is currently 5 ppm (19 mg/m^3), although a proposed revision to 2 ppm is pending. Exposure to aniline is commonly by inhalation of the vapor or by cutaneous absorption of the liquid; probably the latter mode is of the greatest toxicological importance in industry (Piotrowski, 1977).

Blood Concentrations. Aniline has not been measured in blood except in experimental studies with animals. The measurement of blood methemoglobin levels as an index of exposure to aniline will be described.

Metabolism and Excretion. Aniline has not been found in the exhaled air of subjects exposed to it. Less than 1% of an absorbed dose of aniline is excreted unchanged in the urine. From 15 to 60% is oxidized to p-aminophenol, which is excreted in the urine as glucuronide and sulfate conjugates, primarily in the first 24 hours after exposure. The production of this metabolite is more efficient at higher doses of aniline (Piotrowski, 1977). A minor metabolite, phenylhydroxylamine, is apparently responsible for many of the toxic effects produced by aniline (Jenkins et al., 1972). Linch (1974) considers that a urinary p-aminophenol concentration of 10 mg/L is a warning of potentially toxic exposure to aniline and that a concentration of 20 mg/L indicates the need for medical intervention. Piotrowski (1977) has shown that the rate of urinary excretion of p-aminophenol in a timed urine specimen taken at the end of an exposure period may be used to estimate the amount of aniline absorbed by a subject, over a range of 10 - 100 mg. At the current threshold limit value (5 ppm), an 8 hour exposure would result in the absorption of approximately 150 mg of aniline and would lead to a p-aminophenol urinary excretion rate over the last 2 hours of exposure of 13 mg/hour. The urinary p-aminophenol concentration also appears to be directly related to blood methemoglobin levels in workers exposed to aniline (Pacseri, 1961).

Toxicity. Acute or chronic exposure to aniline may produce symptoms of headache, dizziness and nausea. Single oral 15 mg doses of the chemical given to volunteers caused no effects, whereas a dose of 25 mg produced increases of blood methemoglobin of 2% and a dose of 65 mg increased methemoglobin by 16%. Many of the toxic effects of aniline are believed due to the metabolite, phenylhydroxylamine (Jenkins et al., 1972). A methemoglobin level of 15% is consistent with clinical cyanosis, and levels exceeding 60% may be life-threatening.

Biological Monitoring. An increase of blood methemoglobin concentration of 2% over the background level is indicative of significant exposure to aniline. Urine p-aminophenol concentrations greater than 10 mg/L or a urinary excretion rate greater than 13 mg/hr of p-aminophenol represent excessive exposure to aniline.

Analysis. A procedure is presented for the determination of blood methemoglobin content by visible spectrophotometry (Evelyn and Malloy, 1938). This procedure is also useful for assessment of exposure to other amino and nitro compounds which cause methemoglobinemia, such as nitrobenzene. p-Aminophenol may be determined in urine, following acid hydrolysis of conjugates, by a colorimetric procedure (Greenberg and Lester, 1948). It should be noted that urinary p-aminophenol concentrations may reach values as high as 200 mg/L following the ingestion of the drug phenacetin, and therefore the use of this drug must be ruled out when performing aniline exposure tests (Piotrowski, 1977).

References

K. A. Evelyn and H. T. Malloy. Microdetermination of oxyhemoglobin, methemoglobin, and sulfhemoglobin in a single sample of blood. J. Biol. Chem. 126: 655 - 662, 1938.

L. A. Greenberg and D. Lester. The metabolic fate of acetanilid and other aniline derivatives. J. Pharm. Exp. Ther. 88: 87 - 98, 1948.

F. P. Jenkins, J. A. Robinson, J. B. M. Gellatly and G. W. A. Salmond. The no-effect dose of aniline in human subjects and a comparison of aniline toxicity in man and the rat. Food Cosmet. Tox. 10: 671 - 679, 1972.

A. L. Linch. Biological monitoring for industrial exposure to cyanogenic aromatic nitro and amino compounds. Am. Ind. Hyg. Asso. J. 35: 426 - 432, 1974.

J. Pacseri. p-Aminophenol excretion as an index of aniline exposure. Pure Appl. Chem. 3: 313 - 314, 1961.

J. K. Piotrowski. *Exposure Tests for Organic Compounds in Industrial Toxicology,* U.S. Government Printing Office, Washington, D.C., 1977, pp. 70-75.

Blood Methemoglobin by Visible Spectrophotometry

Principle:

Whole blood is diluted with an aqueous buffer and the characteristic absorption of methemoglobin at 635 nm is measured. The change in optical density following the conversion of methemoglobin to cyanmethemoglobin is directly proportional to the concentration of methemoglobin in the specimen. Total hemoglobin must also be determined in order to express the final answer as a percentage.

Reagents:

0.017 mol/L pH 6.6 Phosphate buffer
0.067 mol/L pH 6.6 Phosphate buffer

20% Potassium ferricyanide
10% Sodium cyanide
12% Acetic acid
Neutralized cyanide solution — prepare fresh by adding equal parts of 10% NaCN and 12% acetic acid (prepare and use in hood!)
Concentrated ammonium hydroxide

Instrumental Conditions:

Visible spectrophotometer capable of optical density measurements at 635 and 540 nm

Procedure:

1. Transfer 100 μL whole oxalated blood to a tube containing 10 mL of 0.017 mol/L phosphate buffer. Vortex and allow to stand for 5 min.
2. Determine the optical density of this solution at 635 against a water blank. This reading is L_1.
3. Add 1 drop of neutralized cyanide solution to the solution in the sample cuvette, mix and after two minutes repeat the spectrophotometer determination at 635 nm. This reading is L_2.
4. Add 1 drop conc. NH_4OH to the sample cuvette, mix and transfer 2 mL of this solution to a tube containing 8 mL 0.067 mol/L phosphate buffer. Add 1 drop 20% potassium ferricyanide, vortex and allow to stand for 2 min.
5. Further add 1 drop 10% NaCN and vortex. After 2 min determine the optical density at 540 nm of this solution against a blank containing 10 mL water and 1 drop each of 20% potassium ferricyanide and 10% NaCN. This reading is L_4.

Calculation:

Calculate methemoglobin (M) in the sample using this equation:

$$M\ (\text{g}/100\ \text{mL blood}) = \frac{100\ (L_1 - L_2)}{2.77}$$

Calculate total hemoglobin (T) in the sample using this equation:

$$T\ (\text{g}/100\ \text{mL blood}) = \frac{100 \times L_4}{2.38}$$

Express methemoglobin as a percentage of total hemoglobin using this equation:

$$\%\ M = \frac{M}{T} \times 100\%$$

Quality control materials are not applicable to this procedure.

Evaluation:

Sensitivity: 1% methemoglobin
Linearity: 1 - 70% methemoglobin
C.V.: not established
Relative recovery: not established

Interferences:

Since sulfhemoglobin cannot be converted to cyanmethemoglobin with the reagents used, there is a slight inaccuracy in the total hemoglobin determination if sulfhemoglobin is present in substantial amounts. Other blood pigments do not interfere in the determination of methemoglobin, since the measurement is based on a differential reading, but blood specimens which have been allowed to stand for a period of time may develop methemoglobin spontaneously. Methemoglobinemia in man may be produced by exposure to many industrial chemicals and even certain drugs. In normal healthy subjects, the methemoglobin content of the blood is less than 1%.

Urine p-Aminophenol by Colorimetry

Principle:

Urine is acid-hydrolyzed to free conjugates of p-aminophenol. The cooled solution is extracted with an organic solvent, which is then back-extracted with dilute acid. The acid layer is reacted with α-naphthol and analyzed by spectrophotometry at 620 nm.

Reagents:

Stock solution — 1 mg/mL p-aminophenol in water
Urine standards — 5, 10, 20 and 50 mg/L
6 mol/L Hydrochloric acid
Solid $K_2HPO_4.3H_2O$
Ethylene dichloride
0.1 mol/L Hydrochloric acid
10% α-naphthol in ethanol
10 mol/L Sodium hydroxide

Instrumental Conditions:

Visible spectrophotometer set to 620 nm

Procedure:

1. Transfer 4 mL urine to a 15 mL glass-stoppered tube and add 2 mL 6 mol/L HCl. Stopper lightly and heat in a boiling water bath for 45 min.
2. Transfer 2 mL of the mixture to a 25 mL glass-stoppered graduated cylinder and add 7 g K_2HPO_4. Extract with 10 mL ethylene dichloride.
3. Let mixture stand to separate layers and transfer 5 mL of the solvent layer to a clean 25 mL cylinder. Extract with 15 mL 0.1 mol/L HCl.
4. Transfer 10 mL of the acid layer to a 15 mL centrifuge tube. Add 2 drops 10% α-naphthol and 4 drops 10 mol/L NaOH.
5. Place the tube in a 95° C. water bath for exactly 1 min. Cool immediately in cold water and analyze an aliquot at 620 nm against a urine blank.

Calculation:

Calculation is based on a response factor derived from a standard curve. A quality control specimen containing 10 mg/L p-aminophenol is analyzed daily.

Evaluation:

Sensitivity: 0.2 mg/L
Linearity: 1 - 90 mg/L
C.V.: not established
Relative recovery: not established

Interferences:

Hydrolyzed urine from normal subjects yields a background value of up to 6 mg/L apparent p-aminophenol.

ANTIMONY

Occurrence and Usage. Various salts of both trivalent and pentavalent antimony have been used for centuries as drugs, and they continue to be available as parasiticides for parenteral administration. Inorganic salts of antimony are used as pigments, abrasives and for flame proofing fabrics, whereas metallic antimony is found in a number of alloys. Industrial exposure is usually via inhalation. The current threshold limit value for compounds of antimony is 0.5 mg/m^3 of air, calculated as the metal.

Blood Concentrations. Since trivalent antimony is largely bound to erythrocytes when present in blood, and pentavalent antimony is primarily found in plasma, whole blood is the preferred specimen for assay. Whole blood antimony concentrations in healthy subjects not exposed to the metal rarely exceed 0.01 mg/L. During intravenous therapy with sodium antimony1 tartrate (20 mg antimony administered once every 48 hours for 42 days), blood antimony concentrations averaged 0.52 mg/L at 1 hour after injection and 0.07 mg/L at 48 hours after injection. These levels did not fluctuate significantly throughout the course of therapy (Ozawa, 1956).

Metabolism and Excretion. Soluble forms of trivalent or pentavalent antimony, when administered by inhalation or parenteral injection, appear to be rapidly absorbed and eliminated, largely in urine and to a slight extent in feces. On the other hand, inhalation of insoluble forms or oral ingestion of soluble forms usually results in slow absorption and therefore prolonged elimination from the body. In general, the excretion of pentavalent antimony is more rapid than that of the trivalent form. The liver contains the highest concentration of antimony of any organ in the body during therapeutic administration of antimonials and has the ability to reduce the pentavalent form to the trivalent form. Urine antimony concentrations in persons not exposed to the metal occupationally are usually less than 0.001 mg/L. Occupationally exposed but asymptomatic individuals may develop urine concentrations of up to 0.3 mg/L. During therapy with antimonials, however, urine concentrations may reach 2 mg/L within the first 24 hours after an injection and antimony may still be detectable 100 days after the discontinuation of therapy (Ozawa, 1956; Stemmer, 1976; Taylor, 1966). A smelter worker with antimony pneumoconiosis showed a urine antimony level of 0.05 mg/L seven months after retirement, and a level of 0.03 mg/L over three years later (McCallum, 1963).

Toxicity. The effects of acute or chronic antimony poisoning are similar to those produced by arsenic and include abdominal pain, dyspnea, nausea, vomiting, dermatitis and eye irritation. There is some indication that the body burden of antimony increases with prolonged exposure, although this apparently does not occur to the same extent as with many other toxic metals. Occupational poisoning is most frequently related to the inhalation of antimony compounds, such as the oxide or trichloride, either as fumes or as dusts. In these cases, the air concentrations of antimony have ranged from 5 - 73 mg/m^3 and urine concentrations have reached 5 mg/L (Renes, 1953; Taylor, 1966). Exposure to antimony hydride (stibine) is especially hazardous due to the gaseous nature of this compound and its very rapid pulmonary absorption.

Biological Monitoring. Urine antimony concentrations which exceed 0.01 mg/L are indicative of significant and potentially toxic exposure to antimony. Urine concentrations average 0.7 mg/L in workers exposed to antimony trioxide dust and fume at atmospheric levels of 3 - 5 mg/m^3, 6 to 10 times the current TLV (McCallum, 1963).

Analysis. Urine antimony levels may be useful in the diagnosis of acute or chronic poisoning, and may be determined by colorimetric (Kneip et al., 1976; Taylor, 1977) or atomic absorption procedures (Kneip et al., 1977). The latter technique is also useful for blood level measurements, which are especially recommended during suspected acute intoxication.

References

T. J. Kneip, R. S. Ajemian, J. N. Driscoll et al. Analytical method for antimony in air and urine. Health Lab Sci. 13: 90 - 94, 1976.

T. J. Kneip, R. S. Ajemian, J. N. Driscoll et al. Arsenic, selenium and antimony in urine and air: analytical method by hydride generation and atomic absorption spectroscopy. Health Lab. Sci. 14: 53 - 58, 1977.

R. I. McCallum. The work of an occupational hygiene service in environmental control. Ann. Occ. Hyg. 6: 55 - 64, 1963.

K. Ozawa. Studies on the therapy of schistosomiasis japonica. Tohoku J. Exp. Med. 65: 1 - 9, 1956.

L. E. Renes. Antimony poisoning in industry. Arch. Ind. Hyg. Occ. Med. 7: 99 - 108, 1953.

K. L. Stemmer. Pharmacology and toxicology of heavy metals: antimony. Pharm. Ther. 1: 157 - 160, 1976.

D. G. Taylor. *NIOSH Manual of Analytical Methods*, 2nd ed., National Institute for Occupational Safety and Health, Cincinnati, 1977, pp. 107 - 1 to 107 - 6.

P. J. Taylor. Acute intoxication from antimony trichloride. Brit. J. Ind. Med. 23: 318 - 321, 1966.

Urine Antimony by Colorimetry

Principle:

Urine is first digested with mineral acids, and then treated with perchloric acid in order to oxidize antimony to the pentavalent state. A colored complex is formed with Rhodamine B and the extracted complex is measured colorimetrically.

Reagents:

Stock solution — 1 mg/mL antimony ion (Fisher reference standard)
Aqueous standards — 0.02, 0.05, 0.10 and 0.20 mg/L
Concentrated sulfuric acid
Concentrated nitric acid
70% Perchloric acid
6 mol/L Hydrochloric acid
1 mol/L Phosphoric acid — 70 mL 85% H_3PO_4 per L
Rhodamine B solution — 0.02% in water
Toluene

Instrumental Conditions:

Visible spectrophotometer set to 565 nm

Procedure:

1. Precool in a refrigerator *all* reagents and glassware used in the analysis. Preserve urine samples by adding 5 mg thymol per 100 mL of urine and by refrigeration.
2. Transfer 50 mL urine into a 125 mL Erlenmeyer flask. Add 5 mL conc. H_2SO_4 and 5 mL conc. HNO_3 and heat in a fume hood until white fumes of SO_3 are evolved. Add further 1 mL increments of conc. HNO_3 if necessary to obtain a clear digest.
3. Cool slightly and then add 10 drops of 70% $HClO_4$. Heat until white fumes are evolved and then cool the sample to 4° C. in an ice bath.
4. Add 5 mL 6 mol/L HCl slowly and allow the sample to stand in the ice bath for 15 min.
5. Add 8 mL 1 mol/L H_3PO_4 and 5 mL Rhodamine B solution. Immediately mix this solution and transfer to a 125 mL separatory funnel.
6. Extract the solution with 10 mL toluene by shaking for 1 min. Allow the layers to separate and discard the aqueous layer.
7. Transfer a portion of the toluene layer (centrifuge if necessary to clarify) to a cuvette and measure the absorbance at 565 nm against a water blank treated in the same manner as the urine specimen. If the absorbance is outside the linear range, dilute the sample extract with toluene and correct the final absorbance for the dilution.

Calculation:

Calculation is based on a standard curve prepared each time an analysis is performed. This procedure cannot be controlled by the usual methods due to the instability of antimony in dilute solution.

Evaluation:

Sensitivity: 0.02 mg/L
Linearity: 0.02 - 0.20 mg/L
C.V.: 4 - 5%
Relative recovery: 95 - 103%

Interferences:

The method is relatively specific for antimony when the toluene extraction step is included. All traces of nitric acid must be removed from the final acid digest to insure test validity, and all reagents and glassware must be precooled to insure accuracy.

Urine Antimony by Atomic Absorption Spectrometry

Principle:

Urine is wet ashed to destroy organic matter. Antimony hydride is prepared by adding sodium borohydride to the ashed sample in a generator flask, and is swept into the flame of an atomic absorption spectrometer with argon purge gas. The absorption of antimony at 217.6 nm is measured.

Reagents:

Stock solution — 1 mg/mL antimony ion (Fisher reference standard)
Aqueous standards — 0.01, 0.05, 0.10, 0.20 and 0.50 mg/L (prepare fresh)
Concentrated nitric acid
Concentrated sulfuric acid
Concentrated perchloric acid
Saturated ammonium oxalate
6 mol/L Hydrochloric acid
Sodium borohydride, 8 mm 200 mg pellets

All glassware used in this procedure is to be washed with 50% nitric acid and rinsed several times with distilled water. Urine samples should be preserved with 1 mg/mL NaEDTA and stored refrigerated in acid-washed polyethylene containers.

Instrumental Conditions:

Atomic absorption spectrometer with argon-hydrogen flame and deuterium background correction; a hydride generator flask is placed in series with the argon supply line.
Antimony electrodeless discharge lamp
Measure absorption at 217.6 nm

Procedure:

1. Transfer 25 mL urine to a 125 mL Erlenmeyer flask. Add 3 mL conc. HNO_3, 1 mL conc. H_2SO_4 and $HClO_4$ and heat on a hot plate at 150° C.
2. Add conc. HNO_3 dropwise as needed to render the digest colorless. Additional H_2SO_4 and $HClO_4$ may be added if necessary.
3. Heat until white fumes of SO_3 are evolved. Cool the colorless solution and add 10 mL water and 5 mL saturated ammonium oxalate.
4. Heat again to fumes of SO_3 to remove traces of HNO_3. Cool, transfer solution to a 25 mL volumetric flask and adjust to volume with water.
5. With the argon flow bypassing the generator flask, add 5 mL of the acid digest and 50 mL 6 mol/L HCl to the flask. Close the flask, place on a magnetic stirrer and allow the argon flow to bubble through the solution.
6. Add a 200 mg sodium borohydride pellet through the addition stopcock of the flask and measure the absorption of the generated antimony hydride at 217.6 nm. Compare to standards and reagent blanks analyzed in the same manner.

Calculation:

Calculation is based on a standard curve prepared each time an analysis is performed. This procedure cannot be controlled by the usual methods due to the instability of antimony in dilute solution.

Evaluation:

Sensitivity: 0.002 mg/L
Linearity: 0.01 - 0.50 mg/L
C.V.: not established
Relative recovery: not established

Interferences:

High concentrations of other metals in the specimen may reduce the efficiency of the hydride generation system. The method of standard additions may be employed to correct for this effect. Background correction is necessary in order to compensate for the hydrogen which is swept into the flame during the generation process.

ARSENIC

Occurrence and Usage. Arsenic is the twentieth most abundant element in the earth's crust and is present in all living organisms. In certain areas of the United States and Canada, fresh water supplies contain up to 1.4 mg/L, substantially in excess of the acceptable limit of 0.01 mg/L. Seafood can contain from 2 mg/kg for freshwater fish up to 22 mg/kg for lobsters, most of which is organically bound. The average adult dietary intake of arsenic is 25 - 33 μg/kg/day. The largest source of human exposure to arsenic today is arsenical pesticides, which account for over 80% of the industrial consumption of arsenic. These compounds are derived from arsenic trioxide and include arsenic acid, dimethylarsinic acid (cacodylic acid) and salts of arsenite, arsenate and methanearsonate. Other important uses are in pharmaceuticals, in the ceramic and glass industry and in metallurgy. Arsine gas is occasionally encountered accidentally in industrial processes. Arsenic compounds are absorbed into the body following inhalation, ingestion or dermal contact (especially organo-arsenic compounds). While the threshold limit value for inorganic arsenic compounds is currently set at 0.5 mg/m^3 (expressed as arsenic), this value will probably be lowered to 0.2 mg/m^3 in the near future.

Blood Concentrations. Arsenic is a trace element which is present in all human tissues, probably bound to proteins. In blood, it is evenly distributed between plasma and erythrocytes; blood concentrations in normal subjects vary due to dietary and environmental influence and have been found to range from 0.002 - 0.062 mg/L in some populations (Heydorn, 1970). Asymptomatic workers using dimethylarsinic acid as an herbicide developed maximal blood concentrations of 0.27 mg/L (Wagner and Weswig, 1974).

Metabolism and Excretion. An administered dose of arsenic is distributed throughout the body, with the largest amount found in the muscles; excretion by the kidney is nearly complete within 6 days and accounts for over 90% of a dose, only a trace amount appearing in the feces (Hunter et al., 1942). The majority of a dose of dietary trivalent arsenic is rapidly excreted in urine as dimethylarsinic acid (50%), methylarsonic acid (14%), pentavalent arsenic (8%) and trivalent arsenic (8%); organo-arsenic compounds, as found in crab meat, are excreted unchanged in urine (Crecelius, 1977). Urine arsenic concentrations of unexposed persons may range from 0.01 - 0.30 mg/L. Subjects who ate a sea food meal developed maximal urine arsenic concentrations of 0.2 - 1.7 mg/L within 4 hours. Workers occupationally exposed to arsenic trioxide dust had urine concentrations ranging from 0.02 - 2.00 mg/L (Schrenk and Schreibeis, 1958; Pinto et al., 1976). Concentrations in urine of asymptomatic forest workers applying organic arsenic herbicides averaged 0.36 - 0.62 mg/L, with a range of 0.07 - 2.50 mg/L; the concentrations tended to increase toward the end of the week, but returned to normal by the next Monday (Tarrant and Allard, 1972).

Toxicity. With chronic low-level worker exposure to arsenic, epidemiological evidence suggests that a significant increase in the incidence of respiratory and skin cancers will occur (Pinto and Nelson, 1976). Chronic arsenic poisoning often results in cardiovascular abnormalities and neurological effects and has been attributed to the drinking of contaminated well water or excessive occupational exposure; this is best diagnosed by a measurement of hair or urine arsenic concentrations. Concentrations in hair of normal persons are less than 1 mg/kg (average 0.5), whereas concentrations of subjects with chronic poisoning are often in the 1 - 5 mg/kg region and may range as high as 47 mg/kg (Hindmarsh et al., 1977).

The inhalation of arsine gas may produce rapid death, with massive hemolysis leading to renal failure. The maximum allowable atmospheric concentration of arsine is 0.05 ppm, and a concentration of 25 - 50 ppm is believed to be lethal within 30 minutes. Arsenic concentrations in blood and urine of a subject who survived an arsine exposure were initially as high as 1.6 and 1.9 mg/L, respectively (Pinto, 1976). Concentrations of arsenic in the blood and urine of 3 men who died within 1 hour to 6 days of exposure to arsine fumes averaged 0.4 mg/L (range 0.1 - 0.6) and 0.2 mg/L (range 0.1 - 0.4), respectively (Teitelbaum and Kier, 1969; Pothel and Brosseau, 1976).

The acute ingestion of only 200 mg of arsenic trioxide may be fatal to an adult, death occurring within a few hours or after many days. A 2 year old child who swallowed an unknown amount of sodium arsenite solution was hospitalized and received BAL therapy for 28 days; urine arsenic concentrations on days 6, 10 and 21 were 17.8, 2.3 and 0.1 mg/L, respectively (Petery et al., 1970). A hair concentration of approximately 200 mg/kg was determined in a man who died 6 days after the ingestion of 8 g of arsenic trioxide (Wyttenbach et al., 1967). Blood concentrations of 0.6 - 9.3 mg/L (average 3.3) were observed in a series of 49 fatalities due to accidental or intentional arsenic overdosage (Rehling, 1967).

Biological Monitoring. Urine is most frequently used as an index of industrial arsenic exposure, since hair is easily contaminated by externally deposited arsenic. Urine arsenic concentrations in workers exposed to arsenic at the current 0.5 mg/m^3 limit average about 1 mg/L. Possible dietary or domestic sources of arsenic should be considered when individual urine levels exceed this value.

Analysis. Since most methods of arsenic determination require prior destruction of organic matter, procedures for both wet and dry ashing of biologic specimens will be first presented. Wet ashing does not require special equipment (other than a fume hood) but is suitable only for inorganic arsenic (Taylor, 1977); dry ashing requires a muffle furnace and is the preferred procedure for total arsenic (inorganic plus organic) determination (Stahr, 1977; George, 1973). A colorimetric technique is described which is simple enough to be performed in nearly any laboratory. A more sensitive and specific procedure based on atomic absorption spectrometry is also included (Mushak, 1977).

References

E. A. Crecelius. Changes in the chemical speciation of arsenic following ingestion by man. Env. Health Persp. 19: 147 - 150, 1977.

G. M. Crawford and O. Tavares. Simple hydrogen sulfide trap for the Gutzeit arsenic determination. Anal. Chem. 46: 1149, 1974.

E. H. Daughtrey, Jr., A. W. Fitchett and P. Mushak. Quantitative measurements of inorganic and methyl arsenicals by gas-liquid chromatography. Anal. Chim. Acta 79: 199 - 206, 1975.

H. Freeman, J. F. Uthe and B. Flemming. A rapid and precise method for the determination of inorganic and organic arsenic with and without wet ashing using a graphite furnace. At. Abs. Newsl. 15: 49 - 50, 1976.

G. M. George, L. J. Frahm and J. P. McDonnell. Dry ashing method for the determination of total arsenic in animal tissues: collaborative study. J. Asso. Off. Anal. Chem. 56: 793-797, 1973.

K. Heydorn. Environmental variation of arsenic levels in human blood determined by neutron activation analysis. Clin. Chim. Acta 28: 349-357, 1970.

J. T. Hindmarsh, O. R. McLetchie, L. P. M. Heffernan et al. Electromyographic abnormalities in chronic environmental arsenicalism. J. Anal. Tox. 1: 270-276, 1977.

F. T. Hunter, A. F. Kip and J. W. Irvine, Jr. Radioactive tracer studies on arsenic injected as potassium arsenite. J. Pharm. Exp. Ther. 76: 207 - 220, 1942.

P. Mushak, K. Dessauer and E. L. Walls. Flameless atomic absorption (FAA) and gas-liquid chromatographic studies in arsenic bioanalysis. Env. Health Persp. 19: 5 - 10, 1977.

J. S. Petery, O. M. Rennert, H. Choi and S. Wolfson. Arsenic poisoning in childhood. Clin. Tox. 3: 519 - 526, 1970.

S. S. Pinto. Arsine poisoning: evaluation of the acute phase. J. Occ. Med. 18: 633 - 635, 1976.

S. S. Pinto and K. W. Nelson. Arsenic toxicology and industrial exposure. Ann. Rev. Pharm. 16: 95 - 100, 1976.

S. S. Pinto, M. O. Varner, K. W. Nelson et al. Arsenic trioxide absorption and excretion in industry. J. Occ. Med. 18: 677-680, 1976.

C. Pothel and A. Brosseau. Acute arsine poisoning: report of two cases in the Montreal region. J. Can. Soc. For. Sci. 9: 87-93, 1976.

C. J. Rehling. Poison residues in human tissues. In *Progress in Chemical Toxicology*, Vol. 3 (A. Stolman, ed.), Academic Press, New York, 1967, pp. 363-386.

H. H. Schrenk and L. Schreibeis, Jr. Urinary arsenic levels as an index of industrial exposure. Am. Ind. Hyg. Asso. J. 19: 225 - 228, 1958.

A. U. Shaikh and D. E. Tallman. Determination of sub-microgram per liter quantities of arsenic in water by arsine generation followed by graphite furnace atomic absorption spectrometry. Anal. Chem. 49: 1093 - 1096, 1977.

H. M. Stahr (ed.). Arsenic. In *Analytical Toxicology Methods Manual*, Iowa State University Press, Ames, Iowa, 1977, pp. 80-83.

R. F. Tarrant and J. Allard. Arsenic levels in urine of forest workers applying silvicides. Arch. Env. Health 24: 277 - 280, 1972.

D. G. Taylor (ed.). *NIOSH Manual of Analytical Methods*, 2nd ed., Vol. 1, National Institute for Occupational Safety and Health, Cincinnati, 1977, p. 140 - 1.

D. T. Teitelbaum and L. C. Kier. Arsine poisoning. Arch. Env. Health 19: 133-143, 1969.

S. L. Wagner and P. Weswig. Arsenic in blood and urine of forest workers. Arch. Env. Health 28: 77 - 79, 1974.

A. Wyttenbach, P. Barthe and E. P. Martin. The content of arsenic in the hair in a case of acute lethal arsenic poisoning. J. For. Sci. Soc. 7: 194 - 197, 1967.

Wet Ashing of Biologic Specimens

Principle:

Biologic fluids or tissues are reduced to inorganic matter by heating with nitric, sulfuric and perchloric acids. Inorganic arsenic which is present is oxidized to As_2O_3. The resulting colorless liquid is suitable for analysis by a number of different procedures.

Reagents:

Acid mixture — 3 parts conc. HNO_3, 1 part conc. H_2SO_4 and 1 part conc. $HClO_4$ by volume
Nitric acid — conc. HNO_3
Perchloric acid — conc. $HClO_4$

Procedure:

1. Transfer 5 mL or 5 g of the biologic specimen to a 125 mL Erlenmeyer flask. Add 5 mL of the acid mixture. Perform all following operations in a well-vented safety hood.
2. Warm gently on a hot plate until the frothing subsides.
3. Heat at 130 - 150° C. until solution boils and darkens. Add 1 - 2 mL nitric acid and continue heating.
4. Repeat nitric acid addition until solution remains clear. It may be necessary to occasionally add several drops of perchloric acid if solution does not clarify.
5. Continue heating until white fumes of sulfur trioxide are evolved and the solution is free of nitric acid. The resulting volume should be approximately 5 mL.
6. Transfer the cooled solution quantitatively to a 10 mL volumetric flask, rinsing the walls of the digestion flask with water. Adjust the final volume to 10 mL with water.

Dry Ashing of Biologic Specimens

Principle:

The organic matter of biologic specimens is destroyed by oxidation in a muffle furnace. Both inorganic and organic arsenic are converted to As_2O_3. The ash is dissolved in acid in preparation for analysis by any of the following procedures.

Reagents:

Magnesium oxide
Cellulose powder — Whatman CF-11 (Reeve Angel and Co.)
2 mol/L Hydrochloric acid

Procedure:

1. Transfer 5 mL or 5 g of the biologic specimen to a porcelain evaporating dish and dry in a 95° C. oven for 3 - 4 hours.
2. Add magnesium oxide to cover the specimen (1 - 2 g). Add cellulose powder to cover the magnesium oxide (about 5 mL).
3. Place specimen in cold muffle furnace. Set temperature to 550° C.; when furnace reaches operating temperature allow specimen to ash for 2 - 3 hours.
4. Remove from oven, cool and suspend residue in 5 mL 2 mol/L HCl. Transfer quantitatively to a 10 mL volumetric flask, using water to rinse the dish. Adjust the final volume to 10 mL with water.

Arsenic by Colorimetry

Principle:

A previously ashed specimen is subjected to Zn-HCl arsine generation following conversion of arsenic to the trivalent form. Hydrogen sulfide is removed with a glass wool plug soaked in lead acetate solution. The arsine is chelated with diethyldithiocarbamate and the absorbance of the chelate measured in a spectrophotometer at 540 nm.

Reagents:

Stock solution — 1 mg/mL arsenic (Fisher reference standard SO-A-449 or dissolve 1.32 g As_2O_3 in 10 mL of 40% NaOH and dilute to 1 L with water)
Arsenic standards — 0.5, 2, 5 and 10 mg/L in water
DDC solution — 0.5 g silver diethyldithiocarbamate in 100 mL pyridine (stable if stored in amber bottle)
Concentrated hydrochloric acid
Stannous chloride solution — 40 g $SnCl_2$ in 100 mL conc. HCl
15% Potassium iodide — 15 g KI/100 mL water
10% Lead acetate — 10 g $Pb(C_2H_3O_2)_2$/100 mL water
Zinc — 20 mesh, low arsenic
Arsine generator — Fisher Scientific Co. #1-405

Instrumental Conditions:

Double beam visible spectrophotometer set to 540 nm

Procedure:

1. Transfer 3.0 mL of the previously ashed specimen to the arsine generator flask and dilute to about 35 mL with water. A water blank and four aqueous standards, previously carried through the identical ashing procedure as the specimen, are to be analyzed in the same manner.
2. Add 5 mL conc. HCl, 2 mL 15% KI and 8 drops $SnCl_2$ solution. Swirl and allow to stand for 15 min.
3. Wet a pledget of glass wool in the lead acetate solution and place it loosely into the scrubber tube of the arsine generator. Lubricate all joints with stopcock grease. Add 3.0 mL DDC solution to the absorber tube.
4. Add 3 g zinc to the generator flask and immediately insert the scrubber-absorber assembly. Allow arsine evolution to continue for 2 hours.
5. Transfer the DDC solution to a 3 mL cuvette and measure the absorbance at 540 nm, using the negative control as a reference. (This solution may also be analyzed by graphite furnace atomic absorption spectrometry).

Calculation:

Prepare a standard curve of absorbance versus concentration of the aqueous standards. Determine the specimen concentration from this curve. This procedure cannot be controlled by the usual methods due to the instability of dilute arsenic solutions.

Evaluation:

Sensitivity: 0.2 mg/L
Linearity: 0.2 - 10 mg/L
C.V.: 4 - 9% day-to-day
Relative recovery: 97 - 108%

Interferences:

Antimony will be detected as arsenic if it is present in sufficiently high concentrations, but this is unlikely. The antimony hydride, stibine, forms a chelate which has maximum absorbance at 510 nm. Chromium, copper and molybdenum may interfere with the evolution of arsine if present in high concentrations.

Arsenic by Atomic Absorption Spectrometry

Principle:

A previously ashed specimen is treated to convert arsenic to the trivalent form. Arsenic is chelated with diethyldithiocarbamate, the chelate is extracted into chloroform, partitioned back into water and an aliquot analyzed by graphite furnace atomic absorption spectrometry at 193.7 nm.

Reagents:

Stock solution — 1 mg/mL arsenic (Fisher reference standard SO-A-449)
Arsenic standards — 0.2, 0.5, 1 and 2 mg/L in water
8 mol/L Hydrochloric acid
Saturated potassium iodide
Chloroform
DDC solution — 2% diethylammonium diethyldithiocarbamate in water (prepare fresh)
2 mol/L Nitric acid

Instrumental Conditions:

Atomic absorption spectrometer with graphite furnace
Arsenic electrodeless discharge lamp
Furnace program:
dry 20 sec at 100° C.
char 20 sec at 500° C.
atomize 15 sec at 2100° C.
Measure absorption at 193.7 nm

Procedure:

1. Transfer 0.5 mL of a previously ashed specimen to a 15 mL centrifuge tube. A water blank and four aqueous standards, previously carried through the identical ashing procedure as the specimen, are to be analyzed in the same manner. Add 0.3 mL 8 mol/L HCl and 0.1 mL saturated KI and vortex.
2. Add 2 mL chloroform and 0.1 mL DDC solution. Vortex for 15 sec. and allow layers to separate.
3. Discard the upper layer and transfer 1.0 mL of the lower chloroform layer to a clean tube. Add 1.0 mL 2 mol/L HNO_3 and vortex for 15 seconds.
4. Introduce 10 - 30 μL of the aqueous phase into the graphite furnace.

Calculation:

Prepare a standard curve of absorption versus concentration of the aqueous standards. Determine the specimen concentration from this curve. This procedure cannot be controlled by the usual methods due to the instability of dilute arsenic solutions.

Evaluation:

Sensitivity: 0.1 mg/L
Linearity: 0.2 - 2.0 mg/L
C.V.: 10%
Relative recovery: not established

Interferences:

None known.

BENZENE

Occurrence and Usage. Benzene is a common laboratory and industrial chemical which produces a unique spectrum of acute and chronic toxic effects in man. It is found in gasoline, paint removers and many commercial solvents. The recommended threshold limit value for benzene in the workplace is currently 10 ppm (30 mg/m^3), and the chemical is listed as a potential carcinogen in man. The odor threshold for the compound has been reported as 1.5 - 5 ppm in air.

Blood Concentrations. A 2-hour exposure to 25 ppm benzene produced an average maximal blood benzene concentration of approximately 0.2 mg/L in 3 subjects, measured at the end of exposure (Sato and Fujiwara, 1972).

Metabolism and Excretion. Following human exposure to benzene only about 12% of a dose is exhaled unchanged in the lungs and about 0.1% is excreted unchanged in the urine. The remainder is metabolized in the liver to highly toxic oxidation products. Within 48 hours, from 51% - 87% is excreted in the urine as phenol (Hunter and Blair, 1972), 6% as catechol and 2% as hydroquinone (Teisinger et al, 1952); these phenolic metabolites are eliminated largely in conjugated form. Other minor metabolites, identified in the urine of rabbits but not yet found to be produced in man, include 1,2,4-trihydroxybenzene, muconic acid, phenylmercapturic acid and carbon dioxide (Parke and Williams, 1953). Industrial exposure to benzene is sometimes monitored by determination of urinary phenol levels; normally, these levels are less than 10 mg/L in the nonexposed individual, they do not exceed 30 mg/L in persons chronically exposed to 0.5 - 4.0 ppm of benzene (Roush and Ott, 1977) and they average 200 mg/L during exposure to 25 ppm (Walkley et al., 1961). Certain drugs such as Pepto-Bismol and Chloraseptic are known to elevate urine phenol concentrations to as much as 270 mg/L, obscuring interpretation of urine monitoring results (Fishbeck et al., 1975).

Preliminary investigations have been made into the use of breath concentrations of benzene for monitoring exposure to this chemical (Piotrowski, 1977). Breath concentrations have been found to average 2 ppm at the end of a 4.5 hour sedentary exposure to 25 ppm of benzene, and averaged 0.2 ppm sixteen hours later (Sherwood and Carter, 1970).

Toxicity. Chronic benzene poisoning is manifested by hematopoietic system injury and has been produced by occupational exposure to concentrations as low as 30 ppm. It is estimated that several hundred cases of fatal aplastic anemia due to chronic exposure to benzene at levels of 6 - 470 ppm occurred prior to 1963 (ACGIH, 1971). The acute toxic effects of benzene, however, are due either to central nervous system depression or to myocardial sensitization to epinephrine (Nahum and Hoff, 1934). Atmospheric concentrations of 7500 ppm may cause death within 30 minutes, and concentrations of 20,000 ppm may prove fatal within 5 minutes.

Biological Monitoring. Urine is the most frequently analyzed specimen when monitoring benzene exposure. Urinary phenol concentrations in specimens taken near the end of an exposure which are higher than 75 mg/L indicate exposure to benzene at a level exceeding the current 10 ppm TLV (Haley, 1977).

Blood has been only briefly studied for routine monitoring purposes. Monitoring of breath samples offers a more sensitive method of following exposure to very low atmospheric concentrations of benzene, and warrants further investigation.

Analysis. A gas chromatographic technique is presented for the determination of benzene and other volatile chemicals in blood or breath (Baselt and Barrett, 1975). Procedures are also included for the measurement of urinary phenol levels, by both colorimetry (Walkley et al., 1961) and gas chromatography (Sherwood and Carter, 1970). The colorimetric method is convenient but is not recommended due to numerous interferences by substances in normal urine. With either method, a base-line phenol excretion must be established for each individual prior to exposure to benzene.

References

ACGIH. *Documentation of the Threshold Limit Values*, American Conference of Governmental Industrial Hygienists, Cincinnati, Ohio, 1971, p. 22.

R. Baselt and C. Barrett. Unpublished results, 1975.

W. A. Fishbeck, R. R. Langner and R. J. Kociba. Elevated urinary phenol levels not related to benzene exposure. Am. Ind. Hyg. Asso. J. 36: 820 - 824, 1975.

T. J. Haley. Evaluation of the health effects of benzene inhalation. Clin. Tox. 11: 531 - 548, 1977.

C. G. Hunter and D. Blair. Benzene: pharmacokinetic studies in man. Ann. Occu. Hyg. 15: 193 - 199, 1972.

L. H. Nahum and H. E. Hoff. The mechanism of sudden death in experimental acute benzol poisoning. J. Pharm. Exp. Ther. 50: 336 - 345, 1934.

D. V. Parke and R. T. Williams. Studies in detoxication. 49. The metabolism of benzene containing ($^{14}C_1$) benzene. Biochem. J. 54: 231 - 238, 1953.

J. K. Piotrowski. *Exposure Tests for Organic Compounds In Industrial Toxicology*, U.S. Government Printing Office, Washington, D.C., 1977, pp. 41 - 47.

G. J. Roush and M. G. Ott. A study of benzene exposure versus urinary phenol levels. Am. Ind. Hyg. Asso. J. 38: 67 - 75, 1977.

A. Sato and Y. Fujiwara. Elimination of inhaled benzene and toluene in man. Jap. J. Ind. Health 14: 224 - 225, 1972.

R. J. Sherwood and F. W. G. Carter. The measurement of occupational exposure to benzene vapour. Ann. Occ. Hyg. 13: 125 - 146, 1970.

J. Teisinger, V. Fiserova-Bergerova and J. Kudrna. The metabolism of benzene in man. Prac. Lek. 4: 175 - 188, 1952.

J. E. Walkley, L. D. Pagnotto and H. B. Elkins. The measurement of phenol in urine as an index of benzene exposure. Am. Ind. Hyg. Asso. J. 22: 362-367, 1961.

Blood Solvents by Gas Chromatography

Principle:

Whole blood is diluted with water and the specimen is allowed to equilibrate in a sealed container at a constant temperature. A sample of the headspace vapor is analyzed by flame-ionization gas chromatography. Breath samples may be analyzed by direct injection of 1 - 2 mL, using as standards suitably prepared dilutions of the appropriate chemical in air.

Reagents:

Stock solutions — 1 mg/mL water solutions of benzene, carbon tetrachloride, chloroform, dichloromethane, toluene and trichloroethylene

Blood standards — 0.2, 0.5, 1.0, 2.0 and 5.0 mg/L for each of the above (prepare fresh from stock solution)

Instrumental Conditions:

Gas chromatograph with flame-ionization detector

2 m x 2 mm i.d. glass column containing 2% OV-17 on 100/120 mesh Chromosorb G-HP

Injector, 150° C.; column, 60° C.; detector, 150° C.

Nitrogen flow rate, 20 mL/min

Procedure:

1. Transfer 2 mL blood to a 10 mL serum bottle and add 2 mL water.
2. Seal the bottle by placing aluminum foil over a rubber septum and inserting the septum. Allow the bottle to equilibrate at 37° C. for 10 min (room temperature may be used although sensitivity is diminished).
3. Withdraw 1 mL of the headspace vapor into a 2 mL glass syringe equipped with a 23 gauge metal needle and inject into the gas chromatograph.

	Retention time (min)
dichloromethane	1.3
chloroform	2.0
carbon tetrachloride	2.2
benzene	2.5
trichloroethylene	2.8
toluene	4.9

Calculation:

Calculation is based on a standard curve prepared each time an assay is performed. This procedure cannot be controlled by the usual methods due to the volatility of the analytes.

Evaluation:

Sensitivity: 0.1 mg/L
Linearity: 0.2 - 5.0 mg/L
C.V.: not established
Relative recovery: not established

Interferences:

Normal plasma components do not interfere with the assay. Many other volatile organic compounds are detected with this technique and may interfere. The sensitivity of the assay for any specific chemical may be improved by increasing the column temperature slightly.

Urine Phenol by Colorimetry

Principle:

Phenol is steam-distilled from acidified urine. It is measured in the distillate by reaction with diazotized p-nitroaniline.

Reagents:

Stock solution — 1 mg/mL phenol in 1% HCl
Aqueous standards — 5, 10, 20, 40 and 80 mg/L
50% Sulfuric acid
50% Sodium acetate
5% Sodium nitrite
p-Nitroaniline reagent — dissolve 0.75 g p-nitroaniline in 10 mL water and 20 mL conc. HCl; dilute to 250 mL. Prepare fresh for use by adding 1.5 mL 5% $NaNO_2$ to 25 mL of this solution.
20% Sodium carbonate

Instrumental Conditions:

Visible spectrophotometer set to 525 nm

Procedure:

1. Transfer 10 mL urine to the flask of a steam distillation apparatus. Add 4 mL 50% H_2SO_4 and rinse the sides of the flask with approximately 5 mL water.
2. Begin steam distillation and collect a total volume of 100 mL of distillate. Transfer a 10 mL aliquot to a 20 mL volumetric flask.

3. Add 1 mL 50% sodium acetate and 1 mL p-nitroaniline reagent. After 1 minute, add 2 mL 20% Na_2CO_3 and adjust volume of solution to 20 mL with water.
4. Mix, wait 3 minutes and determine the absorbance of the solution at 525 nm against a reagent blank.

Calculation:

Calculation is based on a response factor derived from a standard curve. A quality control specimen containing 40 mg/L phenol should be analyzed daily.

Evaluation:

Sensitivity: 4 mg/L
Linearity: 5 - 100 mg/L
C.V.: not established
Relative recovery: not established

Interferences:

Cresol, resorcinol and other phenols will react with the color reagent but appear to be removed by the distillation process. A metabolite of p-dichlorobenzene, 2,5-dichlorophenol, will interfere if present in the urine specimen.

Urine Phenol by Gas Chromatography

Principle:

Urine is hydrolyzed to release conjugates of phenol. A single solvent extraction is made and the extract is analyzed directly by flame-ionization gas chromatography.

Reagents:

Stock solution — 1 mg/mL phenol in 1% HCl
Aqueous standards — 5, 10, 20, 40 and 80 mg/L
Perchloric acid
Diisopropyl ether

Instrumental Conditions:

Gas chromatograph with flame-ionization detector
1.5 m x 4 mm i.d. glass column containing 2% polyethylene glycol adipate on Chromosorb W

Injector, 200° C.; column, 150° C.; detector, 250° C.
Nitrogen flow rate, 60 mL/min

Procedure:

1. Transfer 5 mL urine to a 10 mL volumetric flask and add 2 mL perchloric acid. Cap loosely and heat at 95° C. for 2 hours.
2. Cool the solution and add 1 mL of diisopropyl ether to the flask. Adjust the volume to 10 mL with water and shake vigorously for 1 minute.
3. Allow the layers to separate and inject 5 μL of the organic layer into the chromatograph.

	Retention time (min)
phenol	1.7
o-cresol	2.2
m-cresol	5.3
p-cresol	5.3

Calculation:

Calculation is based on a response factor derived from a standard curve. A quality control specimen containing 50 mg/L of phenol is analyzed daily.

Evaluation:

Sensitivity: 2 mg/L
Linearity: 5 - 100 mg/L
C.V.: not established
Relative recovery: not established

Interferences:

None are known. Phenol is present in the urine of normal subjects at an average level of 5 - 8 mg/L (range 2 - 18). The p-cresol content in normal urine averages about 90 mg/L, with a range of 20 - 200 mg/L.

BENZIDINE

Occurrence and Usage. Benzidine, 4,4′-diaminobiphenyl, is widely employed in the manufacture of dyes. Prior to the recognition of its carcinogenic properties, it was a common laboratory reagent. As a carcinogen, benzidine does not have a threshold limit value assigned for its presence in the industrial atmosphere. Dermal absorption is often the major route of entry into the body, although inhalation and ingestion may also occur.

Blood Concentrations. The determination of benzidine or its metabolites in blood is not routinely performed.

Metabolism and Excretion. Of an absorbed dose of benzidine, it has been estimated that urinary excretion accounts for 4 - 10% as the parent compound; another 7 - 16% is excreted as mono- and diacetylbenzidine and much of the remainder as the sulfate conjugate of 3-hydroxybenzidine (Piotrowski, 1977).

The measurement of unchanged benzidine in urine has been used as an index of exposure to the compound. The maximum rate of excretion occurs 2 - 3 hours after an exposure, and urinary levels decline with a half-life of 5 - 6 hours. Urine benzidine concentrations average 9 $\mu g/L$ in workers exposed to air levels of 7 - 11 $\mu g/m^3$; they have ranged from 100 - 200 $\mu g/L$ in workers exposed to air containing 150 - 400 $\mu g/m^3$ of the chemical (Piotrowski, 1977).

Toxicity. Chronic exposure to benzidine is known to produce urinary bladder cancer in man. It is believed that exposure must last for at least six months, and that tumors may appear after a latency period of from 2 to 42 years (Haley, 1975). Workers exhibiting a high incidence of bladder tumors had urine benzidine concentrations of less than 160 $\mu g/L$ (Zavon et al., 1973).

Biological Monitoring. Benzidine concentrations which exceed 10 $\mu g/L$ in random urine specimens are probably indicative of excessive exposure to the chemical, based on industrial experience. As a carcinogen, benzidine or its metabolites should not be detectable in urine or other physiological fluids. In Poland the maximal permissible level for benzidine in urine has been set at 2 $\mu g/L$, which represents the detection limit of the most sensitive method available (Piotrowski, 1977).

Analysis. A colorimetric method for the analysis of unchanged benzidine in urine is described which has a detection limit of 20 $\mu g/L$ (Glassman and Meigs, 1951). A more sensitive and specific liquid chromatographic method is also presented which is applicable as well to the determination of benzidine metabolites (Rice and Kissinger, 1979).

References

J. M. Glassman and J. W. Meigs. Benzidine (4,4′-diaminobiphenyl) and substituted benzidines. Arch. Ind. Hyg. Occ. Med. 4: 519 - 532, 1951.

T. J. Haley. Benzidine revisited: a review of the literature and problems associated with the use of benzidine and its congeners. Clin. Tox. 8: 13 - 42, 1975.

J. K. Piotrowski. *Exposure Tests for Organic Compounds in Industrial Toxicology,* U.S. Government Printing Office, Washington, D.C., 1977, pp. 81 - 85.

J. R. Rice and P. T. Kissinger. Determination of benzidine and its acetylated metabolites in urine by liquid chromatography. J. Anal. Tox. 3: 64 - 66, 1979.

M. R. Zavon, U. Hoegg and E. Bingham. Benzidine exposure as a cause of bladder tumors. Arch. Env. Health 27: 1 - 7, 1973.

Urine Benzidine by Colorimetry

Principle:

Benzidine is extracted from alkalinized urine with an organic solvent and the solvent is concentrated by evaporation. Chloramine-T is used to form a yellow chromophore with the extracted benzidine, and the final solution is analyzed by visible spectrophotometry.

Reagents:

Stock solution — 1 mg/mL benzidine in methanol
Urine standards — 20, 50 and 100 μg/L (prepare fresh)
10 mol/L Sodium hydroxide
Ether
pH 8.4 Buffer — 50 mL 0.2 mol/L H_3BO_3, 50 mL 0.2 mol/L KCl and 8.5 mL 0.2 mol/L NaOH diluted to 200 mL
6 mol/L Hydrochloric acid
10% Chloramine-T in water

Instrumental Conditions:

Visible spectrophotometer set to 440 nm

Procedure:

1. Adjust the urine specimen to pH 8.5 by adding 10 mol/L NaOH dropwise. Centrifuge to remove sediment.
2. Transfer 50 mL urine into a 500 mL separatory funnel. Extract with 150 mL ether by shaking for several minutes.
3. Allow the layers to separate and discard the aqueous layer. Wash the ether layer with 10 mL pH 8.4 buffer and discard the buffer. Reduce the volume of ether to about 1 mL in a rotary evaporator under reduced pressure.

4. To the evaporator flask add 1 mL 6 mol/L HCl, 1 mL water, 1 mL 10% Chloramine-T and 5 mL ether. Swirl the solution and pour into a 60 mL separatory funnel.
5. Rinse the evaporator flask with 5 mL ether and add to the separatory funnel. Shake the mixture in the funnel, allow layers to separate and discard the aqueous phase.
6. Transfer the ether layer to a 10 mL volumetric flask and adjust to volume with ether. Read immediately in the spectrophotometer at 440 nm against a reagent blank.

Calculation:

Calculation is based on a response factor derived from a standard curve. A quality control specimen containing 50 μg/L benzidine is analyzed daily.

Evaluation:

Sensitivity: 20 μg/L
Linearity: 20 - 1000 μg/L
C.V.: 7 - 16%
Relative recovery: not established

Interferences:

Other amines, including β-naphthylamine and o-toluidine, will interfere if present in urine.

Urine Benzidine by Liquid Chromatography

Principle:

Benzidine is extracted from alkalinized urine with an organic solvent. A back-extraction is made into dilute acid and the aqueous layer is analyzed by reversed-phase liquid chromatography with electrochemical detection.

Reagents:

Stock solution — 1 mg/mL benzidine in methanol
Urine standards — 10, 25, 50 and 100 μg/L (prepare fresh)
2.5 mol/L pH 9 NH_4OH/NH_4Cl buffer
Diethyl ether
0.5 mol/L Perchloric acid
Mobile phase — methanol/0.1 mol/L pH 6.2 ammonium acetate, 25:75 by volume

Instrumental Conditions:

Liquid chromatography with a carbon electrochemical detector operated at 450 mv versus an Ag/AgCl reference electrode (Bioanalytical Systems)
15 cm x 4 mm i.d. stainless-steel column containing μBondapak C_{18} (Waters Associates)
Column temperature, ambient
Solvent flow rate, 1 mL/min

Procedure:

1. Transfer 2 mL urine to a 12 mL centrifuge tube. Add 1 mL pH 9 buffer and 1 mL diethyl ether and vortex.
2. Centrifuge and transfer the ether layer to a clean tube. Re-extract the aqueous layer with an additional 1 mL ether and combine the second ether extract with the first.
3. Add 1 mL 0.5 mol/L $HClO_4$ to the combined ether layers and vortex. Centrifuge and inject 20 μL of the aqueous layer into the chromatograph.

	Retention time (min)
benzidine	7
monoacetylbenzidine	13
diacetylbenzidine	30

Calculation:

Calculation is based on a response factor derived from a standard curve. A quality control specimen containing 50 μg/L benzidine is analyzed daily.

Evaluation:

Sensitivity: <1 μg/L
Linearity: 25 - 5000 μg/L
C.V.: 5% at 25 μg/L
Relative recovery: 103%

Interferences:

None are known. The detector must be operated at a potential of 1000 mv in order to detect the acetylated metabolites of benzidine.

BERYLLIUM

Occurrence and Usage. Beryllium and its compounds are important ingredients in the manufacture of alloys, many electrical components and ceramic heat-shields for space vehicles. Exposure is generally via inhalation of beryllium dusts or fumes created during manufacturing processes, and occasionally by dermal contact. The current threshold limit value is 0.002 mg/m^3 of beryllium in the industrial atmosphere, and the metal is listed as a suspected carcinogen.

Blood Concentrations. Beryllium is not routinely measured in blood specimens.

Metabolism and Excretion. Little is known about the disposition of beryllium in the body. When inhaled, the metal or its insoluble salts are deposited in the lung and appear to be slowly absorbed and excreted. It can be found in urine up to ten years after cessation of exposure. The presence of beryllium in lung tissue or urine is indicative of exposure and of potential toxicity. It is not a natural environmental contaminant and is not present in detectable amounts in the tissues or fluids of unexposed persons.

Toxicity. Dermal exposure to beryllium may produce contact dermatitis. Inhalation can cause bronchitis and severe pneumonitis. Chronic beryllium disease is often manifested by dyspnea, cough, fatigue, loss of weight, hepatomegaly and pulmonary granulomatosis. The development of the disease does not appear to be dose related, and may involve a hypersensitivity reaction (Reeves, 1977).

The beryllium contents of lung tissue in 66 individuals with beryllium disease averaged 1.19 mg/kg of dried tissue (range 0.004 - 45.7), whereas in 6 control subjects this averaged 0.005 mg/kg (range 0.003 - 0.010). The finding of beryllium in dried lung tissue at concentrations greater than 0.02 mg/kg is indicative of significant exposure. The test is diagnostically useful, although low or negative results do not preclude the possibility of beryllium disease (Sprince et al., 1976).

The urine of 25 subjects with beryllium disease was found to contain beryllium at concentrations of 0 - 1.7 mg/L, compared to levels of 0 - 0.6 mg/L for six asymptomatic workers. The excretion of beryllium in the urine is quite variable from day to day (Dutra et al., 1949) and does not necessarily correlate with the severity of lung disease or extent of exposure (Klemperer et al., 1951).

Biological Monitoring. For routine industrial monitoring purposes, the determination of beryllium in urine can be a useful adjunct to an occupational hygiene program. The presence of beryllium in urine at concentrations exceeding 0.02 mg/L is confirmation of significant exposure, although these concentrations do not correlate well with extent of exposure or the potential for toxicity.

Analysis. Beryllium may be determined in urine by atomic absorption spectrophotometry, using a nitrous oxide-acetylene flame (Bokowski, 1968). Urine specimens must first be wet-ashed according to a procedure described for arsenic analysis (p. 32).

References

D. L. Bokowski. Rapid determination of beryllium by a direct-reading atomic absorption spectrophotometer. Am. Ind. Hyg. Asso. J. 29: 474 - 481, 1968.

F. R. Dutra, J. Cholak and D. M. Hubbard. The value of beryllium determination in the diagnosis of berylliosis. Am. J. Clin. Path. 19: 229 - 234, 1949.

F. W. Klemperer, A. P. Martin and J. Van Riper. Beryllium excretion in humans. Am. Ind. Hyg. Asso. J. 4: 251 - 256, 1951.

A. L. Reeves. Beryllium in the environment. Clin. Tox. 10: 37 - 48, 1977.

N. L. Sprince, H. Kazemi and H. L. Hardy. Current (1975) problem of differentiating between beryllium disease and sarcoidosis. Ann. N.Y. Acad. Sci. 278: 654 - 664, 1976.

Urine Beryllium by Atomic Absorption Spectrometry

Principle:

Urine is wet-ashed according to a previously described procedure (p. 32). A chelate is formed between beryllium and acetylacetone in aqueous acid solution. The chelate is extracted into methyl isobutyl ketone and the organic layer is analyzed by atomic absorption spectrometry.

Reagents:

Stock solution — 1 mg/mL beryllium ion
Aqueous standards — 0.005, 0.010, 0.020, 0.050 and 0.100 mg/L
Concentrated ammonium hydroxide
10% Disodium ethylenediaminetetraacetic acid
Acetylacetone
Methyl isobutyl ketone

All glassware used in this procedure is to be soaked in 6 mol/L nitric acid overnight and rinsed in distilled water.

Instrumental Conditions:

Atomic absorption spectrometer with a nitrous oxide-acetylene flame
Beryllium hollow cathode lamp
Measure absorption at 234.9 nm

Procedure:

1. Transfer a portion of an ashed urine specimen equivalent to 50 mL of urine to a 100 mL beaker. Adjust the pH to 1.5 by adding concentrated NH_4OH dropwise.
2. Add 10 mL 10% Na_2EDTA solution and 0.5 mL acetylacetone and mix. Adjust the pH to 7 by adding additional conc. NH_4OH.
3. Transfer the solution to a 125 mL separatory funnel. Add 4 mL methyl isobutyl ketone and shake to extract.
4. Allow to stand for 5 minutes and discard the bulk of the lower aqueous layer. Transfer the remainder of the mixture to a 15 mL conical centrifuge tube and centrifuge to separate layers.
5. Transfer the upper organic layer to a clean tube. Aspirate into the flame of the spectrometer and compare the absorbance of the specimen to aqueous standards which have been treated in the same manner.

Calculation:

Calculation is based on a standard curve prepared each time an analysis is performed. This procedure cannot be controlled by the usual methods due to the instability of dilute beryllium solutions.

Evaluation:

Sensitivity: 0.002 mg/L in urine
Linearity: 0.005 - 0.100 mg/L
C.V.: 3%
Relative recovery: 98 - 103%

Interferences:

None are known.

BORATE

Occurrence and Usage. The borate ion is a weak germicide in aqueous solution and has been commonly employed in the household, in medical therapy and in industry for over a century. Boric acid is frequently used as an antiseptic for external use and may be found in eyewashes, mouthwashes, skin powders, ointments and irrigating solutions to the extent of 0.5 - 5%. Sodium borate (borax) is contained in cleaning agents, wood preservatives and fungicides. Borates were once used as food preservatives but have been replaced by less toxic agents for this purpose. Current threshold limit values for the borates range from 1 - 5 mg/ m^3 in the industrial atmosphere.

Blood Concentrations. Borate is found in trace amounts in normal tissue. Blood borate concentrations in 34 children with no known exposure to boric acid averaged 1.43 mg/L (range 0 - 7.15) (Fisher and Freimuth, 1958). Imbus et al. (1963) found that blood boron concentrations, expressed as borate, in normal men averaged 0.6 mg/L with a range of 0.2 - 2.0 . Boric acid is well-absorbed through broken skin surfaces or from mucous membranes, but not from intact skin (Goldbloom and Goldbloom, 1953). No data are available on fluid or tissue concentrations of the ion following human exposure to subtoxic amounts.

Metabolism and Excretion. Borates are excreted unchanged largely by the kidney; from 85 - 100% of a dose may be eliminated in the urine over a period of 5 - 7 days, with small amounts found in sweat and feces (Locksley and Sweet, 1954; Pfeiffer et al., 1945).

Toxicity. Occupational exposure to borax dusts has caused dermatitis, cough, irritation of mucous membranes and shortness of breath in workers (ACGIH, 1977). The remarkable number of human systemic poisonings associated with the borates are undoubtedly due in part to the popular belief that the compounds are relatively innocuous (Valdes-Dapena and Arey, 1962). It is true that relatively large amounts are necessary to produce toxicity in adults. An intravenous dose of 14 - 20 g of sodium borate was administered for the purposes of neutron capture therapy to 10 patients, who experienced immediate nausea, vomiting, defecation, and occasionally seizures and respiratory depression (Locksley and Farr, 1955). The application of boric acid powder for diaper rash has produced neurological disorders, severe erythema of the skin, gastrointestinal symptoms and deaths in infants (Goldbloom and Goldbloom, 1953); one such child developed a serum borate concentration of at least 303 mg/L, which fell to 32 mg/L after 54 hours of peritoneal dialysis with marked improvement in the patient (Baliah et al., 1969). The same manifestations were observed in 11 infants who accidentally ingested boric acid in their formula; from 2 - 4.5 g of the compound was ingested by six of the survivors, who developed serum borate levels of 20 -150 mg/L, while the five infants who ingested larger amounts (4.5 -

14 g) exhibited levels of 200-1600 mg/L and died within 3 days (Wong et al., 1964).

Biological Monitoring. Serum borate concentrations which exceed 20 mg/L are indicative of excessive exposure to borate compounds. Serum concentrations which result from controlled occupational exposure have not been determined.

Analysis. Borate concentrations in biological fluids may be determined using a colorimetric procedure which employs carminic acid (Hatcher and Wilcox, 1950; Rieders and Frere, 1963). The method is not sufficiently sensitive to detect endogenous levels of borate ion.

References

ACGIH. *Documentation of the Threshold Limit Values,* American Conference of Governmental Industrial Hygienists, Cincinnati, Ohio, 1977, pp. 356 - 357.

T. Baliah, H. MacLeish and K. N. Drummond. Acute boric acid poisoning. Can. Med. Asso. J. 101: 166 - 168, 1969.

R. S. Fisher and H. C. Freimuth. Blood boron levels in human infants. J. Invest. Derm. 30: 85 - 86, 1958.

R. B. Goldbloom and A. Goldbloom. Boric acid poisoning. J. Pediat. 43: 631-643, 1953.

J. T. Hatcher and L. V. Wilcox. Colorimetric determination of boron using carmine. Anal. Chem. 22: 567-569, 1950.

H. R. Imbus, J. Cholak, L. H. Miller and T. Sterling. Boron, cadmium, chromium and nickel in blood and urine. Arch. Env. Health 6: 286-295, 1963.

H. B. Locksley and W. H. Sweet. Tissue distribution of boron compounds in relation to neutron-capture therapy of cancer. Proc. Soc. Exp. Biol. Med. 86: 56 - 63, 1954.

H. B. Locksley and L. E. Farr. The tolerance of large doses of sodium borate intravenously by patients receiving neutron capture therapy. J. Pharm. Exp. Ther. 114: 484 - 489, 1955.

C. C. Pfeiffer, L. F. Hallman and I. Gersh. Boric acid ointment. J. Am. Med. Asso. 128: 266 - 274, 1945.

F. Rieders and F. J. Frere. Detection and estimation of toxicologically significant amounts of borate, chlorate and oxalate in biological material. J. For. Sci. 8: 46-53, 1963.

M. A. Valdes-Dapena and J. B. Arey. Boric acid poisoning. J. Pediat. 61: 531 - 546, 1962.

L. C. Wong, M. D. Heimbach, D. R. Truscott and B. D. Duncan. Boric acid poisoning: report of 11 cases. Can. Med. Asso. J. 90: 1018 - 1023, 1964.

Serum Borate by Colorimetry

Principle:

Serum is deproteinized and allowed to react with a chromogen which is relatively specific for borate ion. The absorbance of the solution is measured at 600 nm in a spectrophotometer.

Reagents:

Stock solution — 2 mg/mL borate ion (210 mg boric acid/100 mL water)
Serum standards — 20, 50, 100 and 200 mg/L borate ion
Ammonium sulfate solution — 4 g $(NH_4)_2SO_4$/100 mL water
Sulfuric acid — conc. H_2SO_4
Carminic acid reagent — 20 mg carminic acid/100 mL conc. H_2SO_4 (stable indefinitely)

Instrumental Conditions:

Visible spectrophotometer set to 600 nm

Procedure:

1. Transfer 1 mL serum and 5 mL ammonium sulfate solution to a 15 mL centrifuge tube. Vortex and place into a boiling water bath for 15 min.
2. Centrifuge and decant the supernatant into a 10 mL volumetric flask. Suspend the precipitate in 2 mL water, vortex, centrifuge and add the second supernatant to the first.
3. Adjust the contents of the volumetric flask to 10 mL with water. Transfer 1 mL to a 15 mL centrifuge tube.
4. Add 5 mL sulfuric acid and vortex. Add 5 mL carminic acid solution and vortex.
5. Transfer solution to a cuvette, stopper and allow to stand for 10 min. Determine absorbance at 600 nm, using as reference solution a negative control serum processed in the same manner.

Calculation:

Calculation is based on a response factor derived from a standard curve. A quality control serum containing 50 mg/L borate ion is analyzed daily.

Evaluation:

Sensitivity: 10 mg/L
Linearity: 20 - 200 mg/L
C.V.: 6%
Relative recovery: 92 - 104%

Interferences:

High concentrations of antimony, iron, copper and oxidizing acids may interfere.

CADMIUM

Occurrence and Usage. Exposure to cadmium is a common occurrence in industry, where it is incorporated into a variety of alloys and metal platings; the inhalation of cadmium dust or fumes constitutes a hazard during heating, grinding, welding and soldering operations involving cadmium-containing metal products. The general populace is exposed to cadmium via food, water, air and cigarette smoking, and daily intake of 2 - 200 μg of the metal is normal. Body accumulation of cadmium, which begins from birth, has been suggested to play a role in hypertension. The threshold limit value for cadmium in air, as a dust or fume, is 0.05 mg/m^3.

Blood Concentrations. Mean serum cadmium concentrations in healthy unexposed persons have ranged from 0.0005 - 0.0020 mg/L in separate studies; whole blood contains nearly twice as much cadmium as serum. Although no relationship was observed between age, sex or smoking history and serum cadmium levels, other investigators have found such associations (PetitClerc et al., 1977; Bernard et al., 1977). Blood cadmium concentrations averaged 0.009 mg/L in asymptomatic workers exposed to cadmium fumes, versus 0.004 mg/L in unexposed subjects (Baker et al., 1979).

Metabolism and Excretion. After administration of cadmium by inhalation or injection, the metal is known to accumulate in lungs, liver and kidney, with slow excretion in the urine (Potts et al., 1950). In liver and kidney it is bound to a small protein called metallothionein. Due to this accumulation, kidney cadmium concentrations have been shown to correlate positively with age (Schroeder, 1967). Average concentrations for autopsy specimens in England are 2.0 mg/kg (range 1.2 - 3.7) for liver and 11.7 mg/kg (range 2.1 - 22.0) for kidney (Curry and Knott, 1970), whereas liver concentrations of 23 - 145 mg/kg and kidney concentrations of 13 - 80 mg/kg were observed in 4 workers who died 3 - 9 years after having been occupationally exposed to cadmium for periods of 18 - 26 years (Friberg, 1957). Normal urine cadmium levels are on the order of 0.0001 - 0.0002 mg/L (Perry et al., 1975).

Toxicity. Industrial contamination of water supplies by cadmium, with accumulation of the metal by shellfish, caused an epidemic of cadmium poisoning in Japan known as "itai-itai" disease. Renal damage leading to disturbances in calcium and phosphorus metabolism were believed responsible for the resulting skeletal deformities and severe leg and back pain (Friberg et al., 1971). Early signs of renal damage were observed in 19 cadmium workers whose cadmium levels averaged 0.033 mg/L in blood and 48 μg/g creatinine in urine (Lauwerys et al., 1974). Five men exposed chronically to cadmium fumes at an average air concentration of 0.1 mg/m^3 exhibited symptoms of fatigue, coughing, chest pain and a burning sensation of the throat; urine cadmium levels ranged from 0.01 -

0.05 mg/L in these workers (Hardy and Skinner, 1947). In 5 nonfatal cases of acute exposure to cadmium fumes, blood and urine concentrations ranged from 1.2 - 3.0 mg/L and 0.10 - 0.36 mg/L, respectively (Cotter and Cotter, 1951). In 3 fatal cases related to chronic cadmium poisoning, concentrations of the metal averaged 128 mg/kg (range 5 - 200) in liver and 180 mg/kg (range 70 - 300) in kidney (Curry and Knott, 1970). As little as 4 mg of cadmium may be fatal to an adult when inhaled; by ingestion, the lethal dose is estimated to be several hundred milligrams of a soluble salt.

Biological Monitoring. Urine cadmium levels may be used to estimate cadmium body burden and to monitor chronic exposure to the metal, while blood concentrations offer a better index to recent exposure and acute intoxication (Kjellstrom, 1979). Urine or blood cadmium concentrations which exceed 0.005 mg/L in workers are indicative of excessive exposure to the metal. Lauwerys et al. (1974) suggested that urine cadmium concentrations in workers should not exceed 15 μg/g creatinine.

Analysis. Two atomic absorption procedures are described for the determination of cadmium in body fluids, involving both flame (Berman, 1967) and flameless detection (Perry et al., 1975). The former procedure is more suitable for the detection of elevated levels of the metal, while the latter is sufficiently sensitive to measure blood and urine concentrations of cadmium in healthy unexposed persons. Special precautions must be taken in performing these analyses due to the very low concentrations of cadmium in normal biological specimens and the presence of the metal in common laboratory reagents and glassware.

References

E. L. Baker, W. A. Peterson, J. L. Holtz et al. Subacute cadmium intoxication in jewelry workers: an evaluation of diagnostic procedures. Arch. Env. Health 39: 173 - 177, 1979.

E. Berman. Determination of cadmium, thallium and mercury in biological materials by atomic absorption. At. Abs. Newsl. 6: 57-60, 1967.

A. Bernard, H. A. Roels, J. P. Buchet et al. α_1-Antitrypsin level in workers exposed to cadmium. In *Clinical Chemistry and Chemical Toxicology of Metals* (S. S. Brown, ed.), Elsevier/North Holland, New York, 1977, pp. 161 - 164.

L. H. Cotter and B. H. Cotter. Cadmium poisoning. Arch. Ind. Hyg. Occ. Med. 3: 495 - 504, 1951.

A. S. Curry and A. R. Knott. "Normal" levels of cadmium in human liver and kidney in England. Clin. Chim. Acta 30: 115 - 118, 1970.

L. Friberg. Deposition and distribution of cadmium in man in chronic poisoning. Arch. Ind. Health. 16: 27 - 29, 1957.

L. Friberg, M. Piscator and G. Nordberg. *Cadmium in the Environment*, CRC Press, Cleveland, 1971.

H. L. Hardy and J. B. Skinner. The possibility of chronic cadmium poisoning. J. Ind. Hyg. Tox. 29: 321 - 324, 1947.

T. Kjellstrom. Exposure and accumulation of cadmium in populations from Japan, the United States, and Sweden. Env. Health Persp. 28: 169 - 197, 1979.

R. R. Lauwerys, J. P. Buchet, H. A. Roels et al. Epidemiological survey of workers exposed to cadmium. Arch. Env. Health 28: 145 - 148, 1974.

E. F. Perry, S. R. Koirtyohann and H. M. Perry, Jr. Determination of cadmium in blood and urine by graphite furnace atomic absorption spectrophotometry. Clin. Chem. 21: 626 - 629, 1975.

C. PetitClerc, L. Munan, A. Kelly and M. Cote. Serum cadmium concentrations in patients from a cardiac clinic and in healthy controls. In *Clinical Chemistry and Chemical Toxicology of Metals* (S.S. Brown, ed.), Elsevier/North-Holland, New York, 1977, pp. 157-160.

A. M. Potts, F. P. Simon, J. M. Tobias et al. Distribution and fate of cadmium in the animal body. Arch. Ind. Hyg. Occ. Med. 2: 175 - 188, 1950.

H. A. Schroeder. Cadmium, chromium and cardiovascular disease. Circ. 35: 570 - 582, 1967.

Blood and Urine Cadmium by Flame Atomic Absorption Spectrometry

Principle:

Cadmium is chelated in blood and urine specimens with sodium diethyldithiocarbamate. The chelate is extracted into an organic solvent and the solvent is aspirated into an oxidizing flame. Detection is at 228.8 nm. The sensitivity is adequate for measurement of toxic levels of cadmium.

Reagents:

Stock solution — 1 mg/mL cadmium ion (Fisher reference standard)
Aqueous standards — 0, 0.005, 0.01, 0.05, 0.1 and 0.5 mg/L dilutions of stock solution in 1% nitric acid (prepared weekly)
5% Trichloroacetic acid
2.5 mol/L Sodium hydroxide
DDC solution — 1% sodium diethyldithiocarbamate in water
Methyl isobutyl ketone

Instrumental Conditions:

Atomic absorption spectrophotometer with air-acetylene oxidizing flame
Cadmium hollow cathode lamp
Measure absorption at 228.8 nm

Sample Preparation:

All glassware is to be soaked overnight in 25% nitric acid and rinsed thoroughly in deionized water prior to use.

Blood:

1. Transfer 4 mL blood to a centrifuge tube and add 8 mL 5% trichloroacetic acid. Vortex and let stand 1 hour.
2. Centrifuge and transfer 10 mL supernatant into a 15 mL screw-cap tube. Adjust pH to 6.0 - 7.5 with 2.5 mol/L NaOH.

Urine:

1. Transfer 10 mL urine to a 15 mL screw-cap tube and adjust pH to 6.0 - 7.5 with 2.5 mol/L NaOH.

Procedure:

1. To prepared specimen add 1 mL DDC solution and vortex. Add 2.5 mL methyl isobutyl ketone and shake for 2 min.
2. Centrifuge, transfer the solvent layer to a sample tube and aspirate the solvent into the flame. Determine absorption at 228.8 nm.

Calculation:

Prepare a standard curve of absorption versus concentration of the aqueous standards. Determine the specimen concentration from this curve. This procedure cannot be controlled by the usual methods due to the instability of dilute cadmium solutions.

Evaluation:

Sensitivity: 0.002 mg/L
Linearity: 0.005 - 0.5 mg/L
C.V.: not established
Relative recovery: 98 - 110%

Interferences:

This procedure has high specificity for cadmium. Reagents and glassware must be checked carefully for cadmium contamination by analyzing water blanks. Some investigators have reported better results using plastic tubes which were soaked overnight in 5% Triton X-100 prior to use. Urine specimens which are to be stored prior to analysis should contain 1% conc. HCl to prevent precipitation of cadmium.

Blood and Urine Cadmium by Graphite-Furnace Atomic Absorption Spectrometry

Principle:

Blood and urine specimens are wet-ashed to destroy organic matter. The dry residue is dissolved in dilute nitric acid and analyzed by electrothermal atomic absorption spectrometry at 228.8 nm. Excellent sensitivity is achieved with this procedure.

Reagents:

Stock solution — 1 mg/mL cadmium ion (Fisher reference standard)
Aqueous standards — 0, 0.0002, 0.0005, 0.001 and 0.003 mg/L dilutions of stock solution in 1% nitric acid (prepare weekly)
Nitric acid — conc. HNO_3 (ultrapure grade)
30% Hydrogen peroxide
1% Nitric acid

Instrumental Conditions:

Atomic absorption spectrometer with graphite furnace
Cadmium hollow cathode lamp
Furnace program:
dry 30 sec at 150° C.
char 60 sec at 300° C.
atomize 8 sec at 1950° C.
Argon purge gas in interrupt mode
Measure absorption at 228.8 nm

Procedure:

Pyrex digestion tubes are decontaminated by conducting six blank digestions with 0.5 mL 70% perchloric acid prior to use.

1. Blood — transfer 0.5 mL to a digestion tube and add 1 mL conc. HNO_3.
   Urine — transfer 1 mL to a digestion tube and add 0.2 mL conc. HNO_3.
2. Place tube in a heating block and digest for 3 h at a temperature just below boiling.
3. When the specimen volume is reduced to one-third of the original, add 0.4 mL 30% H_2O_2. Continue heating until sample is evaporated to dryness.
4. Cool tube and dissolve residue in 5 mL (blood) or 2 mL (urine) 1% nitric acid. Inject 20 μL of this solution into the graphite furnace for analysis.

Calculation:

Prepare a standard curve of absorption versus concentration of the aqueous standards. Dilute any specimens which exceed the range of the standard curve. Determine the specimen concentration from this curve. This procedure cannot be controlled by the usual methods due to the instability of dilute cadmium solutions.

Evaluation:

Sensitivity: 0.0001 mg/L
Linearity: 0.0002 - 0.003 mg/L
C.V.: 7 - 14% within-run
Relative recovery: 85 - 110%

Interferences:

This procedure has high specificity for cadmium. Reagents and glassware must be checked carefully for cadmium contamination by analyzing water blanks. Some investigators have reported better results using plastic tubes which were soaked overnight in 5% Triton X-100 prior to use. Urine specimens which are to be stored prior to analysis should contain 1% conc. HCl to prevent precipitation of cadmium.

CARBARYL

Occurrence and Usage. Carbaryl (Sevin) is a carbamate derivative of 1-naphthol which is used as a short-acting insecticide. Human exposure is usually via inhalation, although the compound is also absorbed through the skin. The current threshold limit value is 5 mg/m^3.

Blood Concentrations. Intact carbaryl is not routinely measured in human blood. A method will be presented for blood cholinesterase, the levels of which are frequently used to monitor exposure to carbaryl and other cholinesterase inhibitors.

Metabolism and Excretion. Carbaryl is known to be metabolized by N-demethylation, ring hydroxylation, hydrolysis and conjugation. The hydrolysis pathway results in the urinary excretion of free and conjugated 1-naphthol, which accounts for over 20% of an ingested dose and which may be measured as an index of exposure to the chemical (Knaak et al., 1967). Urine concentrations of 1-naphthol in unexposed subjects average <0.01 mg/L and do not exceed 0.23 mg/L (Kutz et al., 1978). Exposed but asymptomatic workers exhibited 1-naphthol urine concentrations of less than 0.1 to more than 42 mg/L; air concentrations of carbaryl during these exposures ranged from 0.2 to 31 mg/m^3 (Best and Murray, 1962).

Toxicity. The inactivation of cholinesterase by carbaryl produces symptoms of intoxication which include blurred vision, salivation, sweating, nausea, vomiting and convulsions. The effects of the carbamate insecticides in general do not persist as long as those of the organophosphates. Volunteers who ingested doses of carbaryl of up to 0.13 mg/kg daily for 6 weeks were asymptomatic (Wills et al., 1968). Workers exposed to air concentrations of the chemical of up to 31 mg/m^3 were also asymptomatic but did exhibit occasional depression of blood cholinesterase activity (Best and Murray, 1962).

A 1.5 year old child who ingested an unknown amount of carbaryl became moderately intoxicated and was treated with atropine; the urine, collected 18 hours after the incident, contained 31 mg/L 1-naphthol (Best and Murray, 1962). Ingestion of 250 mg has caused severe poisoning in an adult, and at least one death has occurred following intentional ingestion of an unknown amount.

Biological Monitoring. Exposure to anticholinesterase agents such as carbaryl is frequently monitored by determination of blood cholinesterase activity. A pre-exposure cholinesterase level should be obtained for each employee so that the post-exposure level may be expressed as a percentage of that subject's normal cholinesterase activity. A post-exposure blood cholinesterase level which is less than 70% of normal is considered indicative of excessive exposure to carbaryl.

Although standards have not been developed for carbaryl metabolites in urine, it is probable that urinary 1-naphthol concentrations in excess of 4 mg/L represent significant exposure to carbaryl.

Analysis. A method is presented for the determination of cholinesterase activity in whole blood by colorimetry; at least 80% of the activity measured by this technique is erythrocyte cholinesterase, and the method is applicable to all anticholinesterase agents (Fleisher and Pope, 1954). A second procedure is included for the determination of total 1-naphthol in urine by colorimetry (Best and Murray, 1962). Both methods are useful in the routine monitoring of worker exposure to carbaryl.

References

E. M. Best and B. L. Murray. Observations on workers exposed to Sevin insecticide: a preliminary report. J. Occ. Med. 10: 507 - 517, 1962,

J. H. Fleisher and E. J. Pope. Colorimetric method for determination of red blood cell cholinesterase activity in whole blood. Arch. Ind. Hyg. Occ. Med. 9: 323 - 334, 1954.

J. B. Knaak, L. J. Sullivan and J. H. Wills. Metabolism of carbaryl in man. Tox. Appl. Pharm. 10: 390, 1967.

F. W. Kutz, R. S. Murphy and S. C. Strassman. Survey of pesticide residues and their metabolites in urine from the general population. In *Pentachlorophenol*, K. R. Rao (ed.), Plenum Press, New York, 1978, pp. 363 - 369.

J. H. Wills, E. Jameson and F. Coulston. Effect of oral doses of carbaryl in man. Clin. Tox. 1: 265 - 271, 1968.

Blood Cholinesterase by Colorimetry

Principle:

A small volume of blood is incubated with a solution containing 4 μmoles of acetylcholine. Hydroxylamine is added to stop the reaction and to react with the remaining acetylcholine, forming a colored complex. The absorbance of this solution is measured in a spectrophotometer at 540 nm.

Reagents:

0.01% Saponin

0.134 mol/L pH 7.2 Phosphate buffer — add 7 parts of a solution of 23.8 g $Na_2HPO_4 . 2H_2O$ per liter to 3 parts of a solution of 18.2 g KH_2PO_4 per liter and adjust pH to 7.2

0.04 mol/L Acetylcholine — 0.7266 g chloride salt in 100 mL 0.001 mol/L pH 4.5 acetate buffer (stable when refrigerated)

0.004 mol/L Acetylcholine — one volume of above solution diluted with nine volumes of 0.134 mol/L pH 7.2 phosphate buffer fresh as needed

2 mol/L Hydroxylamine hydrochloride — 27.8 g in 200 mL water (stable for 2 weeks when refrigerated)
3.5 mol/L Sodium hydroxide — 28 g in 200 mL water
Hydroxylamine solution — mix equal volumes of 2.5 mol/L NH_2OH . HCl and 3.5 mol/L NaOH fresh as needed
Dilute hydrochloric acid — 1 volume conc. HCl in 2 parts water
0.37 mol/L Ferric chloride — 10 g $FeCl_3 . 6H_2O$ in 100 mL 0.1 mol/L HCl

Instrumental Conditions:

Visible spectrophotometer set to 540 nm

Procedure:

1. Transfer 50 μL whole blood into a tube containing 950 μL 0.01% saponin (tube 1). Prepare a second sample in the same manner for use as a control and set aside (tube 2).
2. Add 1 mL 0.004 mol/L acetylcholine to the first tube and incubate at 25° C. for exactly 10 min. At the same time, incubate 1 mL of 0.004 mol/L acetylcholine in a separate tube (tube 3).
3. Stop the reaction by adding 4 mL hydroxylamine solution to both of the incubated tubes and vortexing. Wait one minute and pour the contents of tube 2 into tube 3.
4. Add 2 mL dilute HCl to tubes 1 and 3 and vortex. Further add 2 mL 0.37 mol/L $FeCl_3$ and vortex.
5. Filter the solutions through Whatman #40 filter paper. After 10 minutes measure the absorbance of each tube at 540 nm, using water as a reference.

Calculation:

The cholinesterase activity of a blood specimen is expressed as the number of micromoles of acetylcholine hydrolyzed during the ten minute incubation, and is calculated using the formula:

$$\mu\text{moles AcCh hydrolyzed} = 4\left(1 - \frac{As}{Ac}\right)$$

where As represents the absorbance of the sample and Ac represents the absorbance of the control. Quality control materials are not applicable to this procedure.

Evaluation:

Sensitivity: 0.2 μmoles
Linearity: 0.2 - 4 μmoles
C.V.: 1%
Relative recovery: not applicable

Interferences:

The average cholinesterase activity in whole blood using this technique is 2.38 μmoles (range 1.93 - 2.83) for adult males and 2.18 μmoles (range 1.73 - 2.63) for females. Approximately 80% of the activity measured by this method is due to erythrocyte cholinesterase, which is less subject to random variation than plasma esterase activity.

Urine 1-Naphthol by Colorimetry

Principle:

Conjugated 1-naphthol in urine is released by acid hydrolysis and the free substance is extracted into an organic solvent. The solvent is removed by evaporation and the residue dissolved in methanolic alkali. The 1-naphthol is reacted with p-nitrobenzene diazonium fluoroborate and the resulting color determined spectrophotometrically.

Reagents:

Stock solution — 1 mg/mL 1-naphthol in methanol
Urine standards — 0.5, 1, 2, 5 and 10 mg/L
Concentrated hydrochloric acid
Dichloromethane
Florisil, 60/80 mesh, packed to a depth of 5.5 cm in a glass column and prewet with water-saturated dichloromethane
PEG solution — 1 mL polyethylene glycol 200 in 100 mL dichloromethane
Methanol
0.1 mol/L Potassium hydroxide in methanol
Color reagent — 25 mg p-nitrobenzene diazonium fluoroborate in 25 mL methanol (prepare fresh)

Instrumental Conditions:

Visible spectrophotometer set to 590 nm

Procedure:

1. Transfer 10 mL urine to a 250 mL Erlenmeyer flask. Add 10 mL conc. HCl and 40 mL water.
2. Attach the flask to a water-cooled condenser. Place on a hot plate and reflux the solution for 20 min.
3. Cool the solution and transfer to a 250 mL separatory funnel. Extract into 25 mL dichloromethane by shaking for 1 min.

4. Allow the layers to separate and pass the organic layer through the Florisil column into a 250 mL Erlenmeyer flask which contains 1 mL PEG solution. Repeat the extraction of the aqueous phase with another 25 mL dichloromethane and again pass the organic layer through the column.
5. Wash the column with 50 mL dichloromethane and collect in the flask. Remove the dichloromethane by evaporation at reduced pressure on a rotary evaporator.
6. Dissolve the residue in 2 mL methanol and transfer this solution with rinsing to a 25 mL volumetric flask. Add 1 mL color reagent and adjust to volume with methanol.
7. Mix the solution by inversion and let stand for 15 min. Measure the absorbance of an aliquot at 590 nm against a urine blank.

Calculation:

Calculation is based on a response factor derived from a standard curve. A quality control specimen containing 2 mg/L 1-naphthol is analyzed daily.

Evaluation:

Sensitivity: 0.2 mg/L
Linearity: 0.5 - 16 mg/L
C.V.: not established
Relative recovery: not established

Interferences:

Urinary 1-naphthol concentrations have not exceeded 0.3 mg/L in healthy unexposed subjects. Concentrations in excess of 4 mg/L may be considered to represent significant exposure to carbaryl.

CARBON DISULFIDE

Occurrence and Usage. Carbon disulfide is widely used as an industrial solvent and as an insecticide. It is also a chemical byproduct in the production of viscose rayon. Exposure is usually via inhalation of the vapor or by dermal contact. The current threshold limit value for carbon disulfide is 20 ppm (60 mg/m^3), although a future revision to 10 ppm is likely.

Blood Concentrations. Carbon disulfide blood concentrations reached maximum levels after 2 hours of exposure to about 30 ppm of the vapor in air and ranged from 0.15 - 0.28 mg/L (Teisinger and Soucek, 1949). Blood concentrations of 0.10 - 0.70 mg/L were observed during exposure to air concentrations on the order of 80 ppm. The half-life for disappearance of the substance from blood is estimated at less than 1 hour (Piotrowski, 1977).

Metabolism and Excretion. From 50 to 90% of an absorbed dose of carbon disulfide is metabolized in the body. From 8 - 20% of the dose may be eliminated unchanged in the exhaled breath and only about 0.5% in the urine. About two-thirds of that which is excreted unchanged in urine is in bound form, and requires acidification and aeration of urine for its release (McKee et al., 1948; Teisinger and Soucek, 1949; Piotrowski, 1977). The metabolized carbon disulfide appears primarily in the urine as inorganic sulfates, thiourea, 2-mercapto-2-thiazolin-5-one and other unidentified products (Pergal et al., 1972a; Pergal et al., 1972b).

Toxicity. Mild exposure to carbon disulfide causes dizziness and headache, while moderate exposure may produce nervousness, fatigue and weight loss. Chronic intoxication has been reported to result in damage to the central and peripheral nervous systems, atherosclerotic tendencies, electrocardiographic abnormalities, and liver and kidney damage (Gordy and Trumper, 1938). Symptoms of moderate to severe intoxication have appeared in individuals chronically exposed to vapor concentrations averaging slightly in excess of 20 ppm (Kleinfeld and Tabershaw, 1955). Exposure to carbon disulfide concentrations of 300 ppm or more can cause serious pathologic changes after only a few days.

Biological Monitoring. Carbon disulfide concentrations in blood, breath and urine have been measured as an approximate index of exposure, using a method which converts the free chemical to a colored complex, copper diethyldithiocarbamate (Teisinger and Soucek, 1949). More recently, the gas chromatographic analysis of carbon disulfide in urine has been reported (Herber, 1976). However, these determinations are not performed routinely.

A widely used exposure test is based on the catalysis of the iodine-azide reaction ($2NaN_3 + I_2 \rightarrow 3N_2 + 2NaI$) by sulfur-containing metabolites of carbon disulfide present in urine specimens. The exposure coefficient determined from urine collected at the end of a work period should exceed 6.5 when a TLV of 20 ppm is in effect (Djuric et al., 1964). Values of less than 6.5 are indicative of excessive exposure to carbon disulfide. The exposure coefficient value correlates well with symptoms of intoxication at higher levels of exposure (10 - 130 ppm), but does not correlate well at lower levels (4 - 11 ppm) (Rosensteel et al., 1974). The determination of this coefficient in urine collected at the beginning of the work day is also recommended in order to (a) detect workers who are still excreting metabolites from the previous day's exposure and who may be at high risk, and (b) to identify spurious results due to the presence of interfering substances, such as metabolites of the drug disulfiram and other industrial thiocarbamates.

Analysis. A method is presented for the determination of a carbon disulfide exposure coefficient by the indirect measurement of urinary metabolites (Djuric et al., 1965). This method requires the prior determination of urinary creatinine, performed by colorimetry (Djuric, 1967).

References

D. Djuric. Determination of carbon disulphide and its metabolites in biological material. In *Toxicology of Carbon Disulphide* (H. Brieger and J. Teisinger, eds.), Excerpta Medica, Amsterdam, 1967, pp. 52 - 61.

D. Djuric, N. Surducki and I. Berkes. Iodine-azide test on urine of persons exposed to carbon disulphide. Brit. J. Ind. Med. 22: 321 - 323, 1965.

S. T. Gordy and M. Trumper. Carbon disulfide poisoning. J. Am. Med. Asso. 110: 1543 - 1549, 1938.

R. F. M. Herber. The application of a new carbon disulfide exposure test in occupational health. Int. Arch. Occ. Env. Health 38: 115 - 120, 1976.

M. Kleinfeld and I. R. Tabershaw. Carbon disulfide poisoning. J. Am. Med. Asso. 159: 677 - 679, 1955.

R. W. McKee, C. Kiper, J. H. Fountain et al. A solvent vapor, carbon disulfide. J. Am. Med. Asso. 122: 217 - 222, 1948.

M. Pergal, N. Vukojevic, N. Cirin-Popov et al. Carbon disulfide metabolites excreted in the urine of exposed workers. Arch. Env. Health 25: 38 - 41, 1972a.

M. Pergal, N. Vukojevic, N. Sad and D. Djuric. II. Isolation and identification of thiocarbamide. Arch. Env. Health 25: 42 - 44, 1972b.

J. K. Piotrowski. *Exposure Tests for Organic Compounds in Industrial Toxicology*, U.S. Government Printing Office, Washington, D.C., 1977, pp. 102 - 106.

R. E. Rosensteel, S. K. Shama and J. P. Flesch. Occupational health case report — no. 1. J. Occ. Med. 16: 22 - 32, 1974.

T. Teisinger and B. Soucek. Absorption and elimination of carbon disulfide in man. J. Ind. Hyg. Tox. 2: 67 - 73, 1949.

Urine Carbon Disulfide Metabolites by the Iodine-Azide Test

Principle:

Urine is treated with a solution containing sodium azide, iodine and potassium iodide. The presence of carbon disulfide metabolites in the sample catalyzes the reduction of iodine to iodide. An exposure coefficient is calculated based on the time required for the disappearance of the iodine color and the creatinine content of the specimen.

Reagents:

Buffer — 110 g/L $NaH_2PO_4 . H_2O$

Iodine-azide reagent — dissolve 3 g NaN_3 in 25 mL water, add 50 mL of a solution containing 24.5 g/L iodine and 50 g/L potassium iodide, and adjust the final volume to 100 mL (prepare fresh)

Procedure:

1. Determine the creatinine concentration of the urine specimen. Discard any specimens which do not contain between 1 and 3 mg/mL creatinine.
2. Transfer 1 mL urine to a clean test tube. Add 0.2 mL buffer and vortex.
3. Add 1 mL iodine-azide reagent and vortex. Measure the elapsed time in seconds from the addition of this reagent until the disappearance of the iodine color.

Calculation:

Calculate the exposure index (E) from the following equation:

$$E = C \log t,$$

where C is the creatinine concentration in mg/L and t is the time in seconds. Quality control materials are not applicable to this procedure.

Evaluation:

Sensitivity: will not detect exposure to carbon disulfide air concentrations of less than 20 ppm

Linearity: not applicable

C.V.: not applicable

Relative recovery: not applicable

Interferences:

This is a non-specific test which responds to the presence of thiols, sulfides, thiosulfates and thiocyanates. The metabolites of disulfiram and other thiocarbamates may give falsely depressed E values. Normal E values for non-exposed subjects, including those on sulfur-rich diets, are in the range of 6 - 10.

Urine Creatinine by Colorimetry

Principle:

Creatinine is measured directly in urine specimens by reaction with picric acid. The chromogen is measured at 530 nm in a visible spectrophotometer.

Reagents:

Stock solution — 100 mg/mL creatinine in 0.1 mol/L hydrochloric acid
Aqueous standards — 1, 2 and 3 mg/mL
1 mol/L Sodium hydroxide
Saturated picric acid

Instrumental Conditions:

Visible spectrophotometer set to 530 nm

Procedure:

1. Transfer 100 μL urine to a 25 mL volumetric flask. Add 1 mL 1 mol/L NaOH and 5 mL saturated picric acid.
2. After 10 minutes, dilute to volume with water. Mix and measure the absorbance of the solution against a reagent blank at 530 nm.

Calculation:

Calculation is based on a response factor derived from a standard curve. A quality control specimen containing 1 mg/mL creatinine is analyzed daily.

Evaluation:

Sensitivity: 0.2 mg/mL
Linearity: 1 - 6 mg/mL
C.V.: not established
Relative recovery: not established

Interferences:

Urine may need to be centrifuged for clarification. Old picric acid solutions may produce a high reagent blank absorbance.

CARBON MONOXIDE

Occurrence and Usage. Carbon monoxide is an odorless, colorless gas which has approximately the same density as air. The compound is produced from the incomplete combustion of organic fuels, and it represents the most abundant air pollutant in the lower atmosphere. Common sources of the gas are cigarette smoke, which contains about 4% carbon monoxide, automobile exhaust, which contains from 0.5 - 10%, and various industrial processes. The metabolism of dichloromethane provides an unexpected source of CO. Atmospheric CO concentrations range from 2 - 50 ppm along expressways and in smoke-filled rooms, and may exceed 100 ppm during temperature inversions and in heavy urban traffic. The current occupational threshold limit value is 50 ppm (55 mg/m^3).

Blood Concentrations. Carbon monoxide is produced endogenously by the catabolism of heme at an average rate of 0.4 mL/hour in resting male subjects; this amount is sufficient to establish a background carboxyhemoglobin (COHb) saturation of 0.4 - 0.7% (Stewart, 1975). COHb averages 1 - 2% in urban nonsmokers and 5 - 6% in smokers (Stewart et al., 1974). Sitting in a smoky room for 1.5 hours caused a 38% increase in the COHb saturation of nonsmokers (Seppanen, 1977). Exposure to a constant air concentration of carbon monoxide results in a constant COHb level after an equilibration period of some hours, the time required being inversely proportional to the CO concentration. Atmospheric concentrations of 50, 100 and 200 ppm produce approximate equilibrium COHb saturations of 8, 16 and 30%, respectively (Peterson and Stewart, 1970).

Metabolism and Excretion. Carbon monoxide is eliminated substantially unchanged by pulmonary excretion, with less than 1% oxidized by metabolic processes to carbon dioxide. The half-life of carboxyhemoglobin in resting adults at sea level is 4 - 5 hours, but may be reduced to approximately 80 minutes by the administration of pure oxygen, and may be further reduced to 24 minutes by using oxygen at 3 atmospheres pressure (Stewart, 1975).

Toxicity. The reversible binding of carbon monoxide with the hemoglobin molecule results in a mild to severe hypoxia, which can produce symptoms of headache, nausea, weakness, confusion, stupor and coma. Blood COHb concentrations of 5 - 10% may aggravate pre-existing heart disease, while concentrations of 15 - 25% often cause dizziness and nausea. Levels of carboxyhemoglobin which exceed 50% saturation are considered as life-threatening.

It has been shown in a number of studies that COHb concentrations of 10% or less adversely affect a person's ability to perform complex tasks as well as strenuous manual labor (Coburn et al., 1977).

Biological Monitoring. The analysis of breath samples for carbon monoxide has been recommended for estimating exposure to this gas (Jones et al., 1958;

Ringold et al., 1962). While this may be a convenient field method, it is not as accurate as a blood determination due to difficulties in obtaining an equilibrated sample and the interindividual variation in the blood/breath partition ratio.

Blood carboxyhemoglobin concentration offers a reliable means of estimating both the extent and the physiologic effect of exposure. Lauwerys (1975) has recommended that the maximum allowable COHb level for workers be set at 5%, corresponding to an 8 hour exposure to 35 ppm of the gas. The current TLV of 50 ppm leads to a COHb level of 8 - 10% in most subjects after 8 hours. A pre-exposure sample must be analyzed to determine the background COHb level resulting from smoking, disease states and non-occupational exposure.

Analysis. Automated visible spectrophotometry using the CO-Oximeter is now a widely used procedure for the determination of carboxyhemoglobin in blood (Dubowski and Luke, 1973), but it requires a specimen volume of 0.4 mL. A manual spectrophotometric technique is presented which is convenient for employee monitoring since it may be performed on a capillary blood specimen (Buchwald, 1969).

References

H. Buchwald. A rapid and sensitive method for estimating carbon monoxide in blood and its application in problem areas. Am. Ind. Hyg. Asso. J. 30: 564 - 569, 1969.

R. F. Coburn, E. R. Allen, S. M. Ayres et al. *Carbon Monoxide*, National Academy of Sciences, Washington, D.C., 1977.

K. M. Dubowski and J. L. Luke. Measurement of carboxyhemoglobin and carbon monoxide in blood. Ann. Clin. Lab. Sci. 3: 53 - 65, 1973.

R. H. Jones, M. F. Ellicott, J. B. Cadigan and E. A. Gaensler. The relationship between alveolar and blood carbon monoxide concentrations during breathholding. J. Lab. Clin. Med. 51: 553 - 564, 1958.

R. Lauwerys. Biological criteria for selected industrial toxic chemicals: a review. Scand. J. Work Env. Health 1: 139 - 172, 1975.

J. E. Peterson and R. D. Stewart. Absorption and elimination of carbon monoxide by inactive young men. Arch. Env. Health 21: 165 - 171, 1970.

A. Ringold, J. R. Goldsmith, H. L. Helwig et al. Estimating recent carbon monoxide exposures. Arch. Env. Health 5: 38 - 48, 1962.

A. Seppanen. Smoking in closed space and its effect of carboxyhaemoglobin saturation of smoking and nonsmoking subjects. Ann. Clin. Res. 9: 281 - 283, 1977.

R. D. Stewart, E. D. Baretta, L. R. Platte et al. Carboxyhemoglobin levels in American blood donors. J. Am. Med. Asso. 229: 1187 - 1195, 1974.

R. D. Stewart. The effect of carbon monoxide on humans. Ann. Rev. Pharm. 15: 409 - 422, 1975.

Blood Carboxyhemoglobin by Visible Spectrophotometry

Principle:

A capillary blood specimen is diluted with ammonium hydroxide and separated into three portions. Portion I is untreated, portion II is saturated with oxygen

(100% oxyhemoglobin standard) and portion III is saturated with carbon monoxide (100% carboxyhemoglobin standard). The absorbances of solutions I and III are measured in the visible region, using solution II as a reference. The calculation of carboxyhemoglobin content is based on absorbance differences at three wavelengths.

Reagents:

Dilute ammonium hydroxide — 1 part conc. NH_4OH in 800 parts water
Oxygen lecture bottle
Carbon monoxide lecture bottle

Instrumental Conditions:

Visible spectrophotometer
Measure absorbance at 414, 421 and 428 nm

Procedure:

1. Collect from 10 - 30 μL of blood in a heparinized capillary tube. Seal the ends with clay or wax and store at 4° C. until analysis.
2. Transfer the blood specimen to a 20 mL serum bottle containing dilute NH_4OH. Fill to the top with dilute NH_4OH and seal the bottle with a plastic snap top in such a way that air is excluded.
3. Mix thoroughly by inversion. Transfer a portion (I) to a 3 mL cuvette and seal the cuvette so that air is excluded.
4. Transfer another portion (II) to a clean serum bottle and bubble oxygen through the solution at the rate of about 50 mL/min for 15 minutes.
5. Bubble carbon monoxide through the final portion (III) at the rate of about 50 mL/min for 2 minutes. Transfer portions II and III to cuvettes.
6. Using solution II as a reference, measure the absorbance of solutions I and III at 414, 421 and 428 nm in the spectrophotometer.

Calculation:

The carboxyhemoglobin content (% COHb) of the specimen is calculated using the following equation:

$$\% \text{ COHb} = \frac{I_{421} - 0.5\,(I_{414} + I_{428})}{III_{421} - 0.5\,(III_{414} + III_{428})} \text{ X } 100$$

where I and III represent the absorbances of solutions I and III at the indicated wavelengths. Quality control materials are not applicable to this procedure.

Evaluation:

Sensitivity: <1% COHb
Linearity: 1 - 40% COHb
C.V.: 1 - 4%
Relative recovery: not applicable

Interferences:

Since each specimen acts as its own reference standard, the determination of total hemoglobin is not necessary. The exact volume of blood used is not critical, although volumes greater than 30 μL may exceed the linearity of the method. Specimens stored at 4° C. for more than a week did not show any appreciable variation in carboxyhemoglobin content.

CARBON TETRACHLORIDE

Occurrence and Usage. Carbon tetrachloride has for years been widely used as a dry-cleaning chemical, degreasing agent and fire extinguisher, although recent United States Food and Drug Administration regulations against its commercial sale have restricted it to laboratory and industrial usage. It is now employed as a grain fumigant, solvent and a chemical intermediate in the manufacture of fluorocarbons. The current threshold limit value for industrial environments is 10 ppm (65 mg/m^3), although this value is pending revision to 5 ppm. The odor threshold of the compound is about 50 ppm.

Blood Concentrations. Using an analytical method which had a 5 mg/L limit of sensitivity, Stewart et al. (1961) were unable to detect carbon tetrachloride in the blood of men exposed to 11 ppm of the vapor for 3 hours or to 49 ppm for 1.2 hours. Monkeys exposed to 46 ppm of the vapor developed maximal blood concentrations of 1.7 mg/L after 4.5 hours (McCollister et al., 1951).

Metabolism and Excretion. The metabolism of carbon tetrachloride has not been studied in man. In monkeys, at least 51% of the absorbed dose was eliminated in the expired air as carbon tetrachloride (40%) and carbon dioxide (11%) in the 29 days after exposure; significant amounts were excreted in urine and feces as metabolic products, including urea and carbonates (McCollister et al., 1951). It is believed that the metabolic conversion of the molecule to a highly reactive free radical accounts for its ability to cause tissue necrosis.

Carbon tetrachloride concentrations in the breath of men exposed to 10 ppm of the vapor for 3 hours averaged 2 - 3 ppm at the end of the exposure, 0.7 ppm after 1 hour and less than 0.3 ppm after 5 hours. Following a 70 minute exposure to 49 ppm, these concentrations were 10 - 20 ppm, less than 2 ppm and less than 0.3 ppm, respectively (Stewart et al., 1961).

Toxicity. Carbon tetrachloride has produced numerous cases of acute and chronic poisoning, by virtue of its central nervous system depressant and nephro- and hepatotoxic effects (Hardin, 1954). Prolonged exposure to vapor concentrations of 25 ppm or more may cause severe kidney and liver damage. Acute renal damage leading to death has resulted from exposure to concentrations of 1000 - 2000 ppm for 30 - 60 minutes. Excessive alcohol usage may potentiate the toxic effects of carbon tetrachloride.

An adult who ingested 30 mL of the chemical and recovered had a serum carbon tetrachloride level of 20 mg/L on admission to the hospital; the first 24 hour urine specimen was found to contain 8 mg/L of the compound (Clarke, 1969). An adult who committed suicide by inhaling carbon tetrachloride vapors had a postmortem blood concentration of 260 mg/L (Cravey, 1978).

Biological Monitoring. The data of Stewart et al. (1961) suggested that carbon tetrachloride breath concentrations should not exceed 3 ppm in workers exposed at the level of the current TLV. This data is based on a 3 hour exposure and has not been confirmed by other authors.

While blood concentrations of carbon tetrachloride have not been used to assess low-level exposure, this approach merits investigation using a suitably sensitive analytical technique.

Analysis. The method described for benzene (p. 39) in blood and breath incorporates headspace sampling with flame-ionization gas chromatography and is applicable to a variety of volatile substances, including carbon tetrachloride.

References

E. G. C. Clarke (ed). *Isolation and Identification of Drugs*, Pharmaceutical Press, London, 1969, p. 240.

R. H. Cravey. Personal communication, 1978.

B. L. Hardin, Jr. Carbon tetrachloride poisoning — a review. Ind. Med. Surg. 23: 93 - 105, 1954.

D. D. McCollister, W. H. Beamer, G. J. Atchison and H. C. Spencer. The absorption, distribution and elimination of radioactive carbon tetrachloride by monkeys upon exposure to low vapor concentrations. J. Pharm. Exp. Ther. 102: 112 - 124, 1951.

R. D. Stewart, H. H. Gay, D. S. Erley et al. Human exposure to carbon tetrachloride vapor. J. Occ. Med. 3: 586 - 590, 1961.

CHLORDANE

Occurrence and Usage. Chlordane is an organochlorine insecticide which has been commercially available since 1949. The technical product is a mixture of 2 chlordane isomers (60 - 75%) and related products (chlordene, heptachlor and nonachlor) and has been widely employed in agriculture and in households. It is frequently used in the form of a dust containing 5% or a solution containing 50% active ingredients. The compound is readily absorbed following inhalation, ingestion or dermal contact. Chlordane, closely related structurally to heptachlor, has come under severe restrictions in some countries due to its persistence in the environment. The current threshold limit value is 0.5 mg/m^3.

Blood Concentrations. Concentrations of chlordane in the blood of nonexposed or occupationally exposed subjects have not been reported.

Metabolism and Excretion. Over a period of 2.5 days, rats excreted 1% of an injected dose of chlordane in the urine and 29% in the feces, primarily as water-soluble metabolites (Poonawalla and Korte, 1964). Oxychlordane, believed to be a human metabolite of chlordane, is found in the adipose tissue of the general population at concentrations of 0.03 - 0.40 mg/kg (Biros and Enos, 1973).

Toxicity. Chlordane is a persistent, fat-soluble central nervous system stimulant. Acute intoxication produces symptoms of confusion, delerium, nausea, convulsions and death. Chronic exposure is known to cause liver and kidney damage.

A 20 month old child ingested chlordane and developed seizures within an hour; after 3 hours, chlordane concentrations of 2.7 mg/L in serum and 3.1 mg/kg in fat were measured, and after 3 months these values had decreased to 0.02 mg/L and increased to 25.5 mg/kg, respectively. Less than 50 μg of chlordane was excreted in the first 24 hour urine specimen (Curley and Garrettson, 1969). A 4 year old child who experienced convulsions after chlordane ingestion exhibited an initial serum concentration of 3.4 mg/L, with a serum half-life of 88 days (Aldrich and Holmes, 1969). In both of these cases the victims recovered within 24 to 48 hours of ingestion, and urine concentrations of unchanged chlordane were very low (0.3 mg/L or less). Two deaths in adults have been due to chlordane poisoning; one occurred about an hour after massive dermal exposure and other 9.5 days after ingestion of 6 g of the compound (Derbes et al., 1955).

Biological Monitoring. Studies have not been made in regard to the assessment of occupational exposure to chlordane through the analysis of biological specimens. By analogy with other chlorinated pesticides, the measurement of blood chlordane concentrations should prove useful in following worker exposure.

Analysis. Concentrations of chlordane in biological material may be determined by the electron-capture gas chromatographic procedure for chlorinated hydrocarbon insecticides which is presented on p. 16.

References

A. D. Aldrich and J. H. Holmes. Acute chlordane intoxication in a child. Arch. Env. Health 19: 129 - 132, 1969.

F. J. Biros and H. F. Enos. Oxychlordane residues in human adipose tissue. Bull. Env. Cont. Tox. 5: 257 - 260, 1973.

A. Curley and L. K. Garrettson. Acute chlordane poisoning. Arch. Env. Health 18: 211 - 215, 1969.

V. J. Derbes, J. H. Dent, W. W. Forrest and M. F. Johnson. Fatal chlordane poisoning. J. Am. Med. Asso. 158: 1367 - 1369, 1955.

N. H. Poonawalla and F. Korte. Metabolism of insecticides, VIII (I): excretion, distribution and metabolism of α-chlordane-^{14}C by rats. Life Sci. 3: 1497 - 1500, 1964.

CHLORDECONE

Occurrence and Usage. Chlordecone (Kepone) is a chlorinated hydrocarbon pesticide, first developed in 1952, which is closely related to mirex. Most of the chlordecone produced in the United States has been exported for the control of agricultural pests, but inadequate precautions during manufacturing led in 1975 to a number of human poisonings and extensive environmental contamination in the manufacturing area. The compound is well absorbed following oral, respiratory or dermal administration. A threshold limit value for occupational exposure has not been set for chlordecone.

Blood Concentrations. Of 216 blood samples obtained from healthy members of the general population living within a one mile radius of a chlordecone manufacturing facility, 40 were found to contain detectable amounts of chlordecone ranging from 0.005 - 0.033 mg/L (Anonymous, 1976). Serum concentrations of chlordecone in 11 occupationally exposed subjects ranged from 0.120 - 2.109 mg/L and averaged 0.734 mg/L. The average serum half-life was found to be 96 days (range 63 - 148) and the average blood/serum concentration ratio, 0.57 (Adir et al., 1978).

Metabolism and Excretion. Metabolites of chlordecone have not been found in human tissues. The compound is primarily eliminated in bile, but is largely reabsorbed, so that the overall elimination rate is only 0.075% of the total body burden per day. Negligible amounts are excreted in urine and sweat (Cohn et al., 1976). A single oral dose administered to rats was slowly excreted over a period of 84 days in feces (66%) and urine (1.6%), apparently as unchanged chlordecone (Egle et al., 1978).

Toxicity. Chronic toxicity due to chlordecone exposure is expressed as neurological, hepatic and hormonal abnormalities. The compound is carcinogenic in animals and is considered a potential human carcinogen.

Chlordecone was found present in blood and biopsy tissues of 32 chemical workers exhibiting symptoms of toxicity in the following concentrations (Cohn et al., 1976):

Chlordecone Concentrations in Nonfatal Poisoning (mg/L or mg/kg)

	Blood	Liver	Fat
Average	5.8	76	22
(Range)	(0.6 - 32)	(13 - 173)	(2.2 - 62)

Biological Monitoring. The blood chlordecone concentration is related to the severity of intoxication and is useful in assessing exposure to chlordecone. Blood concentrations were found to average 0.6 mg/L in asymptomatic exposed workers. In workers exhibiting symptoms of intoxication, including tremor, chest pain, visual disturbances, mental changes and weight loss, chlordecone blood levels averaged 2.5 mg/L (Taylor et al, 1978).

Analysis. An electron-capture gas chromatographic method is described for the determination of chlordecone in blood or serum (Caplan et al., 1979).

References

J. Adir, Y. H. Caplan and B. C. Thompson. Kepone serum half-life in humans. Life Sci. 22: 699-702, 1978.

Anonymous. Preliminary report on Kepone levels found in human blood from the general population of Hopewell, Virginia. Health Effects Research Laboratory, U.S. Environmental Protection Agency, Research Triangle Park, NC, March 3, 1976.

R. V. Blanke, M. W. Fariss, F. D. Griffith, Jr. and P. Guzelian. Analysis of chlordecone (Kepone) in biological specimens. J. Anal. Tox. 1: 57-62, 1977.

Y. H. Caplan, B. C. Thompson and J. H. Hebb, Jr. A method for the determination of chlordecone (Kepone) in human serum and blood. J. Anal. Tox. 3: 202-205, 1979.

W. J. Cohn, R. V. Blanke, F. D. Griffith, Jr. and P. S. Guzelian. Distribution and excretion of Kepone (KP) in humans. Gastroenterology 71: 901, 1976.

J. L. Egle, S. B. Fernandez, P. S. Guzelian and J. F. Borzelleca. Distribution and excretion of chlordecone (Kepone) in the rat. Drug Met. Disp. 6: 91-95, 1978.

R. L. Harless, D. E. Harris, G. W. Sovocool et al. Mass spectrometric analyses and characterization of Kepone in environmental and human samples. Biomed. Mass Spec. 5: 232-237, 1978.

J. R. Taylor, J. B. Selhorst, S. A. Houff and A. J. Martinez. Chlordecone intoxication in man. Neurology 28: 626-630, 1978.

Blood Chlordecone by Electron-Capture Gas Chromatography

Principle:

Chlordecone is extracted from acidified blood into benzene. Dilute alkali is used to back-extract the pesticide from the benzene. After acidification of the aqueous phase, benzene containing an internal standard (dieldrin) is used to extract the chlordecone. An aliquot of this solution is analyzed by electron-capture gas chromatography.

Reagents:

Stock solution — 0.2 mg/mL chlordecone in 95% ethanol
Blood standards — 0.020, 0.050, 0.100, 0.200 and 0.400 mg/L
60% Sulfuric acid
Benzene
1 mol/L Sodium hydroxide
Concentrated sulfuric acid
Internal standard stock solution — 100 mg dieldrin in 10 mL 95% ethanol
Internal standard working solution — 0.75 mL stock solution diluted to 500 mL with benzene

Instrumental Conditions:

Gas chromatograph with electron-capture detector
2 m x 2 mm i.d. glass column containing 10% DC-200 on 100/200 mesh Gas Chrom Q
Injector, 260° C.; column, 230° C.; detector, 300° C.
5% Methane in argon flow rate, 75 mL/min

Procedure:

1. Transfer 1 mL blood to a 25 mL screw-cap tube. Add 1 mL 60% H_2SO_4 and vortex.
2. Extract with 15 mL benzene by shaking for 1 minute. Centrifuge and transfer the benzene layer to a clean tube.
3. Extract with 5 mL 1 mol/L NaOH by shaking for 1 minute. Centrifuge and discard benzene layer.
4. Re-extract with 5 mL benzene, centrifuge and discard the benzene layer. Add 10 drops conc. H_2SO_4 and 1 mL internal standard working solution.
5. Shake for 1 minute and centrifuge. Inject 4 μL of the upper organic layer into the chromatograph.

	Retention time (min)
internal standard	9.8
chlordecone	14.5

Calculation:

Calculation is based on a response factor derived from a standard curve. A quality control specimen containing 0.200 mg/L chlordecone is analyzed daily.

Evaluation:

Sensitivity: 0.010 mg/L
Linearity: 0.020 - 0.400 mg/L
C.V.: 4.1% within-run
Relative recovery: not established

Interferences:

The method is relatively specific for chlordecone since other halogenated pesticides are not extracted by this technique. Background levels of up to 0.005 mg/L apparent chlordecone have been observed in chlordecone-free specimens.

CHLOROFORM

Occurrence and Usage. Chloroform was once used extensively as an anesthetic in man, but is now considered obsolete for this application. It has also been incorporated into many pharmaceutical preparations for its solvent and local anesthetic properties, but its proven carcinogenic potential in laboratory animals has precluded its use in food or drugs in the United States. Chloroform continues to be encountered as a solvent and chemical intermediate in laboratory and industrial situations, for which the current threshold limit value is 10 ppm (50 mg/m^3). The odor threshold of the compound is about 50 ppm.

Blood Concentrations. A single 500 mg dose of chloroform administered to 2 subjects produced maximal blood concentrations of 1 - 5 mg/L at about 1 hour; an average elimination half-life of 1.5 hours was observed (Fry et al., 1972). Blood specimens drawn from 58 patients undergoing chloroform anesthesia exhibited overall concentrations ranging from 20 - 232 mg/L with an average of 92 mg/L; samples from patients in plane 1 of stage III anesthesia averaged 71 mg/L; plane 2, 106 mg/L; plane 3, 122 mg/L; and plane 4, 165 mg/L (Morris et al., 1951).

Metabolism and Excretion. Chloroform undergoes considerable biotransformation in man, with the formation of carbon dioxide and hydrochloric acid. An average of 43% (range 18 - 67) of a single dose is eliminated unchanged in the expired air within 8 hours, and an average of 50% is found as exhaled CO_2 in the same time period. Less than 0.01% of the dose was found in the 8 hour urine (Fry et al., 1972).

Toxicity. Prolonged exposure to chloroform vapor concentrations of 77 - 237 ppm causes weakness, mental dullness and gastrointestinal disturbances (Challen et al., 1958). Chronic exposure to concentrations of up to 205 ppm has produced a high incidence of liver abnormalities in workers (Bomski et al., 1967).

The acute ingestion of as little as 10 mL of chloroform may result in death due to central nervous system depression. Exposure to air concentrations of 100 - 1000 ppm for short periods may cause discomfort and dizziness, and concentrations of 7000 - 20,000 ppm will produce rapid loss of consciousness. In six acute fatalities due to the intentional or forced inhalation of chloroform, blood levels of 10 - 48 mg/L and urine levels of 0 - 60 mg/L were observed (Bidanset, 1973; Bonnichsen and Maehly, 1966).

Biological Monitoring. Blood or breath chloroform concentrations have not been studied in workers exposed to chloroform at or near the level of the TLV. It is likely that breath concentrations offer a convenient means of assessing individual exposure to this compound.

Analysis. The flame-ionization gas chromatographic method described for benzene (p. 39) is applicable to the determination of chloroform in breath and biological fluids.

References

J. Bidanset. Presented at the 25th Annual Meeting of the American Academy of Forensic Sciences, Las Vegas, February 22, 1973.

H. Bomski, A. Sobolewska and A. Strakowski. Toxic damage of the liver by chloroform in chemical industry workers. Arch. Gewerbepath. Gewerbehyg. 24: 127 - 134, 1967.

R. Bonnichsen and A. C. Maehly. Poisoning by volatile compounds. II. Chlorinated aliphatic hydrocarbons. J. For. Sci. 11: 414 - 427, 1966.

P. J. R. Challen, D. E. Hickish and J. Bedford. Chronic chloroform intoxication. Brit. J. Ind. Med. 15: 243 - 249, 1958.

B. J. Fry, T. Taylor and D. E. Hathway. Pulmonary elimination of chloroform and its metabolite in man. Arch. Int. Pharm. Ther. 196: 98 - 111, 1972.

L. E. Morris, E. L. Frederickson and O. S. Orth. Differences in the concentration of chloroform in the blood of man and dog during anesthesia. J. Pharm. Exp. Ther. 101: 56-62, 1951.

CHROMIUM

Occurrence and Usage. Chromium is an essential nutrient for man, being required for the maintenance of normal glucose tolerance. The human diet supplies from 5 - 115 μg/day of the element, of which only 1 - 25% is absorbed from the gastrointestinal tract. Chromium encounters many industrial applications, including its uses in steel and nonferrous alloys, metal-plating, refractory materials, chromate pigments and chromate preservatives. Exposure to the metal and its insoluble and soluble salts is generally via inhalation of dusts or fumes; the current threshold limit values for these compounds range from 0.05 - 0.5 mg/ m^3. Chromite ore processing is listed as having carcinogenic potential, while lead and zinc chromates are suspected carcinogens.

Blood Concentrations. Serum chromium concentrations average about 0.16 μg/L (range 0.04 - 0.35) in healthy subjects (Versieck et al., 1978; Kayne et al., 1978). Literature published prior to 1978 refers to normal serum chromium values ranging from 0.7 to 150 μg/L, due to methodological difficulties in the trace analysis of chromium.

Metabolism and Excretion. Of an absorbed dose of chromium, at least 80% is excreted in the urine and a lesser amount in the feces. Hexavalent chromium, which is generally more soluble and more toxic than the trivalent form, tends to be reduced to trivalent chromium *in vivo*. Chromium does not appear to accumulate in bone or most soft tissues as a result of age, occupation or smoking history. The lung, however, usually contains the highest concentration of any organ in the body and this concentration increases with age, probably as a result of the deposition of insoluble chromium compounds present in air. Normal urinary chromium concentrations average 4 - 5 μg/L and range up to 15 μg/L; the daily urinary output of chromium ranges from 1.6 - 21 μg in healthy young adults (Baetjer et al., 1974). Urine chromium concentrations in one group of welders were found to range from 30 - 200 μg/L (Glyseth et al., 1977).

Toxicity. The inhalation of insoluble chromium compounds has led to pneumoconiosis with impairment of pulmonary function; exposure to the chromite ore roasting process is suspected to have carcinogenic potential. Soluble salts of hexavalent chromium are corrosive and have produced skin ulceration, dermatitis, perforation of the nasal septum, respiratory sensitization and lung cancer. Acute poisoning with soluble salts usually results in local tissue necrosis and severe kidney damage (Baetjer et al., 1974). Electroplaters and paint pigment workers who expressed symptoms of cough, indigestion and dermal itching were found to have urine chromium concentrations of 91 - 1116 μg/L (Tandon et al., 1977).

Biological Monitoring. Urinary chromium concentrations in exposed workers have been found to correlate well with air chromium concentrations and are a good indicator of short-term exposure. A chromium level of 40 - 50 $\mu g/L$, or 30 $\mu g/g$ creatinine, in a urine specimen collected at the end of the working day is consistent with exposure to chromium at the TLV of 0.05 mg/m^3 (Glyseth et al., 1977; Tola et al., 1977). The renal clearance of chromium may be a better indicator of chromium body burden and nephrotoxicity than urine concentrations of the metal (Mutti et al., 1979).

Analysis. A procedure for the analysis of chromium in urine is presented which utilizes atomic absorption spectrometry (Kayne et al., 1978).

References

A. M. Baetjer, D. J. Birmingham, P. E. Enterline et al. *Chromium*, National Academy of Sciences, Washington, D. C., 1974.

B. Glyseth, N. Gundersen and S. Langard. Evaluation of chromium exposure based on a simplified method for urinary chromium determination. Scand. J. Work Env. Health 3: 28 - 31, 1977.

F. J. Kayne, G. Komar, H. Laboda and R. E. Vanderlinde. Atomic absorption spectrophotometry of chromium in serum and urine with a modified Perkin-Elmer 603 atomic absorption spectrophotometer. Clin. Chem. 24: 2151 - 2154, 1978.

A. Mutti, A. Cavatorta, C. Pedroni et al. The role of chromium accumulation in the relationship between airborne and urinary chromium in welders. Int. Arch. Occ. Env. Health 43: 123 - 133, 1979.

S. K. Tandon, A. K. Mathur and J. S. Gaur. Urinary excretion of chromium and nickel among electroplaters and pigment industry workers. Int. Arch. Occ. Env. Health 40: 71 - 76, 1977.

S. Tola, J. Kilpio, M. Virtamo and K. Haapa. Urinary chromium as an indicator of the exposure of welders to chromium. Scand. J. Work Env. Health 3: 192 - 202, 1977.

J. Versieck, J. Hoste, F. Barbier et al. Determination of chromium and cobalt in human serum by neutron activation analysis. Clin. Chem. 24: 303 - 308, 1978.

Urine Chromium by Atomic Absorption Spectrometry

Principle:

Urine is diluted with water and analyzed directly by graphite-furnace atomic absorption spectrometry, using tungsten-halogen background correction.

Reagents:

Stock solution — 1 mg/mL chromium ion (Fisher reference standard)
Aqueous standards — 5, 10, 20, 40 and 80 $\mu g/L$

All solutions should be stored in polyethylene containers which have been washed in 50% nitric acid.

Instrumental Conditions:

Atomic absorption spectrometer with graphite furnace, optical temperature sensor and tungsten-halogen background corrector (Perkin-Elmer Model 5000 with HGA 2200 Graphite Furnace)
Chromium hollow cathode lamp operated at 20 mA
Furnace program:
dry at 110° C. for 100 sec
char at 1100° C. for 60 sec
atomize at 2500° C. for 8 sec
Argon purge gas in interrupt mode, 40 mL/min
Measure absorption at 357.9 nm

Procedure:

1. Dilute 0.5 mL of the urine specimen or aqueous standards to 2.5 mL with deionized water.
2. Inject 20 μL directly into the graphite furnace and begin the temperature program. Measure the absorption at 357.9 nm.

Calculation:

Calculation is based on a standard curve prepared each time an analysis is performed. This procedure cannot be controlled by the usual methods due to the instability of dilute chromium solutions.

Evaluation:

Sensitivity: 0.1 μg/L
Linearity: 5 - 40 μg/L with dilution
C.V.: not established
Relative recovery: not established

Interferences:

None are known. Aqueous blanks should be analyzed frequently to avoid contamination by water or glassware. Use of a deuterium lamp background corrector rather than the tungsten-halogen lamp described may result in large analytical errors.

COBALT

Occurrence and Usage. Cobalt is an essential element for man and is supplied in the diet at an average intake of 280 μg/day. Cobalt as the metal is incorporated into certain grades of steel and into tungsten carbide tools. Compounds of cobalt are used as paint pigments and occasionally as therapeutic agents. Industrial exposure is normally via inhalation of dusts or fumes while working with cobalt-containing tools or alloys. The current threshold limit value for cobalt in air is 0.1 mg/m^3, although revision of this limit to 0.05 mg/m^3 is pending.

Blood Concentrations. Serum cobalt concentrations in normal subjects average 0.11 μg/L and range from 0.04 - 0.27 μg/L (Versieck et al., 1978). Blood cobalt concentrations reached a peak of approximately 30 μg/L in two normal subjects after the oral administration of 50 mg of cobaltous chloride; blood cobalt concentrations in untreated subjects in this study were 0.6 - 1.8 μg/L. Peak blood levels in maintenance hemodialysis patients undergoing daily oral treatment with 50 mg cobaltous chloride for 2 weeks were as high as 800 μg/L, and did not return to normal levels until six months following discontinuation of therapy. Toxicity in these patients was primarily limited to nausea and vomiting, although one patient later died due to suspected cobalt cardiomyopathy (Curtis et al., 1976).

Metabolism and Excretion. Of the cobalt which is ingested in the daily diet, about 86% is excreted in the urine and 14% in the feces (Schroeder et al., 1967). In normal subjects an average of 18% of an oral dose of radioactive cobalt was eliminated in the 24 hour urine (Sorbie et al., 1971). Normal urine cobalt levels range from 1 - 7 μg/L (Hubbard et al., 1966). Cobalt excretion in the 24 hour urine of two normal subjects after an oral dose of 50 mg of cobaltous chloride reached a maximum of 500 - 750 μg during the first day, and fell markedly thereafter (Curtis et al., 1976).

Toxicity. Exposure to cobalt or its compounds has produced an allergic dermatitis in workers. Chronic inhalation of cobalt may result in pulmonary fibrosis, accompanied by cough and dyspnea. Cobalt accumulates in the serum of uremic patients and is believed to contribute to the myocardial failure often observed (Lins and Pehrsson, 1976). The metal has also been implicated in heart disease and polycythemia seen in chronic beer drinkers, at a time when cobalt was a common beer additive (Kesteloot et al., 1968).

Biological Monitoring. The measurement of cobalt in the urine of exposed workers has been proposed as a monitoring tool, although no correlations have been drawn between urinary cobalt concentrations and the extent of exposure.

Analysis. Cobalt in urine may be measured using a colorimetric technique (Hubbard et al., 1966).

References

J. R. Curtis, G. C. Goode, J. Herrington and L. E. Urdaneta. Possible cobalt toxicity in maintenance hemodialysis patients after treatment with cobaltous chloride: a study of blood and tissue cobalt concentrations in normal subjects and patients with terminal renal failure. Clin. Neph. 5: 61 - 65, 1976.

D. M. Hubbard, F. M. Creech and J. Cholak. Determination of cobalt in air and biological material. Arch. Env. Health 13: 190 - 194, 1966.

L. E. Lins and K. Pehrsson. Cobalt intoxication in uraemic myocardiopathy? Lancet 1: 1191 - 1192, 1976.

H. Kesteloot, J. Roelandt, J. Willems et al. An enquiry into the role of cobalt in the heart disease of chronic beer drinkers. Circ. 37: 854 - 864, 1968.

H. A. Schroeder, A. P. Nason and I. H. Tipton. Essential trace elements in man: cobalt. J. Chron. Dis. 20: 869 - 890, 1967.

J. Sorbie, D. Olatunbosun, W. E. N. Corbett and L. S. Valberg. Cobalt excretion test for the assessment of body iron stores. Can. Med. Asso. J. 104: 777 - 782, 1971.

J. Versieck, J. Hoste, F. Barbier et al. Determination of chromium and cobalt in human serum by neutron activation analysis. Clin. Chem. 24: 303 - 308, 1978.

Urine Cobalt by Colorimetry

Principle:

Urine is dry-ashed in a muffle furnace. The residue is treated to diethyldithiocarbamate chelation and chloroform extraction. The extracted cobalt is complexed with Nitroso-R-salt and the resulting color measured in a visible spectrophotometer.

Reagents:

Stock solution — 1 mg/mL cobalt ion (Fisher reference standard)

Aqueous standards — 5, 10, 20 and 40 μg/L

Concentrated nitric acid

Ammonium citrate solution — dissolve 400 g citric acid in 500 mL water, neutralize with ammonium hydroxide and dilute to 1 liter; add 20 mL 10% sodium diethyldithiocarbamate and extract the solution several times with 10 mL portions of chloroform to remove cobalt

Buffer solution — dissolve 247 g ammonium acetate, 109 g sodium acetate and 6 g acetic acid in water and dilute to 1 liter; treat as described above to remove cobalt

Concentrated ammonium hydroxide

DDC solution — dissolve 66 g sodium diethyldithiocarbamate in water and dilute to 500 mL; extract with 10 mL chloroform and store in a polyethylene container

Chloroform
Concentrated hydrochloric acid
10% Nitric acid
0.2% Nitroso-R-salt solution
Sodium acetate

Instrumental Conditions:

Visible spectrophotometer set to 550 nm

Procedure:

1. Transfer 50 mL of urine to a silica evaporation dish and add 10 mL conc. HNO_3. Evaporate to dryness on a hot plate.
2. Ash in a muffle furnace at 500° C. for 1 - 2 hours. Cool and add 95 mL water and 1 mL conc. HNO_3.
3. Heat to dissolve the residue and then cool. Add 20 mL ammonium citrate solution and 10 mL buffer solution.
4. Adjust to pH 6.5 with conc. NH_4OH. Transfer the solution to a 500 mL separatory funnel and add 250 mL water.
5. Add 20 mL DDC solution and extract the mixture with 10 mL chloroform. Allow the layers to separate and transfer the chloroform to a 125 mL separatory funnel.
6. Repeat the chloroform extraction twice, collecting each extract in the 125 mL separatory funnel. Wash the chloroform by shaking with 50 mL of water.
7. Transfer the chloroform layer to a 50 mL centrifuge tube and evaporate to dryness in a water bath. Dissolve the residue in 1 mL conc. HNO_3, heating if necessary, and transfer to a 125 mL beaker.
8. Evaporate to dryness on a hot plate. Cool and add 5 mL water, 0.25 mL conc. HCl and 0.25 mL 10% HNO_3.
9. Heat to dissolve the residue and then cool. Add 0.5 mL 0.2% Nitroso-R-salt and 1 g sodium acetate and boil for 1 min.
10. Add 1 mL conc. HNO_3 and boil again for 1 min. Cool in a dark environment and after 5 min transfer to a 10 mL volumetric flask.
11. Dilute to volume with water and determine the absorbance of an aliquot at 550 nm against a reagent blank.

Calculation:

Calculation is based on a standard curve prepared each time an analysis is performed. This procedure cannot be controlled by the usual methods due to the instability of dilute cobalt solutions.

Evaluation:

Sensitivity: 5 μg/L
Linearity: 5 - 25 μg/L
C.V.: not established
Relative recovery: not established

Interferences:

High concentrations of iron, nickel or copper may interfere with the determination, although the method is designed to avoid these interferences under normal conditions.

COPPER

Occurrence and Usage. Copper is an essential trace metal whose numerous metabolic functions remain to be fully delineated. The daily adult requirement is approximately 2 mg and this is supplied by the diet, which averages 2 - 5 mg per day. Human abnormalities of copper metabolism exist which may result in gradual copper toxicity. Acute copper poisoning is usually a consequence of food contamination by copper utensils, or of the accidental or intentional ingestion of copper salts. Industrial exposure is generally by inhalation of copper fumes or dusts, which have been assigned threshold limit values of 0.2 and 1.0 mg/m^3, respectively.

Blood Concentrations. Total serum copper has been found to average 1.09 mg/L in men and 1.20 mg/L in women; erythrocyte copper averaged 0.89 mg/L of packed cells in both sexes. About 93% of the copper in serum is tightly bound to the copper enzyme, ceruloplasmin, and the remainder is loosely bound to serum protein. Serum copper values for women in the third trimester of pregnancy averaged 2.39 mg/L (Cartwright and Wintrobe, 1964).

Metabolism and Excretion. About one-third of the ingested dietary copper is absorbed. Of this amount, about 80% is excreted into the bile, about 18% passes through the intestinal wall into the bowel and 2 - 4% appears in the urine (Cartwright and Wintrobe, 1964). A small amount of the copper taken up by the liver is incorporated into ceruloplasmin, which is synthesized in the liver, and it soon appears in plasma in this non-diffusible form (Scheinberg and Sternlieb, 1960). Urinary excretion of copper averages only 52 μg daily (range 26 - 64) in normal subjects (Dawson et al., 1968). Urine copper concentrations in 206 asymptomatic workers in copper smelters, where atmospheric copper levels reached as high as 30 - 40 mg/m^3, averaged 79 $\mu g/L$ and ranged up to 1145 $\mu g/L$ (Wagner, 1975).

Toxicity. Chronic copper poisoning generally does not occur in normal subjects who are able to maintain a neutral copper balance over a wide range of dietary and environmental copper intake. In persons with Wilson's disease, however, a progressive copper toxicity develops due to a hereditary metabolic abnormality; serum ceruloplasmin levels are markedly reduced, and excess copper deposits in parenchymal tissues causing damage which is eventually fatal (Scheinberg and Sternlieb, 1960). These patients may have serum copper levels which are only one-half of normal, liver concentrations which are five times normal and urine concentrations which are ten times normal (Fell et al., 1968).

The acute inhalation of copper fume during refining or welding processes may cause typical metal fume fever, with upper respiratory irritation, chills and aching muscles. A number of workers who developed copper fume fever had serum copper levels which averaged 1.26 mg/L (Cohen, 1974). The inhalation of metallic copper dust produces similar symptoms (Gleason, 1968). Chronic copper poisoning in industry is associated with anorexia, nausea, vomiting, nervous manifestations and hepatomegaly; serum copper concentrations have ranged from 0.8 to over 2.0 mg/L in such cases (Suciu et al., 1977).

Moderate gastrointestinal distress is produced by ingestion of several hundred milligrams of a copper salt, and acute symptoms of copper poisoning have been observed in persons using corroded copper utensils for preparing food (Nicholas, 1968). Increases of 15 - 100% in serum copper concentrations of 6 children were measured following the administration of 250 mg of copper sulfate as an emetic (Holtzman and Haslam, 1968). Serum copper levels of up to 5 mg/L were achieved during accidental intoxication by copper sulfate applied to burned skin (Holtzman et al., 1966), and serum concentrations of 13 and 27 mg/L were observed in 2 patients poisoned during hemodialysis with a unit containing a copper heating coil (Klein et al., 1972).

In a study of 48 cases of acute (usually intentional) copper sulfate poisoning, it was found that blood copper levels correlated well with the severity of intoxication, whereas serum levels did not; blood concentrations averaged 2.87 mg/L in mild poisoning cases and 7.98 mg/L in severe cases. Serum ionic copper in these patients averaged 2.57 mg/L when measured within 12 hours of ingestion and 0.23 mg/L after more than 12 hours had elapsed, with concurrent relocation of the copper into erythrocytes (Chuttani et al., 1965). Death usually occurs within 1 - 7 days of the ingestion of 10 - 20 g of copper sulfate and is often preceded by vomiting, hemolysis, liver and kidney damage, and shock. Postmortem blood copper concentrations of 8.7 - 63 mg/L were found in 4 such cases (Grusz-Harday, 1969; Richardson, 1975).

Biological Monitoring. Measurement of copper in a 24 hour urine specimen has been proposed as a routine industrial screening test. Urine copper concentrations appear to relate to the severity of exposure to the metal, but do not necessarily correlate with symptoms of intoxication. If the urine copper level is significantly elevated, a serum copper level determination may provide further confirmation of excessive exposure to the metal (Cohen, 1974).

Analysis. An atomic absorption procedure is described for the analysis of copper in serum and urine (Dawson et al., 1968).

References

G. E. Cartwright and M. M. Wintrobe. Copper metabolism in normal subjects. Am. J. Clin. Nutr. 14: 224 - 232, 1964.

H. K. Chuttani, P. S. Gupta, S. Gulati and D. N. Gupta. Acute copper sulfate poisoning. Am. J. Med. 39: 849 - 854, 1965.

S. R. Cohen. A review of the health hazards from copper exposure. J. Occ. Med. 16: 621 - 624, 1974.

J. B. Dawson, D. J. Ellis and H. Newton-John. Direct estimation of copper in serum and urine by atomic absorption spectroscopy. Clin. Chim. Acta 21: 33-42, 1968.

G. S. Fell, H. Smith and R. A. Howie. Neutron activation analysis for copper in biological material applied to Wilson's disease. J. Clin. Path. 21: 8 - 11, 1968.

K. P. Gleason. Exposure to copper dust. Am. Ind. Hyg. Asso. J. 29: 461 - 462, 1968.

E. Grusz-Harday. Spektrophotometrische Kupferbestimmungen aus Leichenteilen bei drei Fällen von Kupfersulfatvergiftung. Arch. Tox. 24: 338 - 340, 1969.

N. A. Holtzman, D. A. Elliott and R. H. Heller. Copper intoxication. New Eng. J. Med. 275: 347 - 352, 1966.

N. A. Holtzman and R. H. A. Haslam. Elevation of serum copper following copper sulfate as an emetic. Pediat. 42: 189 - 193, 1968.

W. J. Klein, Jr., E. N. Metz and A. R. Price. Acute copper intoxication. Arch. Int. Med. 129: 578 - 582, 1972.

P. O. Nicholas. Food-poisoning due to copper in the morning tea. Lancet 2: 40 - 42, 1968.

A. Richardson. Personal communication, 1975.

H. Scheinberg and I. Sternlieb. Copper metabolism. Pharm. Rev. 12: 355 - 381, 1960.

I. Suciu, V. Lazer, E. Ilea et al. Copper poisoning in the workers from a section of copper electrolysis. In *Environmental Pollution and Human Health* (S. H. Zaidu, ed.), Indian Toxicology Research Centre, Lucknow, India, 1977, p. 211.

W. L. Wagner. *Environmental Conditions in U.S. Copper Smelters,* U.S. Government Printing Office, Washington, DC, 1975.

Serum and Urine Copper by Atomic Absorption Spectrometry

Principle:

Copper is measured directly in acidified urine and after dilution of serum by aspiration into the flame of an atomic absorption spectrometer. Signal suppression by inorganic urinary salts is overcome by preparing standards in a mixed salt solution.

Reagents:

Stock solution — 1 mg/mL copper (Fisher reference standard or dissolve 3.932 g $CuSO_4 . 5H_2O$ per L of water)

Standards for serum — 0.2, 0.5, 1.0 and 2.0 mg/L

Standards for urine — 10, 20, 50 and 100 μg/L in salt solution

Salt solution — 5.08 g NaCl, 2.86 g KCl, 0.31 g $CaCO_3$, 0.42 g $MgCl_2 . 6H_2O$, 0.67 mL conc. H_2SO_4, 8.7 mL conc. HCl and 3.09 g $NH_4H_2PO_4$ per L of water

0.1 mol/L Hydrochloric acid

Concentrated hydrochloric acid — low copper grade (<3 μg/L)

All plasticware used in this procedure should be soaked overnight in 5% nitric acid and rinsed several times in distilled/deionized water

Instrumental Conditions:

Atomic absorption spectrometer with oxidizing air-acetylene flame and three slot burner head

Copper hollow cathode lamp

Measure absorption at 324.8 nm

Procedure:

Serum:

1. Collect blood in a disposable plastic syringe and transfer to a 5 mL plastic tube. Allow to clot, centrifuge and transfer 0.5 mL serum to a 15 mL plastic centrifuge tube. Also transfer 0.5 mL volumes of the serum standards to similar tubes.
2. Dilute serum and appropriate standards to 5 mL with 0.1 mol/L HCl and vortex. Use 0.1 mol/L HCl as a reagent blank.

Urine:

3. Collect a 24 h urine specimen in an acid-washed 2.5 L polyethylene container. Acidify by adding 8.7 mL conc. HCl/L of urine. Urine standards are analyzed directly; the reagent blank for urine determinations consists of the salt solution.

Analysis:

4. Aspirate distilled/deionized water into the flame for 20 seconds, followed by the reagent blank for 20 seconds. Repeat this operation 5 times.
5. Perform a similar cycle but replace the reagent blank with the low standard solution. Repeat these cycles using standards of increasing concentration and finally the unknown. Average the 5 readings for each sample.

Calculation:

Calculation is based on a response factor derived from a standard curve. The value for the reagent blank should be subtracted from the standard and unknown readings prior to preparation of the curve. Quality control specimens consisting of pooled serum and urine are analyzed daily.

Evaluation:

Sensitivity: 0.02 mg/L for serum and 2 μg/L for urine
Linearity: 0.05 - 3.00 mg/L for serum and 10 - 300 μg/L for urine
C.V.: 3% within-run
Relative recovery: 91 - 104%

Interferences:

Care must be taken to minimize copper contamination from reagents and laboratory vessels. Suppression of the copper value in urine by inorganic salts is overcome by preparing urine standards in a synthetic salt mixture. No other interferences were found.

CRESOL

Occurrence and Usage. The three isomers of cresol are used as disinfectants and as chemical intermediates in the production of plasticizers and resins. Industrial exposure is usually by way of inhalation or dermal contact. The current threshold limit value for cresol in air is 5 ppm.

Blood Concentrations. Cresol concentrations in blood are not routinely measured, except in cases of severe poisoning.

Metabolism and Excretion. p-Cresol is found in the excreta of normal individuals, probably as a result of bacterial degradation of amino acids in the intestine. Following intestinal absorption, it is metabolized to glucuronide and sulfate conjugates in the liver and excreted as such in the urine. The other cresol isomers are not normal constituents of human urine (Duran et al., 1973). The p-cresol content in normal urine averages about 90 mg/L, with a range of 20 - 200 mg/L (Van Haaften and Sie, 1965). Whereas only about 5% of the endogenously produced p-cresol is excreted unconjugated in urine, large doses of cresol often result in excretion of substantial amounts of the unconjugated isomers.

Toxicity. Acute or chronic cresol toxicity is manifested by headache, dizziness, vomiting, rapid respiration, dyspnea, weakness, and damage to the lung, liver and kidneys.

A man who ingested at least 25 g of a cresol mixture was hospitalized and died after four days; a maximal serum cresol level of 90 mg/L was achieved on the first day (Arthurs et al., 1977). A 1 year old boy died within 5 hours of accidental dermal application of a cresol antiseptic fluid; the postmortem blood specimen was found to contain 120 mg/L cresols (Green, 1975). Blood and urine cresol concentrations of 190 and 304 mg/L, respectively, were found postmortem in a woman who intentionally ingested a cresol disinfectant (Bruce et al., 1976).

Biological Monitoring. Urinary p-cresol concentrations which substantially exceed the pre-exposure baseline level for an individual are evidence of excessive exposure. Since o- and m-cresol are not normally found in urine, their presence is indicative of occupational or domestic exposure to cresols.

Analysis. The gas chromatographic method described for determination of urinary phenol (p. 41) is also applicable to cresol analysis. Two of the isomers, m- and p-cresol, cannot be distinguished by this procedure.

References

G. J. Arthurs, C. C. Wise and G. A. Coles. Poisoning by cresol. Anaesth. 32: 642 - 643, 1977.

A. M. Bruce, H. Smith and A. A. Watson. Cresol poisoning. Med. Sci. Law 16: 171 - 176, 1976.

M. Duran, D. Ketting, P. K. De Bree et al. Gas chromatographic analysis of urinary volatile phenols in patients with gastro-intestinal disorders and normals. Clin. Chim. Acta 45: 341 - 347, 1973.

M. A. Green. A household remedy misused — fatal cresol poisoning following cutaneous absorption (a case report). Med. Sci. Law 15: 65 - 66, 1975.

R. J. Sherwood and F. W. G. Carter. The measurement of occupational exposure to benzene vapour. Ann. Occ. Hyg. 13: 125 - 146, 1970.

A. B. Van Haaften and S. T. Sie. The measurement of phenol in urine by gas chromatography as a check on benzene exposure. Am. Ind. Hyg. Asso. J. 26: 52 - 58, 1965.

CYANIDE

Occurrence and Usage. Hydrocyanic acid and its sodium and potassium salts are used industrially as fumigants, insecticides, metal polishes and in electroplating solutions. The acid is a volatile liquid which boils at 26° C.; the odor of its vapor can be detected at an air concentration of 1 ppm by some persons. The threshold limit value for hydrogen cyanide is 10 ppm (11 mg/m^3) for an 8 hour day, although as little as 110 ppm may be fatal to an adult after 1 hour. Hydrogen cyanide may be produced in relatively high concentrations in fires which involve nitrogen-containing materials. Another potential source of cyanide are the cyanogenetic glycosides, such as amygdalin, found in seeds of certain fruits, including the apple, apricot, cherry, peach, pear and plum. The threshold limit value for cyanide salts in air is currently 5 mg/m^3.

Blood Concentrations. Cyanide is found in low levels in the tissues of healthy subjects as a result of normal metabolism, eating of cyanogenetic foods and cigarette smoking. Plasma cyanide concentrations in healthy subjects were found to average 0.004 mg/L in nonsmokers and 0.006 mg/L in smokers (Wilson and Matthews, 1966). Whole blood cyanide, most of which is contained in erythrocytes, in 10 nonsmokers was found to average 0.016 mg/L, whereas in 14 smokers the mean level was 0.041 mg/L (Ballantyne, 1977). Thiocyanate, a metabolite of cyanide, normally ranges from 1 - 4 mg/L in the plasma of nonsmokers and 3 - 12 mg/L in smokers (Pettigrew and Fell, 1972).

Metabolism and Excretion. About 80% of a cyanide dose is detoxified by conversion via the liver enzyme rhodanase to thiocyanate, which is subsequently excreted in urine. The remainder is handled by other minor routes, which include pulmonary excretion of unchanged hydrogen cyanide, trapping by hydroxocobalamin with formation of vitamin B_{12}, oxidation of formic acid and carbon dioxide, and reaction with cysteine. Normal urinary cyanide concentrations in 22 nonsmokers averaged 0.067 mg/L (range 0 - 0.300) and in 80 smokers, 0.174 mg/L (range 0.010 - 0.811) (Ansell and Lewis, 1970). Normal urinary thiocyanate concentrations range from 1 - 4 mg/L in nonsmokers and 7 - 17 mg/L in smokers (Maliszewski and Bass, 1955).

Toxicity. Cyanide produces hypoxia by the inhibition of cytochrome oxidase. Chronic cyanide poisoning can produce dizziness, weakness and permanent mental and motor impairment (Hardy et al., 1950). An individual who developed hemiparesis following chronic exposure to cyanide was found to have a blood cyanide concentration of 0.1 mg/L (Sandberg, 1967). Some of the effects of chronic cyanide exposure are similar to those of thiocyanate intoxication (El Ghawabi et al., 1975).

A group of workers chronically exposed to cyanide at levels of 0.2 - 0.8 mg/m^3 who developed symptoms of mild cyanide poisoning was recently studied.

Blood samples drawn at the end of the workshift contained cyanide at an average of 0.18 mg/L (range 0.02 - 0.36) in 15 non-smokers and 0.56 mg/L (range 0.10 - 2.20) in 8 smokers; blood thiocyanate concentrations averaged 4.2 mg/L (range 2.6 - 8.3) and 4.8 mg/L (range 1.6 - 9.2) in the nonsmokers and smokers, respectively. Urine thiocyanate levels in 24 hour specimens averaged 5.7 mg/L (range 1.5 - 12.9) and 6.2 mg/L (1.5 - 16.5) in these two groups. Each of these levels, excluding the urinary thiocyanate of smokers, was substantially elevated over those of equivalent groups of control subjects. It was concluded that the present TLV of 5 mg/m^3 for cyanide aerosols should be reviewed (Chandra et al., 1980).

Acute intoxication occurred in 9 children, 2 of whom died, following the ingestion of apricot seeds capable of releasing 217 mg of cyanide per 100 g of moist seed; the authors cite 9 other poisonings involving fruit seeds (Sayre and Kaymakcalan, 1964). The daily ingestion of 1500 mg of laetrile (amygdalin) by an adult has produced toxicity and a blood cyanide level of 10 mg/L (Smith et al., 1977); the acute ingestion of 500 - 2500 mg by an infant produced a blood cyanide level of 0.29 mg/L at admission, with death after 72 hours (Humbert et al., 1977); and the acute ingestion of 3500 mg by a 17 year old girl caused her death within 24 hours (Sadoff et al., 1978). Blood cyanide concentrations in deaths due to the inhalation of cyanide gas have averaged 7 mg/L (range 1 - 15), whereas in deaths due to cyanide ingestion these concentrations averaged 12 mg/L (range 1 - 53) (Ballantyne, 1974).

Biological Monitoring. Whole blood cyanide concentrations are used primarily in the diagnosis of acute intoxication. Plasma and urine thiocyanate concentrations are useful in monitoring occupational exposure to cyanide, if pre-exposure levels are determined to identify smoking and dietary influences. Urinary thiocyanate in a nonsmoker should not exceed 4 mg/L at the 10 ppm TLV for hydrogen cyanide vapor (Maehly and Swensson, 1970; El Ghawabi et al., 1975).

Analysis. Cyanide may be determined in blood by colorimetry (Feldstein and Klendshoj, 1954) or ion-specific potentiometry (McAnalley et al., 1979), both techniques requiring prior isolation of cyanide by microdiffusion. Plasma and urine thiocyanate levels, more frequently used to monitor chronic exposure to cyanide, may also be determined colorimetrically (Lundquist et al., 1979).

References

M. Ansell and F. A. S. Lewis. A review of cyanide concentrations found in human organs. J. For. Med. 17: 148 - 155, 1970.

B. Ballantyne. The forensic diagnosis of acute cyanide poisoning. In *Forensic Toxicology* (B. Ballantyne, ed.), Wright and Sons, Bristol, 1974, pp. 99 - 113.

B. Ballantyne. In vitro production of cyanide in normal human blood and the influence of thiocyanate and storage temperature. Clin. Tox. 11: 173 - 193, 1977.

H. Chandra, B. N. Gupta, S. K. Bhargava et al. Chronic cyanide exposure — a biochemical and industrial hygiene study. J. Anal. Tox. 4: in press, 1980.

S. H. El Ghawabi, M. A. Gaafar, A. A. El-Saharti et al. Chronic cyanide exposure: a clinical, radioisotope, and laboratory study. Brit. J. Ind. Med. 32: 215 - 219, 1975.

M. Feldstein and N. C. Klendshoj. The determination of cyanide in biologic fluids by microdiffusion analysis. J. Lab. Clin. Med. 44: 166 - 170, 1954.

H. L. Hardy, W. M. Jeffries, M. M. Wasserman and W. R. Waddell. Thiocyanate effect following industrial cyanide exposure. New Eng. J. Med. 242: 968 - 972, 1950.

J. R. Humbert, J. H. Tress and K. T. Braico. Fatal cyanide poisoning: accidental ingestion of amygdalin. J. Am. Med. Asso. 238: 428, 1977.

P. Lundquist. J. Martensson, B. Sorbo and S. Ohman. Method for determining thiocyanate in serum and urine. Clin. Chem. 25: 678 - 681, 1979.

T. F. Maliszewski and D. E. Bass. 'True' and 'apparent' thiocyanate in body fluids of smokers and nonsmokers. J. Appl. Physiol. 8: 289 - 291, 1955.

A. C. Maehly and A. Swensson. Cyanide and thiocyanate levels in blood and urine of workers with low-grade exposure to cyanide. Int. Arch. Arbeitsmed. 27: 195 - 209, 1970.

B. H. McAnalley, W. T. Lowry, R. Oliver and J. C. Garriott. Determination of inorganic sulfide and cyanide in blood using specific ion electrodes. J. Anal. Tox. 3: 111 - 114, 1979.

A. R. Pettigrew and G. S. Fell. Simplified colorimetric determination of thiocyanate in biological fluids, and its application to investigation of the toxic amblyopias. Clin. Chem. 18: 996 - 1000, 1972.

L. Sadoff, K. Fuchs and J. Hollander. Rapid death associated with laetrile ingestion. J. Am. Med. Asso. 239: 1532, 1978.

C. G. Sandberg. A case of chronic poisoning with potassium cyanide? Acta Med. Scand. 181: 233 - 235, 1967.

J. W. Sayre and S. Kaymakcalan. Hazards to health. New Eng. J. Med. 270: 1113 - 1115, 1964.

F. P. Smith, T. P. Butler, S. Cohan and P. S. Schein. Laetrile toxicity: a report of two cases. J. Am. Med. Asso. 238: 1361, 1977.

J. Wilson and D. M. Matthews. Metabolic inter-relationships between cyanide, thiocyanate and vitamin B_{12} in smokers and non-smokers. Clin. Sci. 31: 1 - 7, 1966.

Blood Cyanide by Colorimetry

Principle:

A blood specimen is pipetted into the outer circle of a Conway microdiffusion cell and cyanide is released by the addition of sulfuric acid. The released hydrocyanic acid is captured in sodium hydroxide solution in the central compartment of the dish during a several hour diffusion period. This solution is then reacted with a chromogenic reagent and the resulting color is measured in a spectrophotometer at 580 nm.

Reagents:

Stock solution — 1 mg/mL cyanide (25.0 mg HCN/10 mL water)
Blood standards — 0.5, 1, 2 and 5 mg/L (prepared fresh in whole blood)
0.1 mol/L Sodium hydroxide — 2 g NaOH/500 mL water
0.5 mol/L Sulfuric acid — 14 mL conc. H_2SO_4/500 mL water
1 mol/L Phosphate buffer — 68 g KH_2PO_4/500 mL water
0.25% Chloramine T — 250 mg/100 mL water (REFRIGERATE)

Pyridine-barbituric acid solution — 1.5 g barbituric acid, 7.5 mL pyridine and 1.5 mL conc. HCl in a 25 mL volumetric flask. Dilute to volume with water, warm mixture to dissolve and mix. Prepare fresh.

Instrumental Conditions:

Visible spectrophotometer set to 580 nm.

Procedure:

1. Lubricate edges of Conway diffusion cells with stopcock grease. Add 3.0 mL 0.1 mol/L sodium hydroxide to the center well of all cells.
2. Add 4 mL of one of the following to the outer compartment of each cell: cyanide-free blood, blood standards and patient specimen.
3. Finally add 4 mL of 0.5 mol/L sulfuric acid to the outer compartment and rapidly close the cell. Tilt to mix and leave for 3 - 4 hours at room temperature (or for 1 - 2 h in a 37° oven).
4. Pipet 1 mL of the reagent from the central compartment into a 15 mL centrifuge tube. Add 2 mL 1 mol/L phosphate buffer and 1 mL 0.25% chloramine T. Mix and let stand for 2 - 3 minutes.
5. Add 3 mL pyridine-barbituric acid solution. Mix and allow to stand for 10 minutes. Read in the visible spectrophotometer at 580 nm against the blood blank.

Calculation:

Calculation is based on a response factor derived from a standard curve. This procedure cannot be controlled by the usual methods due to the difficulty in storage of cyanide-containing blood specimens.

Evaluation:

Sensitivity: 0.2 mg/L
Linearity: 0.5 - 5 mg/L
C.V.: not established
Relative recovery: not established

Interferences:

Even freshly drawn whole blood contains a small quantity of cyanide. Both production and loss of cyanide can occur during storage of whole blood. Due to this phenomenon, it is suggested that patient specimens be kept at 4° C. until analysis and that analysis be performed as soon after drawing as is possible.

Blood Cyanide by Ion-Specific Potentiometry

Principle:

Cyanide is isolated from blood by microdiffusion according to the previous procedure. The concentration of the ion in the sodium hydroxide solution is determined by direct potentiometric measurement with a cyanide-specific electrode.

Reagents:

0.1 mol/L Sodium hydroxide
10% Lead acetate solution — 1 g $Pb(C_2H_3O_2)_2$ in 10 mL 0.1 mol/L NaOH

Instrumental Conditions:

pH Meter equipped with cyanide-specific electrode (Orion Research)

Procedure:

1. Process the blood blank, blood standards and patient blood specimen by Conway microdiffusion according to the previous procedure.
2. Stabilize the cyanide electrode by placing in 0.1 mol/L NaOH for 30 minutes or until a constant voltage reading is attained.
3. Determine the electrode response to the sodium hydroxide solution from the center well of the Conway cell of each of the processed specimens.
4. Add 1 drop 10% lead acetate solution to each sodium hydroxide sample after recording the initial reading. A significant change in electrode potential indicates the presence of sulfide as an interfering substance. In this case record the electrode response to each of the solutions after adding lead acetate solution.

Calculation:

Calculation is based on a response factor derived from a standard curve. This procedure cannot be controlled by the usual methods due to the difficulty in storage of cyanide-containing blood specimens.

Evaluation:

Sensitivity: 0.01 mg/L
Linearity: 0.1 - 1.0 mg/L
C.V.: 5% within-run
Relative recovery: 100 - 109%

Interferences:

Although sulfide is known to interfere in this procedure, the addition of lead acetate to the final solution will insure its presence or absence. Since the blood used in the preparation of standards will probably contain a low level of cyanide, a blood blank must be analyzed and the result subtracted from those of the standards and patient specimen.

Plasma and Urine Thiocyanate by Colorimetry

Principle:

Thiocyanate is removed from the specimen by adsorption on an ion-exchange column. The eluate is treated with a halogenating reagent and allowed to react with a pyridine-barbituric acid chromogenic solution. The absorbance of the final solution is measured at 580 nm in the spectrophotometer.

Reagents:

Stock solution — 1 mg/mL thiocyanate ion in water
Aqueous standards — 1, 3, 6 and 12 mg/L
0.1 mol/L Sodium hydroxide — 4 g NaOH per L
1 mol/L Sodium perchlorate — 140 g $NaClO_4 . H_2O$ per L
0.5 mol/L Acetic acid — 28.5 mL conc. acetic acid per L
50 mmol/L Sodium hypochlorite — 5 mL 0.5 mol/L NaClO in 0.1 mol/L NaOH diluted to 50 mL with water (stable for 1 month if refrigerated)
Chromogenic reagent — dissolve 6 g barbituric acid in 30 mL pyridine and 64 mL water; add 6 mL conc. HCl (stable for 1 week if refrigerated)
Ion-exchange column — 4 cm x 0.7 cm i.d. column containing 100/120 mesh Lewatit MP7080 (EM Laboratories, Elmsford, NY 10523)

Instrumental Conditions:

Visible spectrophotometer set to 580 nm

Procedure:

Resin preparation:

1. Wash resin in water and suspend in 1 mol/L HCl. Filter and wash with water until pH of washings exceeds 4.5.
2. Spread resin on a glass plate and dry at 100° C. for 12 h. Suspend in water and let stand 15 min.
3. Decant off water and resuspend resin in 1 mol/L NaOH. Let stand 15 min and wash with water until washings are a neutral pH. Fill resin column to a height of 2.5 cm.

Sample analysis:

1. Dilute 0.5 mL plasma or urine with 5 mL 0.1 mol/L NaOH and apply to the ion-exchange column. Wash column 3 times with 5 mL portions of water.
2. Elute the column with 8 mL 1 mol/L $NaClO_4$. Transfer 4 mL of the eluate to a 12 mL centrifuge tube.
3. Add 0.2 mL 0.5 mol/L acetic acid and vortex. Add 0.1 mL 50 mmol/L NaClO and vortex.
4. Within 1 min add 0.5 mL chromogenic reagent and vortex. After 5 - 15 min measure the absorbance in the spectrophotometer against a water blank which has been processed in the same manner.

Calculation:

Calculation is based on a response factor derived from a standard curve. A quality control specimen consisting of an aqueous solution containing 3 mg/L thiocyanate is analyzed daily.

Evaluation:

Sensitivity: 0.5 mg/L
Linearity: 1 - 12 mg/L
C.V.: 2.3% between-day
Relative recovery: 98 - 105%

Interferences:

Normal plasma components do not interfere with the assay. Cyanide will be measured as thiocyanate if present; normal plasma and urine cyanide concentrations are very low, but this interference may be avoided by washing the column two times with 5 mL of 0.1 mol/L HCl prior to elution with $NaClO_4$. Certain antibiotics, including benzylpenicillin, cloxacillin and cephalothin, interfered when present at very high concentrations (2 g/L); this problem may be avoided by washing the column 3 times with 5 mL of 4 mol/L NH_4Cl prior to elution with $NaClO_4$.

DDT

Occurrence and Usage. DDT (dicophane, chlorophenothane, dichlorodiphenyltrichloroethane) is a chlorinated hydrocarbon which was first synthesized in 1874 and which has been employed as a contact insecticide since 1940. Technical grades of the chemical contain a mixture of p,p′-DDT (67 - 85%), o,p′-DDT (8 - 21%) and related compounds. DDT has come under severe restrictions in some countries since 1970 due to its persistence and accumulation in the food chain. The current threshold limit value for DDT in air is 1 mg/m^3.

Blood Concentrations. Blood concentrations of total DDT (DDT plus DDE, a metabolite) in 44 healthy English adults with no occupational exposure to the chemical averaged 0.013 mg/L, with a range of 0.005 - 0.038 mg/L (Robinson and Hunter, 1966). Two subjects who ingested 10 or 20 mg of technical DDT for 183 days developed maximal serum levels of p,p′-DDT which exceeded 0.200 and 0.500 mg/L, respectively, by the end of the study (Morgan and Roan, 1971). A group of 18 asymptomatic DDT factory workers was found to have total DDT serum concentrations of 0.579 - 2.914 mg/L (average 1.359), consisting largely of nearly equal parts of p,p′-DDT and p,p′-DDE (Poland et al., 1970).

Metabolism and Excretion. DDT is converted to a slight extent to the much less toxic DDE (dichlorodiphenyldichloroethylene) by dehydrochlorination; DDE apparently does not undergo further biotransformation, but is stored for an indefinite period of time in adipose tissues. Most of the p,p′-DDE present in human fat represents preformed dietary DDE rather than endogenously produced DDE. The major detoxification pathway of DDT is via dechlorination to DDD (dichlorodiphenyldichloroethane), an active insecticide, which readily degrades to DDA (dichlorodiphenylacetic acid), a water-soluble, rapidly excreted detoxification product. Urinary DDA represents about 47% of ingested precursor material during low exposure, but DDA excretion becomes quantitatively less important as DDT intake increases (Morgan and Roan, 1971; Roan et al., 1971). Urinary DDA concentrations correlate reasonably well with DDT storage levels in body fat; DDA was undetectable in the urine of members of the general population and ranged from 0.01 - 2.67 mg/L in workers with low to high exposure to DDT (Laws et al., 1967). By contrast, urine concentrations of DDT, DDE and DDD in healthy unexposed persons averaged 0.007, 0.016 and 0.003 mg/L, respectively (Cueto and Biros, 1967), and 0.011, 0.021 and 0.006 mg/L, respectively, in occupationally exposed persons (Laws et al., 1967). Fat concentrations of DDT, DDE and DDD averaged 1.3, 4.5 and 0.025 mg/kg in unexposed persons in Hawaii (Casarett et al., 1968) and 112, 73 and <0.3 mg/kg, respectively, in occupationally exposed workers (Laws et al., 1967). Average fat concentrations of DDT in unexposed persons have ranged from 1.7 - 28 mg/kg in twelve other studies (Matsumura, 1975).

Toxicity. DDT is a central nervous system stimulant which in overdose can cause paresthesia of the tongue and lips, tremor, confusion and convulsions. Several instances of fatal DDT poisoning have been reported in humans, although the hydrocarbon vehicle involved in these cases probably contributed significantly to the deaths (Hill and Robinson, 1945; Hill and Damiani, 1946; Reingold and Lasky, 1947; Smith, 1948). In general, the compound is felt to be relatively safe, having an estimated lethal dose of 30 g in an adult. Men who received 35 mg daily oral doses of recrystallized DDT for a period of 21.5 months and who developed body fat concentrations of 129 - 659 mg/kg of DDT and 51 - 142 mg/kg of DDE exhibited no definite clinical or laboratory abnormalities (Hayes et al., 1971). A healthy person who self-administered an acute oral 5 g dose of technical DDT developed nausea, insomnia and excitability which diminished over a period of one week (Rappolt, 1973).

Biological Monitoring. The most meaningful measurements for monitoring exposure to DDT are of DDT itself in serum or adipose tissue, or of DDA in urine. Each of these levels has been shown to be proportional to the extent of DDT exposure. A 10 mg daily dose of DDT results, after an equilibrium period of 6 - 12 months, in steady-state levels of 0.15 - 0.20 mg/L DDT in serum, 100 mg/kg DDT in biopsy fat, and 0.5 - 2.0 mg/L DDA in urine (Piotrowski, 1977). Preexposure levels are necessary to determine the degree of environmental DDT accumulation in each individual.

Analysis. Biological fluids and tissues may be assayed for DDT, DDE and DDD by electron-capture gas chromatography as described in the section on aldrin (p. 16). A method is presented for the determination of DDA in urine by electron-capture gas chromatography of a methyl derivative (Cranmer et al., 1969).

References

L. J. Casarett, G. C. Fryer, W. L. Yauger, Jr. and H. W. Klemmer. Organochlorine pesticide residues in human tissue — Hawaii. Arch. Env. Health 17: 306 - 311, 1968.

M. F. Cranmer, J. J. Carroll and M. F. Copeland. Determination of DDT and metabolites, including DDA, in human urine by gas chromatography. Bull. Env. Cont. Tox. 4: 214 - 223, 1969.

C. Cueto, Jr. and F. J. Biros. Chlorinated insecticides and related materials in human urine. Tox. Appl. Pharm. 10: 261 - 269, 1967.

W. J. Hayes, Jr., W. E. Dale and C. I. Pirkle. Evidence of safety of long-term, high oral doses of DDT for man. Arch. Env. Health 22: 119 - 135, 1971.

K. R. Hill and G. Robinson. A fatal case of D.D.T. poisoning in a child. Brit. Med. J. 2: 845 - 847, 1946.

W. R. Hill and C. R. Damiani. Death following exposure to DDT. New Eng. J. Med. 235: 897 - 899, 1946.

E. R. Laws, Jr., A. Curley and F. J. Biros. Men with intensive occupational exposure to DDT. Arch. Env. Health 15: 766 - 775, 1967.

F. Matsumura. *Toxicology of Insecticides*, Plenum, New York, 1975, p. 453.

D. P. Morgan and C. C. Roan. Absorption, storage, and metabolic conversion of ingested DDT and DDT metabolites in man. Arch. Env. Health 22: 301 - 308, 1971.

J. K. Piotrowski. *Exposure Tests for Organic Compounds in Industrial Toxicology,* U.S. Government Printing Office, Washington, D.C., 1977, pp. 115 - 121.

A. Poland, D. Smith, R. Kuntzman et al. Effect of intensive occupational exposure to DDT on phenylbutazone and cortisol metabolism in human subjects. Clin. Pharm. Ther. 11: 724 - 731, 1970.

R. T. Rappolt, Sr. Use of oral DDT in three human barbiturate intoxications: hepatic enzyme induction by reciprocal detoxicants. Clin. Tox. 6: 147 - 151, 1973.

I. M. Reingold and I. I. Lasky. Acute fatal poisoning following ingestion of a solution of DDT. Ann. Int. Med. 26: 945 - 947, 1947.

C. Roan, D. Morgan and E. H. Paschal. Urinary excretion of DDA following ingestion of DDT and DDT metabolites in man. Arch. Env. Health 22: 309 - 315, 1971.

J. Robinson and C. G. Hunter. Organochlorine insecticides: concentrations in human blood and adipose tissue. Arch. Env. Health 13: 558 - 563, 1966.

N. J. Smith. Death following accidental ingestion of DDT. J. Am. Med. Asso. 136: 469 - 471, 1948.

Urine DDA by Electron-Capture Gas Chromatography

Principle:

DDA is extracted from urine with acidified hexane. The extract is treated with boron trifluoride in methanol to form the methyl derivative of DDA, which is re-extracted and analyzed by electron-capture gas chromatography.

Reagents:

Stock solution — 1 mg/mL DDA in methanol
Urine standards — 0.05, 0.1, 0.2, 0.5 and 1.0 mg/L
2% Acetic acid in nanograde hexane
Methylation reagent — 10% boron trifluoride in nanograde methanol (prepare fresh)
Hexane (nanograde)

Instrumental Conditions:

Gas chromatograph with electron-capture detector
1.8 m x 4 mm i.d. glass column containing 5% QF-1 on 80/100 mesh Gas Chrom Q
Injector, 220° C.; column, 170° C.; detector, 350° C.
Nitrogen flow rate, 80 mL/min

Procedure:

1. Transfer 5 mL urine to a 15 mL screw-cap tube. Extract with 5 mL 2% acetic acid in hexane by shaking for 2 minutes.
2. Centrifuge and transfer the upper organic layer to a clean tube. Re-extract the aqueous phase twice more in a like manner, centrifuging each time and combining the organic layers.

3. Evaporate the hexane extract to dryness at 50° C. under a stream of nitrogen. Add 2 - 3 mL methylation reagent and heat at 50° C. for 30 min.
4. Add 5 mL water to the tube and vortex. Extract the solution three times with 5 mL hexane, centrifuging and transfering the hexane layer to a 15 mL conical centrifuge tube each time.
5. Evaporate the combined hexane layers to dryness at 50° C. under a stream of nitrogen. Dissolve the residue in 1.0 mL hexane, vortex and inject 10 μL into the gas chromatograph.

	Relative retention time
p,p'-DDA derivative	1.0
p,p'-DDD derivative	1.3
p,p'-DDT derivative	1.4

Calculation:

Calculation is based on a response factor derived from a standard curve. A quality control specimen containing 0.2 mg/L DDA is analyzed daily.

Evaluation:

Sensitivity: 0.04 mg/L
Linearity: 0.05 - 1.0 mg/L
C.V.: not established
Relative recovery: not established

Interferences:

Specimens are occasionally encountered which produce many interfering peaks on the chromatogram. In these cases, the use of a microcoulometric detector will improve the sensitivity of detection for DDA while not responding to most contaminants.

DIAZINON

Occurrence and Usage. Diazinon is an organothiophosphate derivative widely used as an agricultural and household insecticide since its synthesis in 1953. The concentrated commercial form contains 25% diazinon and is intended to be used outdoors in a 0.05% dilution. The compound is inactivated by photochemical oxidation and therefore does not accumulate in the environment. Occupational exposure is generally by dermal contact or inhalation. The current threshold limit value for diazinon is 0.1 mg/m^3.

Blood Concentrations. Diazinon itself is not routinely measured in blood specimens except in cases of acute intoxication. Blood cholinesterase levels are generally used to monitor exposure to diazinon and other cholinesterase inhibitors. Oral doses of diazinon given to volunteers for 37 days at the rate of 0.02 mg/kg/day reduced plasma cholinesterase levels to 86% of pre-exposure levels; 0.05 mg/kg/day for 28 days reduced the levels to 60 - 65%, but neither dosage regimen affected erythrocyte cholinesterase levels (ACGIH, 1971).

Metabolism and Excretion. The metabolism of diazinon has not been specifically studied in man, but it is known to be rapidly and extensively biotransformed in animals. It is activated by oxidation to diazoxon, a potent cholinesterase inhibitor, and both this compound and its parent are inactivated by hydrolysis to the corresponding phosphoric acid derivatives, diethylphosphoric acid and diethylphosphorothioic acid. Minor metabolites include hydroxy derivatives formed by oxidation of the isopropyl side chain; hydroxydiazinon is a toxic compound which is found in blood to the extent of 25 - 70% of the diazinon content. Diazinon itself accumulates in fat in concentrations over 100 times those in blood. Over 80% of a dose is eliminated as products of hydrolysis in the 24 hour urine of experimental animals (Nakatsugawa et al., 1969; Janes et al., 1973; Iverson et al., 1975). Urinary concentrations of diethylphosphoric acid and diethylphosphorothioic acid in members of the general population average less than 0.02 mg/L of each (Kutz et al., 1978).

Toxicity. The estimated fatal dose of diazinon in man is 25 g by oral ingestion. Contaminated food caused the acute intoxication of 8 children, who were treated with atropine for the relief of sweating, nausea, abdominal cramps and muscle weakness; diethylphosphoric acid was found in urine specimens collected 23 and 58 days after the incident in concentrations of up to 0.22 mg/L (Reichert et al., 1977). Two subjects who survived the intentional ingestion of 60 and 100 mL of 25% diazinon solution were noted to have red blood cell cholinesterase levels within a short time of ingestion which were depressed to 19% and 39% of normal, respectively; maximal plasma diazinon concentrations noted shortly after ingestion in these two patients were 0.1 and 1.7 mg/L, while urine metabolite levels peaked within the first two days at 85 and 41 mg/L for diethylphosphoric acid and 101 and 35 mg/L for diethylphosphorothioic acid (Klemmer et al., 1978). At least one fatality has been reported due to the suicidal ingestion of diazinon (Heyndrickx et al., 1974).

Biological Monitoring. Blood cholinesterase determinations are the most useful index for monitoring exposure to diazinon and other cholinesterase inhibitors; a blood cholinesterase level which is less than 70% of the pre-exposure level is indicative of excessive exposure to diazinon.

The measurement of organic phosphates in urine is a useful adjunct to cholinesterase determination in diazinon-exposed workers. Total urinary organic phosphate levels in excess of 0.1 mg/L represent significant exposure to organophosphate insecticides (Knaak et al., 1979).

Analysis. A method for blood cholinesterase determination was presented in the section on carbaryl (p. 60). The phosphoric acid metabolites of diazinon may be assayed in urine by a colorimetric procedure which is also applicable for monitoring exposure to dichlorvos, malathion, methylparathion, and parathion (Mattson and Sedlak, 1960).

References

ACGIH. *Documentation of the Threshold Limit Values,* American Conference of Governmental Industrial Hygienists, Cincinnati, Ohio, 1971, pp 70 - 71.

A. Heyndrickx, F. Van Hoof, L. De Wolf and C. Van Peteghem. Fatal diazinon poisoning in man. J. For. Sci. Soc. 14: 131 - 133, 1974.

F. Iverson, D. L. Grant and J. Lacroix. Diazinon metabolism in the dog. Bull. Env. Cont. Tox. 13: 611 - 618, 1975.

N. F. Janes, A. F. Machin, M. P. Quick et al. Toxic metabolites of diazinon in sheep. J. Agr. Food Chem. 21: 121 - 124, 1973.

H. W. Klemmer, E. R. Reichert and W. L. Yauger, Jr. Five cases of intentional ingestion of 25 percent diazinon with treatment and recovery. Clin. Tox. 12: 435 - 444, 1978.

J. B. Knaak, K. T. Maddy and S. Khalifa. Alkyl phosphate metabolite levels in the urine of field workers giving blood for cholinesterase test in California. Bull. Env. Cont. Tox. 21: 375 - 380, 1979.

F. W. Kutz, R. S. Murphy and S. C. Strassman. Survey of pesticide residues and their metabolites in urine from the general population. In *Pentachlorophenol,* K. R. Rao (ed.), Plenum Press, New York, 1978, pp. 363 - 369.

A. M. Mattson and V. A. Sedlak. Ether-extractable urinary phosphates in man and rats derived from malathion and similar compounds. J. Agr. Food Chem. 8: 107 - 110, 1960.

T. Nakatsugawa, N. M. Tolman and P. A. Dahm. Oxidative degradation of diazinon by rat liver microsomes. Biochem. Pharm. 18: 685 - 688, 1969.

E. R. Reichert, W. L. Yauger, Jr., M. N. Rashad et al. Diazinon poisoning in eight members of related households. Clin. Tox. 11: 5 - 11, 1977.

Urine Organic Phosphates by Colorimetry

Principle:

The organic phosphate metabolites of the organophosphate pesticides are extracted from acidified urine with ether. Following evaporation of the solvent and oxidation of the organic matter, a chromogenic reagent is added and the resulting color is measured at 820 nm.

Reagents:

Stock solution — 1 mg/mL diethylphosphoric acid in methanol
Urine standards — 0.5, 1, 2 and 4 mg/L
Hydrochloric acid — conc. HCl
Ether
Sodium sulfate — anhydrous Na_2SO_4
0.1 mol/L Hydrochloric acid
Ethanol (absolute)
0.1 mol/L Potassium hydroxide
60% Perchloric acid
Ascorbic acid reagent — 10 mL 6 mol/L H_2SO_4, 20 mL water and 10 mL 2.5% ammonium molybdate are mixed together; add 10 mL 10% ascorbic acid and mix (prepare fresh)

Instrumental Conditions:

Visible spectrophotometer set to 820 nm

Procedure:

1. Transfer 20 mL urine to a 125 mL separatory funnel. Adjust pH to about 2 with conc. HCl and extract with 40 mL ether.
2. Discard lower aqueous layer. Add sufficient Na_2SO_4 to ether to break any emulsion and shake vigorously.
3. Filter the ether through a glass wool plug inserted in the funnel stem into a clean separatory funnel. Wash ether with 1 mL 0.1 mol/L HCl.
4. Add sufficient Na_2SO_4 to absorb the aqueous layer, shake and filter ether as before into a 50 mL centrifuge tube. Add 5 mL ethanol and 0.5 mL 0.1 mol/L KOH.
5. Heat at 50° C. for 10 min and then evaporate to dryness under a stream of nitrogen. Dissolve the residue in 2 mL water.
6. Transfer the solution to a small test tube, add 0.5 mL 60% perchloric acid and heat at 190 - 210° C. until a colorless dry residue remains. Cool the tube.
7. Add 4 mL ascorbic acid reagent and incubate at 37° C. for 0.5 - 1 hour. Read against a negative urine control at 820 nm in the spectrophotometer.

Calculation:

Calculation is based on a response factor derived from a standard curve. A quality control specimen containing 1 mg/L diethylphosphoric acid is analyzed daily.

Evaluation:

Sensitivity: 0.2 mg/L
Linearity: 0.5 - 4 mg/L
C.V.: not established
Relative recovery: not established

Interferences:

Normal urine may contain small amounts of organic phosphorus compounds. The use of a control urine as a blank for the reference cell will help to eliminate false positive results. The phosphate metabolites of organophosphate pesticides are known to be unstable in stored specimens and therefore analysis should be conducted soon after sampling. A number of organophosphate insecticides, including diazinon, dichlorvos, malathion, methylparathion and parathion, are degraded to organic phosphate metabolites which will be detected by this procedure.

p-DICHLOROBENZENE

Occurrence and Usage. p-Dichlorobenzene has been widely used as a deodorant, disinfectant and insecticide. Occupational exposure usually occurs during manufacturing processes and results from inhalation of the vapor or particulate matter. The current threshold limit value is 75 ppm (450 mg/m^3) in the industrial atmosphere.

Blood Concentrations. p-Dichlorobenzene is not routinely measured in blood specimens.

Metabolism and Excretion. In rats, p-dichlorobenzene is metabolized by oxidation to 2,5-dichlorophenol and 2,5-dichloroquinol; these metabolites account for 60% and 6% of the dose, respectively, as urinary sulfate and glucuronide conjugates within six days of a single dose (Azouz et al., 1955).

Workers employed in the manufacture of p-dichlorobenzene and exposed to air concentrations of the chemical ranging from 7 - 49 ppm had urinary 2,5-dichlorophenol levels of 10 - 233 mg/L. The urine metabolite concentrations were reasonably well correlated with the degree of exposure, averaging about 90 - 100 mg/L at p-dichlorobenzene air concentrations of 33 ppm. 2,5-Dichlorophenol urine concentrations reach a maximum at the end of an exposure, decline rapidly at first and then more slowly, with excretion continuing for a period of some weeks after a single exposure (Pagnotto and Walkley, 1965).

Toxicity. p-Dichlorobenzene causes eye and nose irritation at air concentrations of 80 - 160 ppm, and only slight skin irritation upon dermal contact (Hollingsworth et al., 1956). Exposure to higher concentrations has caused headache, nausea, malaise, jaundice, anemia and hepatic necrosis and cirrhosis (Cotter, 1953).

Biological Monitoring. The measurement of 2,5-dichlorophenol concentrations in urine provides a useful index of exposure to p-dichlorobenzene. However, the levels to be expected during exposure at the 75 ppm TLV have not been ascertained.

Analysis. 2,5-Dichlorophenol has been determined in urine by colorimetry, but this method is subject to interference by other phenolic substances (Pagnotto and Walkley, 1965). A more specific procedure is presented which involves gas chromatography with electron-capture detection (McKinney et al., 1970).

References

W. M. Azouz, D. V. Parke and R. T. Williams. The metabolism of halogenobenzenes. Ortho- and para-dichlorobenzenes. Biochem. J. 59: 410 - 415, 1955.

L. H. Cotter. Paradichlorobenzene poisoning from insecticides. N.Y. State J. Med. 53: 1690 - 1692, 1953.

R. L. Hollingsworth, V. K. Rowe, F. Oyen et al. Toxicity of paradichlorobenzene. Arch. Hyg. Occ. Med. 14: 138 - 147, 1956.

C. E. Fletcher and W. F. Barthel. The electron-capture gas chromatography of paradichlorobenzene metabolites as a measure of exposure. Bull. Env. Cont. Tox. 5: 354 - 361, 1970.

L. D. Pagnotto and J. E. Walkley. Urinary dichlorophenol as an index of para-dichlorobenzene exposure. Am. Ind. Hyg. Asso. J. 26: 137 - 142, 1965.

Urine 2,5-Dichlorophenol by Electron-Capture Gas Chromatography

Principle:

Urine is treated with concentrated acid to hydrolyze conjugated 2.5-dichlorophenol. The free chemical is extracted into benzene and a portion of this extract is analyzed directly by electron-capture gas chromatography.

Reagents:

Stock solution — 1 mg/mL 2,5-dichlorophenol in methanol
Urine standards — 20, 50, 100 and 200 mg/L
Concentrated hydrochloric acid
Benzene (nanograde)
Anhydrous sodium sulfate

Instrumental Conditions:

Gas chromatograph with electron-capture detector
1.8 m x 2 mm i.d. glass column containing 15% FFAP on 60/80 mesh Chromosorb W
Injector, 225° C.; column, 170° C.; detector, 250° C.
Nitrogen flow rate, 45 mL/min

Procedure:

1. Transfer 5 mL urine to a 15 mL screw-cap tube and add 0.5 mL conc. HCl. Shake in a mechanical shaker at room temperature for 30 min.
2. Extract the solution twice with 5 mL portions of benzene, centrifuging and transfering the organic layer to a 15 mL conical centrifuge tube each time.
3. Add 0.5 g anhydrous Na_2SO_4 to the benzene and vortex. Centrifuge and inject 1 μL into the chromatograph.

	Retention time (min)
2,5-dichlorophenol	7.3

Calculation:

Calculation is based on a response factor derived from a standard curve. A quality control specimen containing 100 mg/L 2,5-dichlorophenol is analyzed daily.

Evaluation:

Sensitivity: 5 mg/L
Linearity: 20 - 200 mg/L
C.V.: not established
Relative recovery: not established

Interferences:

Normal urinary constituents do not interfere with the analysis.

DICHLOROMETHANE

Occurrence and Usage. Dichloromethane (methylene chloride) is commonly employed commercially and industrially as a paint remover, degreaser, aerosol propellant and solvent. Prior to 1972 it was thought that the major toxic effect of the chemical in normal usage was narcosis, and the threshold limit value was accordingly set at 500 ppm. It is now recognized that dichloromethane inhalation at this level may lead to accumulation of dangerous quantities of carbon monoxide, and an atmospheric concentration of 200 ppm (700 mg/m^3) has been adopted for industrial purposes. This value is currently scheduled for revision to 100 ppm.

Blood Concentrations. Subjects exposed to 200 ppm of dichloromethane vapor for 2 hours achieved maximal blood concentrations of approximately 2 mg/L; the blood levels declined with a half-life of 40 minutes after the cessation of the exposure (DiVincenzo et al., 1972). Average blood concentrations of 3.1 and 12.5 mg/L were achieved by subjects exposed to 500 ppm of the vapor for 30 minutes during rest and heavy physical exertion, respectively (Astrand et al., 1975). Carboxyhemoglobin (COHb) saturation levels of 7% and 10% were observed in volunteers exposed to dichloromethane at concentrations of 250 and 500 ppm, respectively, for 7.5 hours (Peterson, 1978). The COHb saturation in 3 subjects exposed to 986 ppm of the vapor for 2 hours ranged from 7 - 15% at one hour post-exposure, with a mean value of 10% (Stewart et al., 1972).

Metabolism and Excretion. DiVincenzo et al. (1972) have estimated that as much as 40% of an absorbed dose of dichloromethane is not eliminated in the expired air. A portion of this retained amount is known to be metabolized to carbon monoxide; the half-life of excretion of the CO so produced is approximately 13 hours, or 2.5 times that of inhaled carbon monoxide. This effect may be due to the continued metabolism of accumulated dichloromethane (Ratney et al., 1974). Only a small fraction of a dose is excreted unchanged in the urine; an average of 22 μg was eliminated in the 24 hour urine following a 2 hour exposure to 100 ppm of the chemical (DiVincenzo et al., 1972). Rats metabolize only 7% of an administered dose of dichloromethane, as much as 5% being converted to carbon monoxide, and excrete 92% unchanged in the breath (DiVincenzo and Hamilton, 1975).

Toxicity. Toxic reactions to dichloromethane have been limited for the most part to acute exposures, and have resulted from either its direct CNS depressant effects, its *in vivo* conversion to carbon monoxide or its oxidation to phosgene in an open flame (Gerritsen and Buschmann, 1960). This latter property is shared with many other chlorinated hydrocarbons. The use of dichloromethane as a paint remover has produced carboxyhemoglobin levels of 26 and 40% in 2 healthy persons (Langehennig et al., 1976) and death in a person with a history of coronary disease (Stewart and Hake, 1976). The narcotic effects of this chemical have been held accountable for only a few fatalities, 2 of which were industrial accidents (Moskowitz and Shapiro, 1952; Baselt, 1978). The dichloromethane blood concentration in a death by inhalation following home usage of a paint remover was 510 mg/L (Bonventre et al., 1977).

Biological Monitoring. Dichloromethane exposure in workers may be monitored by the analysis of dichloromethane in blood or breath, or carbon monoxide in blood.

Blood dichloromethane concentrations measured during exposure probably should not exceed 2 mg/L in subjects exposed at the 200 ppm level for 8 hours (DiVincenzo et al., 1972). Breath dichloromethane concentrations average about 33 ppm during exposure to air containing 100 ppm of the chemical, and about 75 ppm during exposure to 250 ppm. Blood and breath concentrations plateau after 2 hours of exposure, and decline rapidly after the cessation of exposure (Astrand et al., 1975; Stewart et al., 1976). It should be noted that physical exertion during exposure can dramatically increase the blood and breath content of dichloromethane.

For medical reasons, blood carboxyhemoglobin saturation should not exceed 5% in workers exposed to dichloromethane, and this level is probably not exceeded at the 200 ppm TLV in resting nonsmokers (Astrand et al., 1975). Preexposure specimens should be analyzed to establish background carboxyhemoglobin levels for each individual.

Analysis. Dichloromethane is conveniently assayed in blood and breath by flame-ionization gas chromatography as described in the section on benzene (p. 39). A method for blood carboxyhemoglobin determination was described on p. 69.

References

I. Astrand, P. Ovrum and A. Carlsson. Exposure to methylene chloride. Scand. J. Work Env. Health 1: 78 - 94, 1975.

R. C. Baselt. Unpublished results, 1978.

J. Bonventre, O. Brennan, D. Jason et al. Two deaths following accidental inhalation of dichloromethane and 1,1,1-trichloroethane. J. Anal. Tox. 1: 158 - 160, 1977.

G. D. DiVincenzo, F. J. Yanno and B. D. Astill. Human and canine exposures to methylene chloride vapor. Am. Ind. Hyg. Asso. J. 33: 125 - 135, 1972.

G. D. DiVincenzo and M. L. Hamilton. Fate and disposition of (^{14}C) methylene chloride in the rat. Tox. Appl. Pharm. 32: 385 - 393, 1975.

W. B. Gerritsen and C. H. Buschmann. Phosgene poisoning caused by the use of chemical paint removers containing methylene chloride in ill-ventilated rooms heated by kerosene stoves. Brit. J. Ind. Med. 17: 187 - 189, 1960.

P. L. Langehennig, R. A. Seeler and E. Berman. Paint removers and carboxyhemoglobin. New Eng. J. Med. 295: 1137, 1976.

S. Moskowitz and H. Shapiro. Fatal exposure to methylene chloride vapor. Arch. Ind. Hyg. Occ. Med. 6: 116 - 123, 1952.

J. E. Peterson. Modeling the uptake, metabolism and excretion of dichloromethane by man. Am. Ind. Hyg. Asso. J. 39: 41 - 47, 1978.

R. S. Ratney, D. H. Wegman and H. B. Elkins. In vivo conversion of methylene chloride to carbon monoxide. Arch. Env. Health 28: 223 - 226, 1974.

R. D. Stewart, T. N. Fisher, M. J. Hosko et al. Carboxyhemoglobin elevation after exposure to dichloromethane. Science 176: 295 - 296, 1972.

R. D. Stewart and C. L. Hake. Paint-remover hazard. J. Am. Med. Asso. 235: 398 - 401, 1976.

R. D. Stewart, C. L. Hake and A. Wu. Use of breath analysis to monitor methylene chloride exposure. Scand. J. Work Env. Health 2: 57 - 70, 1976.

2,4-DICHLOROPHENOXYACETIC ACID

Occurrence and Usage. The chlorinated phenoxyacid derivatives, 2,4-dichlorophenoxyacetic acid (2,4-D) and its congener, 2,4,5-trichlorophenoxyacetic acid (2,4,5-T), have been used increasingly as herbicides over the last 30 years. The two compounds are often found combined in commercial preparations, which may contain up to 50% of active ingredients, in the form of the dimethylamine salts or various alkyl esters. These hormonal agents produce their effects by overstimulating plant growth. Dioxin (2,3,7,8-tetrachlorodibenzodioxin), a contaminant in some preparations of 2,4-D and 2,4,5-T, is one of the most potent teratogenic agents known. The current threshold limit value for both 2,4-D and 2,4,5-T is 10 mg/m^3.

Blood Concentrations. The oral ingestion of 5 mg/kg (350 mg/70 kg) of 2,4-D by 6 healthy subjects resulted in an average peak plasma concentration of about 35 mg/L at 12 hours; the average plasma half-life in these asymptomatic volunteers was 33 hours (Kohli et al., 1974).

Metabolism and Excretion. Metabolites of 2,4-D other than conjugates have not been detected in human urine. An average of 77% of a dose was eliminated unchanged in the urine during the 4 days following a single oral dose (Kohli et al., 1974). Asymptomatic workers involved in the application of 2,4-D were found to have urine 2,4,-D concentrations of 0.2 - 1.0 mg/L (Shafik et al, 1971).

Toxicity. The mean lethal dose of 2,4-D in man is estimated to be 28 g. Instances of neuritis and peripheral neuropathy with incomplete recovery have been reported following dermal exposure to the agent (Berkley and Magee, 1963; Goldstein et al., 1959). A terminally ill coccidioidomycosis patient received a total of 16.3 g of the sodium salt of 2,4-D by intravenous injection over a period of a month; injection of as much as 2.0 g had no apparent effects, but an infusion of 3.6 g over a period of 2 hours produced fibrillary twitching, stupor and hyporeflexia (Seabury, 1963). One person has survived the gastritis, hyperthermia and respiratory muscle paralysis associated with the accidental ingestion of 7.2 g of 2,4-D (Berwick, 1970). Another nonfatal case which involved intentional ingestion and absorption of about 7 g of the amine salt of 2,4-D was treated with forced alkaline diuresis. An initial 2,4-D plasma concentration of 400 mg/L was noted to decline with a half-life of 220 hours, but the enhancement of renal elimination brought about by urinary alkalinization reduced the plasma half-life to 4.7 hours (Park et al., 1977). Maximal concentrations of 1031 mg/L in serum and 1900 mg/L in urine were observed during the first and third days, respectively, of a nonfatal overdosage with 2,4-D (Rivers et al., 1970). Two adults who died following the intentional ingestion of 2,4-D exhibited blood concentrations of 669 and 826 mg/L (Nielsen et al., 1965; Coutselinis et al., 1977).

Biological Monitoring. 2,4-D may be determined in either plasma or urine of exposed workers. Concentrations produced by the 10 mg/m^3 TLV have not been established; however, no untoward effects have been noted in subjects who developed plasma and urine levels of up to 40 and 100 mg/L, respectively, after the ingestion of 2,4-D at a dose of 5 mg/kg (Kohli et al., 1974).

Analysis. The determination of 2,4-D and related compounds in biological specimens may be conveniently performed by flame-ionization gas chromatography using on-column methylation (Park et al., 1977).

References

M. C. Berkley and K. R. Magee. Neuropathy following exposure to a dimethylamine salt of 2,4-D. Arch. Int. Med. 111: 351 - 352, 1963.

P. Berwick. 2,4-Dichlorophenoxyacetic acid poisoning in man. J. Am. Med. Asso. 214: 1114 - 1117, 1970.

A. Coutselinis, R. Kentarchou and D. Boukis. Concentration levels of 2,4-D and 2,4,5-T in forensic material. For. Sci. 10: 203 - 204, 1977.

N. P. Goldstein, P. H. Jones and J. R. Brown. Peripheral neuropathy after exposure to an ester of dichlorophenoxyacetic acid. J. Am. Med. Asso. 171: 1306 - 1309, 1959.

J. D. Kohli, R. N. Khanna, B. N. Gupta et al. Absorption and excretion of 2,4-dichlorophenoxyacetic acid in man. Xenobiotica 4: 97 - 100, 1974.

K. Nielsen, B. Kaempe and J. Jensen-Holm. Fatal poisoning in man by 2,4-dichlorophenoxyacetic acid (2,4-D): determination of the agent in forensic materials. Acta Pharm. Tox. 22: 224 - 234, 1965.

J. Park, I. Darrien and L. F. Prescott. Pharmacokinetic studies in severe intoxication with 2,4-D and mecoprop. Proc. Eur. Soc. Tox. 18: 154 - 155, 1977.

J. B. Rivers, W. L. Yauger and H. W. Klemmer. Simultaneous gas chromatographic determination of 2, 4-D and dicamba in human blood and urine. J. Chrom. 50: 334 - 337, 1970.

J. H. Seabury. Toxicity of 2,4-dichlorophenoxyacetic acid for man and dog. Arch. Env. Health 7: 202 - 209, 1963.

M. T. Shafik, H. C. Sullivan and H. F. Enos. A method for determination of low levels of exposure to 2,4-D and 2,4,5-T. Int. J. Env. Anal. Chem. 1: 23 - 33, 1971.

Plasma and Urine 2,4-Dichlorophenoxyacetic Acid by Gas Chromatography

Principle:

2,4-D and the internal standard, 2,4,5-T, are extracted from acidified plasma or urine with ether. A back extraction is performed into a methylating reagent and the methyl esters are chromatographed on OV-17, with detection by flame-ionization.

Reagents:

Stock solution — 10 mg/mL dichlorophenoxyacetic acid in methanol
Aqueous standards — 25, 50, 100 and 200 mg/L

Internal standard — 400 mg trichlorophenoxyacetic acid in 100 mL methanol
1 mol/L Hydrochloric acid
Ether
Methylating reagent — 1:1 mixture of water and 0.2 mol/L trimethylanilinium hydroxide in methanol (prepared fresh)

Instrumental Conditions:

Gas chromatograph with flame-ionization detector
4′ x 2 mm i.d. glass column containing 10% OV-17 on 100/200 mesh Gas Chrom Q
Injector, 310° C.; column, 200° C.; detector, 300° C.
Nitrogen flow rate, 60 mL/min

Procedure:

1. Transfer 1 mL plasma or urine to a 15 mL screw-cap tube and add 100 μL internal standard and 2 mL 1 mol/L HCl. Vortex.
2. Add 5 mL ether and shake to extract. Centrifuge.
3. Transfer the ether layer to a 15 mL glass-stoppered conical centrifuge tube. Add 100 μL of the methylating reagent and vortex for 30 seconds.
4. Centrifuge and inject 2 μL of the lower aqueous layer into the gas chromatograph.

	Retention time (min)
2,4-D	5
internal standard	7

Calculation:

Calculation is based on a response factor derived from a standard curve. A quality control specimen containing 50 mg/L 2,4-D is analyzed daily.

Evaluation:

Sensitivity: 1 mg/L
Linearity: 10 - 400 mg/L
C.V.: 5.3% within-run
Relative recovery: not established

Interferences:

The specimen should be analyzed with and without the internal standard to insure that 2,4,5-T is not one of the constituents of the ingested herbicide. Other chemical substances have not been studied for potential interference. This method is also applicable to the determination of 2,4,5-T, using 2,4-D as internal standard.

DIELDRIN

Occurrence and Usage. The epoxide of aldrin is known as dieldrin (HEOD), an organochlorine insecticide which has seen widespread usage since its development nearly 30 years ago. Technical grades of the chemical contain at least 85% dieldrin and are available in the form of powders, solutions and bait granules. Dieldrin, a stereoisomer of endrin, has been banned from most uses in the United States due to its persistence and accumulation in the environment and its chronic toxicity potential. The threshold limit value is currently 0.25 mg/m^3 for industrial exposure to dieldrin, which is known to be well absorbed after inhalation or dermal contact.

Blood Concentrations. Blood concentrations of dieldrin in some United States residents resulting from dietary intake were found to average 0.0015 mg/L; approximately 25% of whole blood dieldrin was present in erythrocytes (Radomski et al., 1971). The same value for whole blood dieldrin was reported by Dale and coworkers (1966), who also determined that plasma dieldrin concentrations in persons occupationally exposed to varying amounts of the chemical averaged 0.0094 - 0.0270 mg/L. Adults who were orally administered either 50 or 211 μg of dieldrin daily for 24 months developed steady-state blood levels averaging 0.007 and 0.020 mg/L, respectively; these concentrations had no apparent effect on the subjects and the levels declined with an average half-life of 1 year upon termination of dieldrin intake (Hunter et al., 1969). Half-lives of 50 and 97 days have also been reported (Garrettson and Curley, 1969; Brown et al., 1964).

Metabolism and Excretion. Dieldrin is not thought to undergo appreciable metabolic degradation in man, but this has not been definitely established. A major fecal detoxification product in rats has been identified as 9-hydroxydieldrin, which bears a hydroxyl group on the carbon of the methylene bridge (Baldwin et al., 1970), whereas the major urinary metabolite is 2-ketodieldrin, a product of oxidative dechlorination (McKinney et al., 1972). Adipose tissue is a major body depot for dieldrin storage; the average fat concentration in the general population of southern England was found to be 0.21 mg/kg (Hunter et al., 1963), while the mean value for United States residents was 0.14 mg/kg (Hoffman et al., 1967). Fat concentrations of dieldrin in subjects ingesting 50 or 211 μg of the chemical daily for 24 months reached maximum levels of 1.59 and 4.94 mg/kg, respectively (Hunter et al., 1969). Industrially exposed asymptomatic workers had an average fat concentration of 6.12 mg/kg (Hayes and Curley, 1968). Only negligible amounts of unchanged dieldrin, if any, are excreted in human urine (Cueto and Hayes, 1962).

Toxicity. The acute lethal dose of dieldrin in man is on the order of 1.5 - 5 g. Clinical signs of poisoning, including headache, dizziness, nausea, sweating, myoclonic limb movements and convulsive seizures, may be evident when the blood dieldrin concentration exceeds 0.15 - 0.20 mg/L (Brown et al., 1964). A 4-year old boy who survived the ingestion of dieldrin was found to have concentrations of 0.27 mg/L in serum and 47 mg/kg in fat 3 days after the incident (Garrettson and Curley, 1969). Several dieldrin fatalities have occurred, in both children and adults, although chemical determinations on tissue specimens were not performed (Conley, 1960; Pribilla, 1963; Weinig et al., 1966; Garrettson and Curley, 1969).

Dieldrin is a known liver carcinogen in animals and is believed to be teratogenic as well; its tendency to accumulate in the body during constant exposure makes it especially hazardous in these regards.

Biological Monitoring. Dieldrin may be determined in blood or biopsy fat as an index of exposure to the chemical. While levels to be expected during exposure at the 0.25 mg/m^3 TLV have not been established, it is known that systemic toxicity is generally manifested in workers with blood concentrations exceeding 0.15 mg/L and fat concentrations exceeding 60 mg/kg. Persons with values in excess of these should be removed from exposure to dieldrin (Brown et al., 1964).

Analysis. Dieldrin concentrations in biologic specimens may be estimated using the electron-capture gas chromatographic technique presented in the section on aldrin (p. 16).

References

M. K. Baldwin, J. Robinson and R. A. G. Carrington. Metabolism of HEOD (dieldrin) in the rat: examination of the major faecal metabolites. Chem. Ind.: 595 - 597, 1970.

V. K. H. Brown, C. G. Hunter and A. Richardson. A blood test diagnostic of exposure to aldrin and dieldrin. Brit. J. Ind. Med. 21: 283 - 286, 1964.

B. E. Conley. Occupational dieldrin poisoning. J. Am. Med. Asso. 172: 2077 - 2080, 1960.

C. Cueto, Jr. and W. J. Hayes, Jr. The detection of dieldrin metabolites in human urine. J. Agr. Food Chem. 10: 366 - 369, 1962.

W. E. Dale, A. Curley and C. Cueto, Jr. Hexane extractable chlorinated insecticides. Life Sci. 5: 47 - 54, 1966.

L. K. Garrettson and A. Curley. Dieldrin. Studies in a poisoned child. Arch. Env. Health 19: 814 - 822, 1969.

W. J. Hayes, Jr. and C. Curley. Storage and excretion of dieldrin and related compounds. Arch. Env. Health 16: 155 - 162, 1968.

W. S. Hoffman, H. Adler, W. I. Fishbein and F. C. Bauer. Relation of pesticide concentrations in fat to pathological changes in tissues. Arch. Env. Health 15: 758 - 765, 1967.

C. G. Hunter, J. Robinson and A. Richardson. Chlorinated insecticide content of human body fat in southern England. Brit. Med. J. 1: 221 - 224, 1963.

C. G. Hunter, J. Robinson and M. Roberts. Pharmacodynamics of dieldrin (HEOD). Arch. Env. Health 18: 12 - 21, 1969.

J. D. McKinney, H. B. Matthews and L. Fishbein. Major fecal metabolite of dieldrin in rat. Structure and chemistry. J. Agr. Food Chem. 20: 597 - 602, 1972.

O. Pribilla. Akute tödliche Dieldrinvergiftung. Arch. Tox. 20: 61 - 71, 1963.

J. L. Radomski, W. B. Deichmann, A. A. Rey and T. Merkin. Human pesticide blood levels as a measure of body burden and pesticide exposure. Tox. Appl. Pharm. 20: 175 - 185, 1971.

W. Weinig, G. Machbert and P. Zink. Über den Nachweis des Dieldrins bei einer Dieldrinvergiftung. Arch. Tox. 22: 115 - 124, 1966.

DIMETHYLFORMAMIDE

Occurrence and Usage. Dimethylformamide is a common laboratory and industrial solvent, which is readily absorbed following inhalation of the vapor or skin contact with the liquid. The current threshold limit value for occupational exposure is 10 ppm (30 mg/m^3) in the industrial atmosphere.

Blood Concentrations. Dimethylformamide reached an average level of 2.8 mg/L in the blood of subjects exposed to 21 ppm of the vapor for 4 hours, and was undetectable at 4 hours after the exposure; the metabolite, methylformamide, averaged between 1 and 2 mg/L in the blood and this level was maintained for at least 4 hours after exposure. Maximal blood levels of about 14 mg/L and 8 mg/L were observed for dimethylformamide and methylformamide, respectively, at 0 and 3 hours after a 4 hour exposure to 87 ppm of the vapor. Repeated daily exposures to 21 ppm of dimethylformamide did not result in accumulation of the chemical or its metabolite in blood (Kimmerle and Eben, 1975).

Metabolism and Excretion. It is known that dimethylformamide is metabolized in man by sequential N-demethylation to methylformamide and formamide, which are largely eliminated in the urine. Dimethylformamide is only detectable in urine after acute exposure to higher concentrations of the chemical (Kimmerle and Eben, 1975). Although quantitative data have not been obtained, it is likely that a substantial portion of an absorbed dose of dimethylformamide is excreted unchanged in the expired breath.

After a 4 hour exposure to 26 ppm of dimethylformamide, methylformamide and formamide excretion in the 24 hour urine of 4 persons averaged 24 and 6.9 mg, respectively. The corresponding values for an 87 ppm exposure were 97 and 17 mg, respectively (Kimmerle and Eben, 1975).

Toxicity. Exposure to dimethylformamide by inhalation, dermal contact or ingestion can produce nausea and vomiting at lower levels of exposure, and severe abdominal pain, hepatomegaly and hepatic necrosis at higher levels. Liver and kidney damage are frequently observed in animal toxicity testing (Massmann, 1956; Clayton et al., 1963; Potter, 1973).

Biological Monitoring. The determination of a dimethylformamide metabolite, methylformamide, in the urine of exposed workers has been recommended as a guide to monitoring worker exposure. The fluctuation in the rate of excretion of this metabolite requires that methylformamide determinations be carried out on 24 hour urine specimens. The 24 hour urinary excretion of 50 mg or less of methylformamide is consistent with occupational exposure to 20 ppm of dimethylformamide vapor (Kimmerle and Eben, 1975).

Analysis. Methylformamide concentrations in urine may be determined by flame-ionization gas chromatography, involving direct sample introduction (Barnes and Henry, 1974).

References

J. R. Barnes and N. W. Henry. The determination of N-methylformamide and -methylacetamide in urine. Am. Ind. Hyg. Asso. J. 35: 84 - 87, 1974.

J. W. Clayton, Jr., J. R. Barnes, D. B. Hood and G. W. H. Schepers. The inhalation toxicity of dimethylformamide. Am. Ind. Hyg. Asso. J. 24: 144 - 154, 1963.

G. Kimmerle and A. Eben. Metabolism studies of N, N-dimethylformamide. Int. Arch. Arbeitsmed. 34: 127 - 136, 1975.

W. Massman. Toxicological investigations on dimethylformamide. Brit. J. Ind. Med. 13: 51 - 54, 1956.

H. P. Potter. Dimethylformamide-induced abdominal pain and liver injury. Arch. Env. Health 27: 340 - 341, 1973.

Urine Methylformamide by Gas Chromatography

Principle:

Urine is injected directly into the gas chromatograph. Methylformamide is quantitated by flame-ionization detection.

Reagents:

Stock solution — 1 mg/mL methylformamide in water
Urine standards — 10, 20, 40 and 80 mg/L

Instrumental Conditions:

Gas chromatograph with flame-ionization detector
1.5 m x 2 mm i.d. glass column containing 80/100 mesh Chromosorb W
Injector, 200° C; column, 180° C.; detector, 200° C.
Helium flow rate, 45 mL/min

Procedure:

1. Centrifuge a portion of the urine specimen. Inject 2 μL of the clear supernatant into the gas chromatograph.

Calculation:

Calculation is based on a response factor derived from a standard curve. A quality control specimen containing 40 mg/L methylformamide is analyzed daily.

Evaluation:

Sensitivity: 8 mg/L
Linearity: 10 - 100 mg/L
C.V.: 3 - 8%
Relative recovery: 94 - 104%

Interferences:

Occasionally interfering peaks appear on the chromatogram at heights representing traces of methylformamide (<2 mg/L). It may be necessary to allow 25 minutes between injections for the elution of normal urinary components.

DINITRO-o-CRESOL

Occurrence and Usage. Dinitro-o-cresol (DNOC) is used primarily as a blossom-thinning agent and as a fungicide and insecticide on fruit trees. Occupational exposure generally is a result of inhalation or skin contact with the aerosol. The current threshold limit value is 0.2 mg/m^3 in the environmental air.

Blood Concentrations. Plasma levels of DNOC measured one day after exposure in asymptomatic workers exposed to 0.2 mg/m^3 of the chemical for periods of 5 - 48 hours ranged from 1.4 to 4.3 mg/L (Batchelor et al., 1956). Volunteers given 75 mg of DNOC orally once daily for five days exhibited accumulation of the substance in the blood, with no symptoms of toxicity apparent until the third or fourth day when the blood concentrations had risen to a level of 15 - 20 mg/L. The chemical was still detectable in the blood at a level of about 1 mg/L 40 days after the experiment (Harvey et al., 1956).

Metabolism and Excretion. The metabolism of DNOC has not been investigated in man, but it is known that about 2% of an ingested dose is excreted unchanged in the 24 hour urine (Harvey et al., 1951), and that the urinary concentration of the substance is a poor index of the blood concentration (Bidstrup et al., 1952).

In the sheep, about 34% of an intraperitoneal dose is eliminated in the 72 hour urine as free DNOC (4%), conjugated DNOC (7%), conjugated 6-amino-4-nitro-o-cresol (23%) and traces of 4,6-diamino-o-cresol (Jegatheeswaran and Harvey, 1970).

Toxicity. DNOC is known to have a mild corrosive effect on skin, to cause moderate CNS stimulation and to cause severe systemic poisoning by uncoupling oxidative phosphorylation. In volunteers administered daily oral doses of the chemical, a sense of well-being appeared at blood DNOC levels of 20 mg/L, while symptoms of headache, malaise and yellow coloration of the sclera developed at levels around 40 mg/L (Harvey et al., 1951). Blood concentrations of 44 - 60 mg/L have produced serious intoxication in exposed workers, and a level of 75 mg/L caused death in one subject (Bidstrup et al., 1952). A number of deaths have occurred as a result of occupational exposure, preceded by hyperthermia, rapid respiration and coma. Rigor mortis sets in rapidly after death, and autopsy findings include pulmonary edema and liver and kidney congestion (Bidstrup and Payne, 1951).

Biological Monitoring. Blood from exposed workers should be analyzed weekly for DNOC. The specimen should be drawn no sooner than 8 hours after the end of the weekly exposure, since transient peak levels often appear during the exposure period. A blood DNOC concentration of 10 mg/L is considered a warning level and a call for corrective action, while a concentration of 20 mg/L requires removal of the affected employee from the workplace and placement under medical observation (Smith et al., 1978).

Analysis. DNOC may be conveniently analyzed in blood specimens by a colorimetric procedure (Smith et al., 1978).

References

G. S. Batchelor, K. C. Walker and J. W. Elliot. Dinitroorthocresol exposure from apple-thinning sprays. Arch. Ind. Health 13: 593 - 596, 1956.

P. L. Bidstrup and D. J. H. Payne. Poisoning by dinitro-ortho-cresol. Brit. Med. J. 2: 16 - 19, 1951.

P. L. Bidstrup, J. A. L. Bonnell and D. G. Harvey. Prevention of acute dinitro-ortho-cresol (D.N.O.C.) poisoning. Lancet 1: 794 - 795, 1952.

D. G. Harvey, P. L. Bidstrup and J. A. L. Bonnell. Poisoning by dinitro-ortho-cresol. Some observations on the effects of dinitro-ortho-cresol administered by mouth to human volunteers. Brit. Med. J. 2: 13 - 16, 1951.

T. Jegatheeswaran and D. G. Harvey. The metabolism of DNOC in sheep. Vet. Rec. 87: 19 - 20, 1970.

D. L. Smith, J. R. May, R. A. Rhoden et al. *NIOSH Criteria for a Recommended Standard – Occupational Exposure to Dinitro-ortho-Cresol.* U.S. Dept. of HEW Pub. No. 78 - 131, 1978.

Blood Dinitro-o-Cresol by Colorimetry

Principle:

DNOC is extracted from blood, in the presence of sodium chloride and sodium bicarbonate, into an organic solvent. The yellow color which is produced in the organic layer is measured by visible spectrophotometry.

Reagents:

Stock solution — 1 mg/mL dinitro-o-cresol in 0.5% Na_2CO_3 (heat to dissolve)
Aqueous standards — 5, 10, 20 and 40 mg/L
Methyl ethyl ketone
Salt mixture — 1 part sodium chloride and 9 parts sodium bicarbonate by weight
Concentrated hydrochloric acid

Instrumental Conditions:

Visible spectrophotometer set to 430 nm

Procedure:

1. Transfer 1 mL blood to each of two 15 mL screw-cap tubes labeled *blank* and *sample.* Add 5 mL methyl ethyl ketone to each and vortex briefly.

2. Add 1 - 2 g of the salt mixture to each tube, cap and shake to extract. Centrifuge and transfer the upper layers to clean tubes.
3. Add 1 drop conc. HCl to the blank tube and vortex. Centrifuge to clear the solution.
4. Transfer the contents of the tubes to cuvettes. Zero the spectrophotometer with methyl ethyl ketone, and determine the absorbance of the blank and sample solutions at 430 nm.

Calculation:

Subtract the blank reading from the sample reading, and estimate the DNOC concentration by comparing this value to a standard curve of absorbance vs. concentration for the aqueous standards. A quality control specimen consisting of 20 mg/L DNOC in water is analyzed daily.

Evaluation:

Sensitivity: 0.5 mg/L
Linearity: 5 - 50 mg/L
C.V.: not established
Relative recovery: not established

Interferences:

2,4-Dinitrophenol is known to interfere in this procedure. Abnormally high blood concentrations of β-carotene or bilirubin may yield non-specific absorbance causing a false elevation of the DNOC level. Interference by blood pigments is present if the blank absorbance exceeds 0.15.

DIOXANE

Occurrence and Usage. Dioxane is a widely used laboratory and industrial solvent which is well-absorbed following inhalation and skin contact. The current threshold limit value is 50 ppm (180 mg/m^3), although this value is pending revision to 25 ppm.

Blood Concentrations. Subjects exposed to 50 ppm of dioxane for a period of 6 hours developed an average steady-state plasma dioxane concentration of 12 mg/L; at the end of exposure this level declined with a half-life of 1 hour and it was predicted that no accumulation of dioxane would occur with repeated daily exposure. A dioxane metabolite, β-hydroxyethoxyacetic acid, attained a peak plasma level of about 10 mg/L at 1 hour after the end of the exposure, declining with a half-life of about 3 hours (Young et al., 1977).

Metabolism and Excretion. Dioxane is metabolized in man by oxidation to β-hydroxyethoxyacetic acid (HEAA), which accumulates in blood and which is extensively excreted in urine. The total elimination of dioxane from the human body has not been studied, and it is probable that a substantial portion of a dose is eliminated unchanged in the expired breath; however, of that portion which is eliminated as known metabolites in urine, the vast majority is HEAA and only a fraction is found as unchanged dioxane.

The highest urinary concentrations of both dioxane and HEAA occur during the latter portion of an exposure period. Workers exposed to dioxane vapor for 7.5 hours at a level of 1.6 ppm had end-of-shift urine concentrations which averaged 0.3 mg/L for dioxane and 50 mg/L for HEAA; these concentrations are estimated at 8 mg/L and 813 mg/L, respectively, in subjects exposed to 50 ppm of dioxane for 6 hours (Young et al., 1976; Young et al., 1977).

In the rat, between 40 and 60% of a labeled dose of dioxane is eliminated in the 48 hour urine. About 11% of the dose was found as unchanged dioxane in the urine and 33% as p-dioxane-2-one; the latter compound is the lactone of HEAA and is the form which Woo et al. (1977) believe predominates in urine, probably due to the spontaneous rearrangement of HEAA.

Toxicity. Dioxane is irritating to the eyes, nose and throat at an air concentration of 300 ppm, and to the skin upon contact. Prolonged exposure to high concentrations of the vapor may produce severe intoxication characterized by anorexia, nausea, vomiting, abdominal pain, convulsions and unconsciousness; autopsy of several victims has shown evidence of cerebral edema, bronchopneumonia and necrosis of the liver and kidneys (Johnstone, 1959).

Studies in animals have shown that dioxane can cause malignant tumors of the lung, liver, kidney and nasal cavity.

Biological Monitoring. Although not established as a routine method, it is evident that the measurement of dioxane (or its metabolite, HEAA) in plasma would provide a useful index to human exposure. A more convenient procedure involves the determination of dioxane and HEAA in urine specimens collected at the end of a shift, the concentrations of which are proportional to the extent of dioxane exposure. According to the kinetics of dioxane elimination, dioxane should not be detectable and HEAA should be present at very low levels in urine specimens collected just before the start of a shift in workers who are exposed on a daily basis to 50 ppm of dioxane (Young et al., 1977).

Analysis. Dioxane in plasma or urine may be analyzed by the gas chromatographic method described in the section on benzene (p. 39). A method for the determination of HEAA in urine is presented which involves flame-ionization gas chromatography (Braun, 1977).

References

W. H. Braun. Rapid method for the simultaneous determination of 1,4-dioxan and its major metabolite, β-hydroxyethoxyacetic acid, concentrations in plasma and urine. J. Chrom. 113: 263 - 266, 1977.

R. T. Johnstone. Death due to dioxane? Arch. Ind. Health 20: 445 - 447, 1959.

T. Woo, J. C. Arcos, M. F. Argus et al. Structural identification to p-dioxane-2-one as the major urinary metabolite of p-dioxane. Arch. Pharm. 299: 283 - 287, 1977.

J. D. Young, W. H. Braun, P. J. Gehring et al. 1,4-Dioxane and β-hydroxyethoxyacetic acid excretion in urine of humans exposed to dioxane vapors. Tox. App. Pharm. 38: 643 - 646, 1976.

J. D. Young, W. H. Braun, L. W. Braun et al. Pharmacokinetics of 1,4-dioxane in humans. J. Tox. Env. Health 3: 507 - 520, 1977.

Urine HEAA by Gas Chromatography

Principle:

The methyl derivative of β-hydroxyethoxyacetic acid is formed in urine by heating in the presence of methanol and acid. Water is removed by the addition of acetic anhydride to force the reaction to completion. The solution is diluted with methanol and an aliquot is analyzed by flame-ionization gas chromatography.

Reagents:

Stock solution — 1 mg/mL HEAA (Dow Chemical Co., Midland, Michigan) in methanol
Urine standards — 50, 100, 200, 500, and 1000 mg/L
Concentrated hydrochloric acid
Methanol
Acetic anhydride

Instrumental Conditions:

Gas chromatograph with flame-ionization detector
1.8 m x 2 mm i.d. glass column containing 3% OV-17 on 80/100 mesh Supelcoport
Injector, 250° C.; detector, 250° C.
Column temperature program:
initial, 80° C.
20°C./min increase
final, 150° C.
Helium flow rate, 30 mL/min

Procedure:

1. Transfer 0.5 mL of the specimen to a 12 mL centrifuge tube. Add 100 μL conc. HCl and 1 mL methanol and vortex.
2. Incubate at 60° C. for 5 minutes. Add slowly, while the solution is still warm, 2 mL of acetic anhydride.
3. Dilute to 5.0 mL with methanol, vortex and inject 1 μL of the solution into the chromatograph.

	Retention time (min)
HEAA derivative	4.3

Calculation:

Calculation is based on a response factor derived from a standard curve. A quality control specimen consisting of 50 mg/L HEAA in water is analyzed daily.

Evaluation:

Sensitivity: 50 mg/L
Linearity: 50-1000 mg/L
C.V.: 10-11%
Relative recovery: not established

Interferences:

The direct injection of urine tends to cause peak broadening after a period of time. Replaceable glass sleeves should be used in the injection port and changed daily, and the first several inches of the column packing may need to be changed occasionally.

ENDRIN

Occurrence and Usage. Endrin, a stereoisomer of dieldrin, is considered one of the most toxic of the chlorinated hydrocarbon insecticides. It has seen widespread usage in agriculture against soil and foliage pests since 1950, although its use has been recently curtailed in some countries due to its environmental persistence. Industrial exposure is generally via inhalation or dermal absorption. The current threshold limit value is 0.1 mg/m^3 in the occupational environment.

Blood Concentrations. Endrin was not found present in the plasma, fat or urine of members of the general population or of occupationally exposed workers in amounts measurable by a technique with detectability limits of 0.003, 0.03 and 0.002 mg/L, respectively (Hayes and Curley, 1968).

Metabolism and Excretion. The disposition of endrin in man has not been investigated, although it is likely handled in a manner similar to that of dieldrin. In rats endrin is oxidized on the methylene bridge carbon atom to 9-hydroxyendrin, the major fecal metabolite, which undergoes further oxidation to 9-ketoendrin, the major urinary excretion product (Baldwin et al., 1970).

Toxicity. The contamination of foodstuffs by endrin has resulted in several mass poisonings, with multiple fatalities; the onset of symptoms, which included vomiting, convulsions and unconsciousness, ranged from 0.5 - 10 hours after ingestion of the poison (Davies and Lewis, 1956; Weeks, 1967). Death often occurs within 1 - 2 hours after ingestion of 6 g of endrin (Reddy et al., 1966). One subject who ate endrin contaminated bread and suffered a convulsion exhibited a serum endrin concentration of 0.053 mg/L within 30 minutes of the convulsion; this concentration fell to 0.038 mg/L after 20 hours, while a urine concentration of only 0.020 mg/L was observed for the first 24 hour specimen. A serum concentration of 0.004 mg/L was determined for the patient's husband, who had also eaten the bread but failed to develop symptoms (Coble et al., 1967). In the surviving victims of several mass endrin poisonings, blood concentrations of 0.007 - 0.032 mg/L and urine concentrations of <0.004 - 0.007 mg/L were measured on the day of onset of symptoms; samples of blood and urine taken 29 - 31 days after the outbreak of poisoning were uniformly negative for endrin. Concentrations of 0.685 mg/kg in liver and 0.116 mg/kg in kidney were found in one fatal case (Curley et al., 1970).

Biological Monitoring. Plasma is the only tissue or fluid for which a reasonable correlation has been established between the endrin concentration and the degree of intoxication. Plasma endrin concentrations have been less than 0.003 mg/L in asymptomatic exposed workers (Hayes and Curley, 1968).

Analysis. Endrin is measured in biological specimens using the electron-capture gas chromatography techniques presented in the section on aldrin.

References

M. K. Baldwin, J. Robinson and D. V. Parke. Metabolism of endrin in the rat. J. Agr. Food Chem. 18: 1117 - 1123, 1970.

Y. Coble, P. Hildebrandt, J. Davis et al. Acute endrin poisoning. J. Am. Med. Asso. 202: 489 - 493, 1967.

C. Cueto, Jr. and F. J. Biros. Chlorinated insecticides and related materials in human urine. Tox. Appl. Pharm. 10: 261 - 269, 1967.

A. Curley, R. W. Jennings, H. T. Mann and V. Sedlak. Measurement of endrin following epidemics of poisoning. Bull. Env. Cont. Tox. 5: 24 - 29, 1970.

W. E. Dale, A. Curley and C. Cueto, Jr. Hexane extractable chlorinated insecticides in human blood. Life Sci. 5: 47 - 54, 1966.

G. M. Davies and I. Lewis. Outbreak of food-poisoning from bread made of chemically contaminated flour. Brit. Med. J. 2: 393 - 398, 1956.

W. J. Hayes, Jr. and C. Curley. Storage and excretion of dieldrin and related compounds. Arch. Env. Health 16: 155 - 162, 1968.

D. B. Reddy, V. D. Edward, G. J. S. Abraham and K. V. Rao. Fatal endrin poisoning. J. Ind. Med. Asso. 46: 121 - 124, 1966.

D. E. Weeks, Endrin food-poisoning. Bull. WHO 37: 499 - 512, 1967.

ETHANOL

Occurrence and Usage. Ethanol is widely encountered as a manufactured product and as a solvent in industry, where many employees are exposed to the compound by inhalation of the vapor. Ethanol is incorporated into many elixirs, mouthwashes and other medicinal liquids in appreciable amounts. It is also present to the extent of 3 - 6% by volume in naturally fermented beers and ales, 10 - 12% in wines and 20 - 60% in distilled beverages. The current threshold limit value for industrial exposure is 1000 ppm (1900 mg/m^3).

Blood Concentrations. Because ethanol distributes evenly throughout the body water, its concentration in blood following a known dose may be estimated on the basis of the subject's sex, body weight and degree of adiposity. Ethanol is present as an endogenous substance in the blood of man, probably produced in the intestinal tract, at an average level of 1.5 mg/L (Lester, 1962). Resting subjects develop blood ethanol concentrations of less than 100 mg/L when exposed to vapor concentrations of 7500 - 8500 ppm for 3 hours, while an exercising subject developed a blood level of 450 mg/L under the same conditions (Lester and Greenberg, 1951), A single oral dose of 0.5 mL/kg (35 mL/70 kg) of pure ethanol given to 4 fasting men produced an average maximal blood concentration of about 400 mg/L at 2 hours; a dose of 1.4 mL/kg (98 mL/70 kg) produced a level of 1200 mg/L at 1 hour; and 2.0 mL/kg (140 mL/70 kg), a level of 2000 mg/L at 1 hour. The levels declined at a mean rate for the 21 subjects of 189 mg/L per hour (Sidell and Pless, 1971). The presence of food in the stomach may cause up to 70% reduction in the peak blood ethanol concentration attained after a measured oral dose; this effect is due to a reduction in both the efficiency and rate of absorption of the ethanol (Lin et al., 1976; Wilkinson et al., 1977).

Metabolism and Excretion. The metabolism of alcohol proceeds at a rate which has been assumed to be essentially independent of the dose (zero-order); this is a valid approximation at higher concentrations, but at concentrations less than 200 mg/L the kinetics of elimination become first-order and therefore non-linear (Wagner et al., 1976). There is evidence that first-order kinetics also apply at very high blood ethanol concentrations (Bogusz et al., 1977; Hammond et al., 1973). Ethanol is biotransformed to acetaldehyde and then to acetic acid by liver enzymes; these enzymes are induced during chronic ethanol administration, which may result in an increase of up to 72% in the rate of ethanol disappearance from the blood of naive subjects (Misra et al., 1971). Other authors have found that this effect is not consistent in all subjects (Vesell et al., 1971). Acetaldehyde accumulates to a slight extent in the blood of normal persons after ethanol administration, and to a greater extent in alcoholic subjects; these concentrations are on the order of a thousandth of the ethanol levels (Korsten et al., 1975). About 95% of a dose undergoes metabolism and the remainder is excreted unchanged in the breath, urine, sweat and feces.

At equilibrium, the concentration of ethanol in any tissue or fluid is a function of the water content of that specimen. It has been determined that the plasma/whole blood ratio varies from 1.10 - 1.35 with an average of 1.18 (Payne et al., 1968). Urine concentrations of alcohol are often used to estimate blood concentrations; during the elimination phase the urine/blood ratio of 1.3 applies and provides a valid estimate in most cases (Heise, 1967). The blood/breath ratio during the elimination phase averages 2180, with a range of 1837 - 2863 (Jones, 1978).

Toxicity. Inhalation of ethanol at levels of 5,000 - 10,000 ppm produces eye and throat irritation, followed by increasing degrees of central nervous system depression with continued exposure. Blood ethanol concentrations as high as 500 mg/L may be produced during physical exertion in subjects exposed to vapor levels as low as 8000 ppm for 6 - 8 hours; at this blood concentration, the central depressant effect of ethanol is sufficient to cause an industrial hazard.

Toxic reactions, including flushing of the face and increased pulse rate, have been observed in subjects undergoing therapy with disulfiram when exposed to ethanol at air concentrations of 8000 ppm for short periods of time (Lester and Greenberg, 1951).

Biological Monitoring. The determination of ethanol in blood, breath or urine sampled during or just after the work period can provide a useful index to exposure. Lester and Greenberg (1951) indicate that the blood alcohol concentration should not exceed 200 - 300 mg/L in exposed workers. Pre-exposure specimens should be taken to rule out non-occupational sources of ethanol.

Analysis. Since ethanol is both formed and destroyed in biological specimens *in vitro,* the proper preservation of these specimens is important for analytical purposes. The formation of alcohol by microorganisms is inhibited by fluoride, mercuric ion and cold storage; ethanol loss occurs by volatilization and destruction by microorganisms, both of which are retarded by the above conditions, and by hemoglobin-catalyzed oxidation, which may be inhibited by sodium azide (Bradford, 1966; Brown et al., 1973; Christopoulos et al., 1973; Smalldon and Brown, 1973). The gas chromatographic method presented in the section on acetone (p. 9) is applicable to the determination of ethanol in biological specimens.

References

M. Bogusz, J. Pach and W. Stasko. Comparative studies on the rate of ethanol elimination in acute poisoning and in controlled conditions. J. For. Sci. 22: 446 - 451, 1977.

L. W. Bradford. Preservation of blood samples containing alcohol. J. For. Sci. 11: 214 - 216, 1966.

G. A. Brown, D. Neylan, W. J. Reynolds and K. W. Smalldon. The stability of ethanol in stored blood. Anal. Chim. Acta 66: 271 - 283, 1973.

G. Christopoulos, E. R. Kirch and J. E. Gearien. Determination of ethanol in fresh and putrefied post mortem tissues. J. Chrom. 87: 455 - 472, 1973.

K. B. Hammond, B. H. Rumack and D. O. Rodgerson. Blood ethanol. J. Am. Med. Asso. 226: 63 - 64, 1973.

H. A. Heise. Concentrations of alcohol in samples of blood and urine taken at the same time. J. For. Sci. 12: 454 - 462, 1967.

A. W. Jones. Variability of the blood:breath alcohol ratio in vivo. J. Stud. Alc. 39: 1931 - 1931, 1978.

M. A. Korsten, S. Matsuzaki, L. Feinman and C. S. Lieber. High blood acetaldehyde levels after ethanol administration. New Eng. J. Med. 292: 386 - 389, 1975.

Y. J. Lin, D. J. Weidler, D. C. Garg and J. G. Wagner. Effects of solid food on blood levels of alcohol in man. Res. Comm. Chem. Path. Pharm. 13: 713 - 722, 1976.

D. Lester and L. A. Greenberg. The inhalation of ethyl alcohol by man. Quart. J. Stud. Alc. 12: 167 - 178, 1951.

D. Lester. The concentration of apparent endogenous ethanol. Quart. J. Stud. Alc. 23: 17 - 25, 1962.

P. S. Misra, A. LeFevre, H. Ishii et al. Increase of ethanol, meprobamate and pentobarbital metabolism after chronic ethanol administration in man and in rats. Am. J. Med. 51: 346 - 351, 1971.

J. P. Payne, D. W. Hill and D. G. L. Wood. Distribution of ethanol between plasma and erythrocytes in whole blood. Nature 217: 963 - 964, 1968.

F. R. Sidell and J. E. Pless. Ethyl alcohol: blood levels and performance decrements after oral administration to man. Psychopharm. 19: 246 - 261, 1971.

K. W. Smalldon and G. A. Brown. The stability of ethanol in stored blood. Part II. The mechanism of ethanol oxidation. Anal. Chim. Acta 66: 285 - 290, 1973.

E. S. Vesell, J. G. Page and G. T. Passananti. Genetic and environmental factors affecting ethanol metabolism in man. Clin. Pharm. Ther. 12: 192 - 201, 1971.

J. G. Wagner, P. K. Wilkinson, A. J. Sedman et al. Elimination of alcohol from human blood. J. Pharm. Sci. 65: 152 - 154, 1976.

P. K. Wilkinson, A. J. Sedman, E. Sakmar et al. Fasting and nonfasting blood ethanol concentrations following repeated oral administration of ethanol to one adult male subject. J. Pharm. Biopharm. 5: 41 - 52, 1977.

ETHER

Occurrence and Usage. Ether (diethyl ether, ethyl ether) is a volatile and flammable liquid which is utilized as a solvent in the manufacture of synthetic dyes and plastics. Although it was the first successful surgical anesthetic agent, due to its flammability and irritating odor it is rarely used today. The current threshold limit value for occupational exposure is 400 ppm (1200 mg/m^3) in the workroom air.

Blood Concentrations. Blood ether concentrations in workers exposed at the current TLV have been estimated to reach 18 mg/L (ACGIH, 1971). Subanesthetic doses of ether, which produce analgesia but not unconsciousness, result in arterial blood concentrations of 100 - 150 mg/L. During surgical anesthesia these concentrations vary between 500 and 1500 mg/L, with an average deep surgical anesthesia concentration of 1200 mg/L in arterial blood (Faulconer, 1952).

Metabolism and Excretion. Over 90% of a dose of ether is exhaled unchanged after exposure ceases; a small amount is excreted in urine and there is a minor degree of biotransformation via oxidation to water and carbon dioxide (Price, 1975). The following partition coefficients are exhibited by ether at normal body temperature (Wollman and Smith, 1975).

Blood:Gas	Brain:Blood	Liver:Blood	Kidney:Blood	Fat:Blood
12	1.0-1.1	0.9	0.8	4.2

Toxicity. Inhalation of ether at the TLV may cause nose and throat irritation. Exposure to higher concentrations produces central nervous system depression, with nausea, irregular respiration, and lowering of body temperature and pulse rate. Concentrations of 2000 ppm are known to cause dizziness in some individuals and are associated with a blood ether concentration of about 90 mg/L; a level of 100,000 ppm may be rapidly fatal. Reports of toxicity due to chronic exposure to ether indicate that symptoms include loss of appetite, headache, exhaustion and psychic disturbances (ACGIH, 1971).

Relatively little data is available regarding tissue concentrations of ether in overdosage, although persons have died following the intentional ingestion of as little as 30 mL of the liquid. Postmortem blood ether concentrations of 600 - 3750 mg/L were observed in 3 surgical patients who died within 2.5 hours of cessation of ether administration (Campbell, 1960).

Biological Monitoring. Blood ether concentrations have been found to correlate with both the degree of worker exposure and the extent of intoxication; these concentrations should not exceed a level of about 20 mg/L in asymptomatic workers.

The levels of ether in breath or urine corresponding to occupational exposure at the TLV have not been established. However, it is probable that the ether content of these specimens is proportional to the magnitude and extent of exposure and that the concentrations would be useful in monitoring the exposure status of individual workers.

Analysis. Ether may be measured in biological specimens using the following gas chromatographic technique devised for the analysis of several common inhalation anesthetics (Yokota et al., 1967).

References

ACGIH. *Documentation of the Threshold Limit Values,* American Conference of Governmental Industrial Hygienists, Cincinnati, Ohio, 1971, p. 106.

J. E. Campbell. Deaths associated with anesthesia. J. For. Sci. 5: 501 - 549, 1960.

A. Faulconer, Jr. Correlation of concentrations of ether in arterial blood with electro-encephalographic patterns occurring during ether-oxygen and during nitrous oxide, oxygen and ether anesthesia of human surgical patients. Anesthesiol.13: 361 - 369, 1952.

H. L. Price. General anesthetics. In *The Pharmacological Basis of Therapeutics,* 5th ed. (L. S. Goodman and A. Gilman, eds.), MacMillan, New York, 1975, pp. 89 - 96.

H. Wollman and T. C. Smith. Uptake, distribution, elimination and administration of inhalational anesthetics. In *The Pharmacological Basis of Therapeutics,* 5th ed. (L. S. Goodman and A. Gilman, eds.), MacMillan, New York, 1975, pp. 71 - 80.

T. Yokota, Y. Hitomi, K. Ohta and F. Kosaka. Direct injection method for gas chromatographic measurement of inhalation anesthetics in whole blood and tissues. Anesthesiol. 28: 1064 - 1073, 1967.

Blood and Urine Inhalation Anesthetics by Gas Chromatography

Principle:

Ether in biological fluids is analyzed by direct injection of the specimen into a gas chromatograph equipped with a flame-ionization detector and a molecular sieve column. The method is rapid and applicable to the measurement of other anesthetic gases and liquids as well.

Reagents:

Stock solution — 1 mg/mL ether in water
Blood or urine standards — 10, 20, 50, 100 and 200 mg/L

Instrumental Conditions:

Gas chromatograph with replaceable glass injector sleeve and flame-ionization detector

0.75 m x 3 mm i.d. stainless steel column containing 0.3% diethylene glycol succinate on 60/80 mesh molecular sieve type 5A (liquid phase may be omitted with little effect on peak shape)
Injector, 200° C.; column, 120° C., detector, 150° C.
Nitrogen flow rate, 90 mL/min

Procedure:

1. With a 5 μL direct-injection syringe (Hamilton #7105 N) draw up 0.5 μL of water. Then draw up exactly 1 μL of specimen.
2. Wipe off the needle of the 5 μL syringe and inject the contents into the gas chromatograph. Withdraw the needle and immediately rinse the syringe with water.

	Retention time (sec)
cyclopropane	17
halothane	23
methoxyflurane	35
ether	73

Calculation:

Calculation is based on a standard curve of peak height versus concentration of the standards. This procedure cannot be controlled by the usual methods due to the difficulty in storage of quality control specimens containing these volatile substances.

Evaluation:

Sensitivity: 10 mg/L
Linearity: 10 - 200 mg/L
C.V.: 3 - 5% within-run
Relative recovery: 96 - 100%

Interferences:

The injection technique must be practiced and standardized in order to obtain consistent results. The glass insert for the injector should be replaced with a clean insert (used injectors may be cleaned by soaking in chromic acid solution overnight) after every 15 - 20 injections, replacing the septum at the same time. After several months of usage it may be necessary to replace the column packing in the first 1 - 2 cm of the column. The molecular sieve column should be reactivated by heating to 200° C. overnight after several months of use to remove absorbed water.

Specimens should be stored at 4° C. and analyzed as soon as possible. Breath samples may be analyzed by direct injection of 1 - 2 mL, using as standards suitably prepared dilutions of the appropriate chemical in air.

ETHYLBENZENE

Occurrence and Usage. Ethylbenzene is employed commercially as a solvent, fuel additive and chemical intermediate in the production of styrene. It is readily absorbed by the pulmonary route and after direct application to the skin. The current threshold limit value for ethylbenzene in the industrial atmosphere is 100 ppm (435 mg/m^3).

Blood Concentrations. Ethylbenzene has not been measured in the blood of exposed workers.

Metabolism and Excretion. Ethylbenzene is metabolized in man by oxidation of the side-chain to methylphenylcarbinol, which accounts for about 5% of a dose as a urinary glucuronide conjugate. Further oxidation of this first metabolite produces mandelic acid and phenylglyoxylic acid, compounds which are also major metabolites of styrene and which represent 64 and 25% of a dose of ethylbenzene as urinary excretion products. Mandelic acid is an endogenous urinary substance found in normal urine at levels of up to 5 mg/L (Van Roosmalen and Drummond, 1978). Only a minor portion of a dose is eliminated unchanged in the expired breath and urine (Bardodej and Bardodejova, 1970).

The urinary excretion of mandelic acid reaches a maximum during the last 2 hours of an 8 hour exposure, and then declines with a half-life of 4 - 7 hours following the termination of exposure. Mandelic acid concentrations in the urine of resting subjects exposed to 92 ppm of ethylbenzene for 8 hours average about 900 mg/L (Piotrowski, 1977).

Toxicity. Exposure to ethylbenzene at an air concentration of 1000 ppm causes eye and nose irritation. Concentrations of 2000 ppm may produce lacrimation and dizziness, while higher levels cause increasing degrees of central nervous system depression.

Biological Monitoring. The excretion of mandelic acid in urine during the last 2 hours of an 8 hour exposure to ethylbenzene is proportional to the air concentration of the chemical. It has been determined that under these conditions a level of 100 ppm ethylbenzene produces a maximal urinary mandelic acid concentration of 2000 mg/L at a specific gravity of 1.025, or 1.5 mg mandelic acid per mg creatinine. This value has been proposed as a biological threshold limit for exposure to ethylbenzene (Bardodej and Bardodejova, 1970).

Analysis. Mandelic acid may be analyzed in urine by the following gas chromatographic procedure, which is also applicable to the determination of phenylglyoxylic acid, hippuric acid, and m- and p-methylhippuric acid (Van Roosmalen and Drummond, 1978). Phenylglyoxylic acid is unstable in urine unless the specimen is frozen.

References

Z. Bardodej and E. Bardodejova. Biotransformation of ethyl benzene, styrene, and alpha-methylstyrene in man. Am. Ind. Hyg. Asso. J. 31: 206 - 209, 1970.

J. K Piotrowski. *Exposure Tests for Organic Compounds in Industrial Toxicology*, U.S. Government Printing Office, Washington, D.C., 1977, pp. 58 - 59.

P. B. Van Roosmalen and I. Drummond. Simultaneous determination by gas chromatography of the major metabolites in urine of toluene, xylenes and styrene. Brit. J. Ind. Med. 35: 56 - 60, 1978.

Urine Aromatic Acids by Gas Chromatography

Principle:

Several of the acidic metabolites of aromatic solvents, including hippuric acid, mandelic acid, methylhippuric acid and phenylglyoxylic acid, are extracted from acidified urine with ethyl acetate. The extract is evaporated to dryness and the residue treated with a reagent to form trimethylsilyl derivatives of the metabolites.

Reagents:

Stock solutions —
- 1 mg/mL hippuric acid in methanol
- 1 mg/mL mandelic acid in methanol
- 1 mg/mL m-methylhippuric acid in methanol
- 1 mg/mL phenylglyoxylic acid in methanol

Aqueous standards — 500, 1000 and 2000 mg/L for each of the above
Internal standard — 10 mg/mL heptadecanoic acid (Eastman Kodak) in methanol
Ammonium sulfate
5% Sulfuric acid
Ethyl acetate
Tri-sil (Pierce Chemical Co.)

Instrumental Conditions:

Gas chromatograph with flame-ionization detector
1.2 m x 2 mm i.d. glass column containing 3% OV-1 on 80/100 mesh Gas Chrom Q
Injector, 250° C.; detector, 250° C.
Column temperature program:
- initial, 130° C. (6 min)
- 12° C./min increase
- final, 215° C.

Nitrogen flow rate, 20 mL/min

Procedure:

1. Transfer 1 mL urine to a 15 mL screw-cap tube. Add 100 μL internal standard, 1 g ammonium sulfate, and 0.2 mL 5% H_2SO_4.
2. Extract with 4 mL ethyl acetate by shaking for 2 minutes. Centrifuge to separate layers and transfer 2 mL of the upper organic layer to a 5 mL glass-stoppered conical centrifuge tube.
3. Evaporate the extract to dryness under a stream of nitrogen at 40° C. Add 100 μL Tri-sil, stopper and heat at 75° C. for 5 min.
4. Cool and inject 1 μL of the solution into the chromatograph.

	Retention time (min)
phenylglyoxylic acid derivative	1.8
mandelic acid derivative	2
hippuric acid derivative	8
m-methylhippuric acid derivative	10
internal standard derivative	13

Calculation:

Calculation is based on a response factor derived from a standard curve. A quality control specimen containing 1000 mg/L of each of the appropriate acids is analyzed daily.

Evaluation:

Sensitivity: 2 - 4 mg/L
Linearity: 200 - 2000 mg/L
C.V.: 1.5 - 5%
Relative recovery: 97 - 99%

Interferences:

Normal urinary levels of hippuric acid are from 500 to 1200 mg/L while mandelic acid concentrations are less than 5 mg/L. Phenylglyoxylic acid and m- and p-methylhippuric acid have not been detected in the urine of normal subjects. Salicyluric acid, an aspirin metabolite, elutes just before the internal standard and does not interfere in the procedure.

FLUORIDE

Occurrence and Usage. Hydrogen fluoride and its inorganic salts find wide application in industry. Sodium fluoride, sodium fluosilicate (Na_2SiF_6) and cryolite (Na_3AlF_6) are employed as insecticides, rodenticides and delousing powders. Fluoride minerals are used in the manufacture of glass, aluminum, steel and fertilizer. The presence of fluoride in drinking water promotes resistance to tooth decay in children, and thus in many geographic areas where water supplies are lacking in this anion, it is added at a recommended level of 1 ppm. It is also incorporated into some dentrifrices as stannous fluoride (SnF_2), is often applied topically to the teeth in dental treatment programs, and may be administered to children in daily oral doses of 2.2 mg of sodium fluoride on a chronic basis. Since fluoride increases the density and calcification of bone, its use for patients with osteoporosis has been recommended, in a daily dose of 33 - 220 mg as the sodium salt. The average daily dietary fluoride intake for an adult ranges from 0.5 - 5 mg as the anion. Industrial exposure to fluoride is generally the result of inhalation of dust produced during the processing of fluoride-containing minerals in many different industries. The current threshold limit value for fluoride in air is 2.5 mg/m^3 (expressed as F).

Blood Concentrations. Background plasma fluoride concentrations in 3 subjects on a low fluoride diet (<0.4 mg F/day) were on the order of 0.010 mg/L. Following single oral doses of 1.5 - 10 mg of fluoride (3.3 - 22 mg as NaF) given to healthy subjects, plasma fluoride concentrations reached peaks of 0.06 - 0.4 mg/L within 30 minutes of administration and declined with half-lives of 2.0 - 9.0 hours. Plasma contains about 72% of whole blood fluoride (Carlson et al., 1960); fluoride occurs as a free ion in plasma and is not protein bound (Ekstrand et al., 1977).

Metabolism and Excretion. In both healthy and osteoporotic subjects, about half of the ingested fluoride is excreted unchanged in the daily urine, about 6 - 10% in the feces, and from 13 - 23% in sweat. Retention in bone probably accounts for much of the balance, and this percentage is relatively unaffected by the extent of daily intake (McClure et al., 1945; Spencer et al., 1975; Ekstrand et al., 1977). Urine concentrations of fluoride in normal subjects have been found to range from 0.2 - 3.2 mg/L, being largely dependent on the dietary intake. Urine fluoride concentrations in a group of asymptomatic workers averaged 4.5 mg/L (range 2.1 - 14.7) during chronic exposure to air fluoride levels averaging 2.65 mg/m^3 (Derryberry et al., 1963).

Toxicity. Low-level exposure to airborne fluoride is first expressed as irritation of mucous membranes of the eyes, nose and throat. Continued exposure may produce symptoms of early fluoride toxicity which include respiratory distress, neurological abnormalities, gastrointestinal pain and muscular fibrillation.

The daily absorption of 10 - 80 mg of fluoride over a period of years can lead to a condition known as crippling skeletal fluorosis, in which excessive calcification of bone results in stiffening of ligaments and fusion of joints (Hodge and Smith, 1977; Waldbott, 1979).

Numerous instances of acute fluoride poisoning have occurred as a result of the accidental or intentional ingestion or inhalation of fluorides. One mass poisoning involved 263 persons, 47 of whom died, following the inadvertent addition of sodium fluoride to food (Lidbeck et al., 1943). The acute ingestion of 1.5 g of hydrofluoric acid has caused death in an adult (Curry, 1962), while it is felt that 5 - 10 g represents a minimal lethal dose of sodium fluoride. Blood fluoride concentrations averaged 8.0 mg/L (range 2.6 - 16) in 10 fatal cases resulting from both ingestion and inhalation (Gettler and Ellerbrook, 1939; Curry, 1962; Greendyke and Hodge, 1964; Cranston and Bastos, 1975; Speaker, 1976).

Biological Monitoring. The fluoride concentration in urine is a useful index to fluoride intake in workers, and has been found to average about 4 mg/L in an end-of-shift specimen following an 8 hour exposure at the current TLV of 2.5 mg/m^3. While plasma fluoride concentrations may also be used as an index of exposure, this is not routinely done.

A biological threshold limit value of 5 mg/L for urinary fluoride has been proposed, when measured in a pre-shift specimen collected after two days off work and corrected to a specific gravity of 1.024. This value is considered to represent an individual's body burden of fluoride (Smith, 1971).

Analysis. Inorganic fluoride is measured directly in plasma or urine specimens using a fluoride-specific electrode (Cernik et al., 1970; Singer and Ophaug, 1979).

References

C. H. Carlson, W. D. Armstrong and L. Singer. Distribution and excretion of radiofluoride in the human. Proc. Soc. Exp. Biol. Med. 104: 235 - 239, 1960.

A. A. Cernik, J. A. Cooke and R. J. Hall. Specific ion electrode in the determination of urinary fluoride. Nature 227: 1260 - 1261, 1970.

D. Cranston and M. L. Bastos. Personal communication, 1975.

A. S. Curry. Twenty-one uncommon cases of poisoning. Brit. Med. J. 1: 687 - 689, 1962.

O. M. Derryberry, M. D. Bartholomew and R. B. L. Fleming. Fluoride exposure and worker health. Arch. Env. Health 6: 503 - 511, 1963.

J. Ekstrand, G. Alvan, L. O. Boreus and A. Norlin. Pharmacokinetics of fluoride in man after single and multiple oral doses. Eur. J. Clin. Pharm. 12: 311 - 317, 1977.

A. O. Gettler and L. Ellerbrook. Toxicology of fluorides. Am. J. Med. Sci. 197: 625 - 638, 1939.

R. M. Greendyke and H. C. Hodge. Accidental death due to hydrofluoric acid. J. For. Sci. 9: 383 - 390, 1964.

H. C. Hodge and F. A. Smith. Occupational fluoride exposure. J. Occ. Med. 19: 12 - 39, 1977.

W. L. Lidbeck, I. B. Hill and J. A. Beeman. Acute sodium fluoride poisoning. J. Am. Med. Asso. 121: 826 - 827, 1943.

F. J. McClure, H. H. Mitchell, T. S. Hamilton and C. A. Kinser. Balances of fluorine ingested from various sources in food and water by five young men. J. Ind. Hyg. Tox. 27: 159 - 170, 1945.

L. Singer and R. H. Ophaug. Concentrations of ionic, total, and bound fluoride in plasma. Clin. Chem. 25: 523 - 525, 1979.

F. A. Smith. Biological monitoring guides — fluoride. Am. Ind. Hyg. Asso. J. 32: 274 - 279, 1971.

J. H. Speaker. Determination of fluoride by specific ion electrode and report of a fatal case of fluoride poisoning. J. For. Sci. 21: 121 - 126, 1976.

H. Spencer, D. Osis and E. Waitrowski. Retention of fluoride with time in man. Clin. Chem. 21: 613 - 618, 1975.

G. L. Waldbott. Preskeletal fluorosis near an Ohio enamel factory: a preliminary report. Vet. Hum. Tox. 21: 4-8, 1979.

Plasma and Urine Fluoride by Ion-Specific Potentiometry

Principle:

Plasma and urine specimens are diluted with a pH 5 buffer solution. Ionic fluoride is determined by direct ion-specific electrode potentiometry.

Reagents:

Stock solution — 100 mg/L fluoride (dissolve 221 mg NaF in one liter of water; store in a polyethylene container)

Aqueous standards — 0.05, 0.10, 0.20 and 0.40 mg/L for plasma determinations (prepare fresh); 1.0, 2.0, 4.0 and 8.0 mg/L for urine determinations (prepare fresh)

Buffer solution — dissolve 6.4 g NaCl in 1 L 0.05 mol/L pH 5.0 acetate buffer (store in a polyethylene container)

Instrumental Conditions:

Digital pH meter (Orion Research model 801) with fluoride-specific electrode (Orion Research model 94-09) and KCl reference electrode (Corning Glass Works)

Procedure:

1. Plasma: Dilute 1 mL plasma with 1 mL buffer solution.
   Urine: Dilute 1 mL urine with 9 mL buffer solution.
2. Place the electrode into the solution and allow several minutes for equilibration prior to recording the ion potential. Treat aqueous standards in the same manner as specimens.

Calculation:

Calculation is based on a standard curve which is prepared each time an analysis is performed. This procedure cannot be controlled by the usual methods due to the instability of dilute fluoride solutions.

Evaluation:

Sensitivity: 0.04 mg/L
Linearity: 0.04 - 10 mg/L
C.V.: 5.6% within-run
Relative recovery: average 97%

Interferences:

Fluoride contamination by chemicals, water and glassware may be minimized by using high-purity reagents and polyethylene containers. Specimen containers should be checked for contamination by adding a volume of the buffer solution to the containers, allowing equilibration for several hours and analyzing the solutions for fluoride. Total fluoride concentrations in both plasma and urine are approximately twice those of ionic fluoride which is measured by this technique; total fluoride may be determined by first treating specimens with an equal volume of 1 mol/L perchloric acid and heating at 100° C. for 15 min prior to following this procedure.

FORMALDEHYDE

Occurrence and Usage. Formaldehyde is a gas at room temperature, but is commonly used in the laboratory as a 37% aqueous solution known as formalin. As much as 15% methanol may be added to this solution to prevent polymerization of the chemical. Formaldehyde is employed in the manufacture of synthetic resins, fabrics, paper, wood products, preservatives and disinfectants. Occupational exposure is usually by inhalation of the gas or direct contact with the liquid. Significant residential exposures have occurred as a result of the release of formaldehyde fumes from synthetic foam insulation used in exterior walls. The current threshold limit value for occupational exposure is 2 ppm in air (3 mg/m^3), and the odor threshold is about 1 ppm.

Blood Concentrations. Workers exposed to formaldehyde at a concentration of 7 mg/m^3 developed blood levels of 0.6 - 4.0 mg/L (Piotrowski, 1977).

In animals administered 35 mg/kg of formaldehyde by intravenous infusion, a blood formaldehyde concentration of about 25 mg/L was produced which declined to about 1 mg/L by one hour after the end of the infusion. About four times as much formaldehyde was found in erythrocytes as in plasma. The peak plasma concentration of formic acid, a metabolite, was 144 mg/L at the end of the infusion, and this level declined with a half-life of 1.5 hours (Malorny et al., 1965).

Metabolism and Excretion. Formaldehyde is a highly reactive substance which probably combines rapidly with cellular constituents in all exposed tissues, including the mucous membranes of the respiratory tract. It is known to be oxidized to formic acid in erythrocytes and in the liver, and this metabolite is further oxidized to carbon dioxide and water (Malorny et al., 1965). A portion of the formic acid which is produced by metabolism of formaldehyde is excreted in urine. Formic acid is also an endogenous substance, being formed by the degradation of glycine, and its concentration in the urine of normal unexposed subjects averages 17 mg/L (Triebig et al., 1978).

Toxicity. Formaldehyde vapor causes mild irritation of the mucous membranes of the eyes and respiratory passages at a level of 2 - 3 ppm, while levels of 10 - 20 ppm result in moderate to severe irritation after only a few minutes. Lacrimation, cough, inflammation of the bronchi, pulmonary edema and death have resulted from exposure to very high concentrations of the chemical. Direct contact with formalin may produce dermatitis, with sensitization occurring in some persons upon repeated exposure.

The ingestion of formalin has caused several deaths, preceded by severe corrosive damage to the stomach and small intestine, circulatory collapse and kidney damage (Gosselin et al., 1976).

Biological Monitoring. Concentrations of formaldehyde in blood and urine have been used to monitor worker exposure to the chemical in preliminary investigations (Piotrowski, 1977). A more promising indicator is the level of formic acid in urine, which has not as yet been correlated with the extent of formaldehyde exposure in man, but which has been proposed as a routine monitoring technique. Pre-exposure specimens would need to be analyzed to assess the contribution of endogenous formic acid to the total value (Triebig et al., 1978).

Analysis. Formic acid may be measured in urine by flame-ionization gas chromatography of the benzyl derivative (Triebig et al., 1978). This procedure is relatively simple to perform but has the disadvantage of requiring the synthesis of the derivatization reagent.

References

R. E. Gosselin, H. C. Hodge, R. P. Smith and M. N. Gleason, *Clinical Toxicology of Commercial Products,* 4th ed., Williams and Wilkins, Baltimore, 1976, pp. 166 - 168 (Section III).

G. Malorny, N. Rietbrock and M. Schneider. Die Oxydation des Formaldehyds zu Ameisensäure im Blut, ein Beitrag zum Stoffwechsel des Formaldehyds. Naunyn-Schmiedebergs Arch. Exp. Path. Pharm. 250: 419 - 436, 1965.

J. K. Piotrowski. *Exposure Tests for Organic Compounds in Industrial Toxicology,* U.S. Government Printing Office, Washington, D.C., 1977, p. 122.

G. Triebig, K. H. Schaller and K. Gobler. Eine einfache und zuverlässige gas-chromatographische Bestimmung von Ameisensäure im Urin. Fresenius Z. Anal. Chem. 290: 114, 1978.

Urine Formic Acid by Gas Chromatography

Principle:

Formic acid and an internal standard, propionic acid, are extracted from acidified urine into ethyl acetate. The compounds are esterified with phenyldiazomethane reagent and analyzed as the benzyl esters by flame-ionization gas chromatography.

Reagents:

Stock solution — 1 mg/mL formic acid in water
Aqueous standards — 10, 20, 50 and 100 mg/L
Internal standard — 1 mg/mL propionic acid in water
1 mol/L Hydrochloric acid
Ethyl acetate
Derivatization reagent — ethereal phenyldiazomethane prepared as follows:

Preparation of p-tosylbenzylamide

Dissolve 20 g benzylamine in dry pyridine and cautiously and slowly add 40 g p-toluenesulfonyl chloride with constant stirring. Let the hot, red mixture stand for 1 hour and then pour into cool water. Collect the oily precipitate and recrystallize from alcohol (yield, 94%; m.p. 114° C.).

Preparation of p-tosyl-N-nitrosobenzylamide

Mix together 26.1 g p-tosylbenzylamide with 200 mL acetic anhydride and 300 mL glacial acetic acid, stirring for a period of 3 hours at 5° C.; add slowly over this period of time 25 g of sodium nitrite. Place the green reaction mixture into a cold room overnight and then pour into a liter of cold water. Filter the colorless crystalline solid and dry in a vacuum dessicator (yield, 97%, m.p. 87 - 89° C.).

Preparation of phenyldiazomethane

Suspend 14.5 g p-tosyl-N-nitrosobenzylamide in 100 mL ether and, after cooling in ice-water, add with stirring a solution of 2.25 g KOH in 30 mL methanol. After 5 minutes of stirring, allow the solution to stand in a cold room for 30 minutes. Shake the red solution five times with an equal volume of ice-cold water in a separatory funnel, discarding the water layer each time. Add several grams of anhydrous sodium sulfate to the ether layer and gently shake. Filter the solution into a 100 mL glass-stoppered graduated cylinder and make up to volume with ether (yield 38%; stable for one month at −20° C.).

Instrumental Conditions:

Gas chromatograph with flame-ionization detector

1.6 m x 2 mm i.d. glass column containing 10% Carbowax 20M on 80/100 mesh Chromosorb P

Injector, 250° C.; column, 190° C.; detector 250° C.

Nitrogen flow rate, 30 mL/min

Procedure:

1. Transfer 5 mL urine to a 15 mL screw-cap tube. Add 100 μL internal standard and 1 mL 1 mol/L HCl and vortex.
2. Extract with 2 mL ethyl acetate by shaking vigorously. Centrifuge to separate layers and transfer 1 mL of the upper organic layer to a 5 mL glass-stoppered conical centrifuge tube.
3. Add 0.2 mL derivatization reagent to the extract, stopper and let stand for 20 hours at room temperature. Inject 1 μL of the solution into the gas chromatograph.

	Retention time (min)
formic acid derivative	6.1
acetic acid derivative	6.8
internal standard derivative	8.4

Calculation:

Calculation is based on a response factor derived from a standard curve. A quality control specimen containng 20 mg/L formic acid is analyzed daily.

Evaluation:

Sensitivity: 10 mg/L
Linearity: 10 - 100 mg/L
C.V.: 4.9%
Relative recovery: 80 - 113%

Interferences:

Normal urine contains an average 17 mg/L formic acid. Formic acid is a metabolite of methanol, formic acid esters and certain halogenated methane derivatives, as well as formaldehyde. Normal urine constituents do not interfere with the assay.

HEXACHLOROBENZENE

Occurrence and Usage. Hexachlorobenzene (HCB) is used as a fungicide for the control of smut diseases in cereal grains, primarily seed wheat. The chemical is an aromatic benzene derivative, and is not to be confused with benzene hexachloride (lindane, hexachlorocyclohexane), which is actually a cyclohexane derivative. Occupational exposure to HCB occurs during manufacturing, application and transport of chemical wastes. Environmental exposure occurs as a result of dietary intake of contaminated food or water; at one time the feeding of HCB-treated seed grain to livestock or its incorporation into bread was a common practice in certain areas of the world. HCB has no assigned threshold limit value.

Blood Concentrations. Hexachlorobenzene concentrations in the whole blood of German children were found to range from 2.6 - 78 μg/L in 1975 (Richter and Schmid, 1976). In New Zealand adults with no known occupational exposure, these values ranged from 0 - 95 μg/L and averaged 22 μg/L, whereas a group of occupationally exposed but asymptomatic subjects showed whole blood values of 0 - 410 μg/L with an average of 56 μg/L (Siyali, 1972). Some otherwise unexposed U.S. citizens living near a chemical factory had background plasma HCB concentrations of 0 - 1.8 μg/L (average 0.5) (Burns and Miller, 1975), while a group of vegetable spraymen using an HCB-contaminated herbicide developed plasma HCB levels which averaged 40 μg/L and which ranged from 0 - 310 μg/L (Burns et al., 1974).

Metabolism and Excretion. Very little information regarding the disposition of HCB in humans is available. It is known to be stored in body fat, and has been found in amounts from a trace to 8.2 mg/kg (average 1.3) in the fat of residents of Australia, where the feeding of HCB-contaminated grain to livestock was once practiced (Brady and Siyali, 1972). The half-life of HCB in adipose tissue of sheep is approximately 16 weeks (Avrahami, 1972).

Toxicity. Several episodes of mass poisoning have occurred due to the chronic ingestion of HCB-contaminated food, with an estimated daily intake of 50 - 200 mg of the compound continuing for some months before the onset of symptoms. The primary toxic effect is cutaneous porphyria, involving blistering and epidermolysis of the face and hands (De Matteis et al., 1961; Schmid, 1960).

Biological Monitoring. The measurement of hexachlorobenzene in specimens of whole blood, plasma or biopsy fat should provide a useful index to the body burden and thus the extent of exposure to the chemical in workers. It has been suggested that whole blood HCB levels in the range of 50 - 100 μg/L represent excessive recent exposure, beyond that normally encountered environmentally (Siyali, 1972).

Analysis. Hexachlorobenzene may be determined in biological specimens by the general procedure for chlorinated hydrocarbon pesticides presented in the section on aldrin (p. 16). HCB elutes in this electron-capture gas chromatographic assay at about the same retention time as α-BHC, which has not been detected in blood specimens and is only infrequently encountered in fat.

References

M. Avrahami. Hexachlorobenzene. New Zealand J. Agr. Res. 15: 476 - 481, 1972.

M. N. Brady and D. S. Siyali. Hexachlorobenzene in human body fat. Med. J. Aust. 1: 158 - 161, 1972.

J. E. Burns, F. M. Miller, E. D. Gomes and R. A. Albert. Hexachlorobenzene exposure from contaminated DCPA in vegetable spraymen. Arch. Env. Health 29: 192 - 194, 1974.

J. E. Burns and F. M. Miller. Hexachlorobenzene contamination: its effects in a Louisiana population. Arch. Env. Health 30: 44 - 48, 1975.

F. De Matteis, B. E. Prior and C. Rimington. Nervous and biochemical disturbances following hexachlorobenzene intoxication. Nature 191: 363 - 366, 1961.

E. Richter and A. Schmid. Hexachlorbenzolgehalt im Vollblut von Kindern. Arch. Tox. 35: 141 - 147, 1976.

D. S. Siyali. Hexachlorobenzene and other organochloride pesticides in human blood. Med. J. Aust. 2: 1063 - 1066, 1972.

R. Schmid. Cutaneous porphyria in Turkey. New Eng. J. Med. 263: 397 - 398, 1960.

HEXACHLOROPHENE

Occurrence and Usage. Hexachlorophene (hexachlorophane) is an antibacterial agent which was first synthesized in 1939 and which has been used extensively in various commercial hygienic products. It has been found in concentrations of up to 0.2% in cosmetics, up to 0.5% in mouthwashes and up to 3% in soaps and antiseptic solutions. Many of these products have recently been withdrawn from the U.S. market due to accumulation of the agent in users. Hexachlorophene does not have an assigned threshold limit value. Occupational exposure may be via dermal absorption, inhalation or ingestion.

Blood Concentrations. Blood concentrations of hexachlorophene in fifty infants averaged 0.022 mg/L (range 0.003 - 0.182) at birth and 0.109 mg/L (range 0.009 - 0.646) upon discharge from the hospital, after 1 - 11 days of daily washing with diluted 3% hexachlorophene solution. The baseline blood levels of hexachlorophene in normal adults averaged 0.028 mg/L (range 0 - 0.089) (Curley et al., 1971). Adults who used a mouthwash containing 0.5% hexachlorophene once daily for 3 weeks developed blood concentrations which averaged 0.06 mg/L; those who performed whole-body washing once daily for 3 - 6 weeks with a 3% soap attained concentrations which averaged 0.24 mg/L (range 0.10 - 0.38) (Ulsamer et al., 1973). Other workers have reported mean blood values as high as 0.655 mg/L after similar whole body washing by adults (Calesnick et al., 1975).

Metabolism and Excretion. The disposition of hexachlorophene in man has not been studied. A brief report indicated that up to 10% of a single oral 20 mg/kg dose is eliminated in the urine over a 4 - 5 day period (Chung et al., 1963). Concentrations of the chemical in human milk have been found to range from trace amounts to 0.009 mg/L (West et al., 1975) and in adult adipose tissue, from 0.00 - 0.05 mg/kg (Ulsamer et al., 1973).

Toxicity. Repeated exposure of newborns to high concentrations of hexachlorophene is associated with vacuolar encephalopathy of the brainstem reticular formation (Shuman et al., 1974). Premature infants and patients with burned or abraded skin are most sensitive to dermal use of the compound. A 10-year old boy with first and second degree burns was given multiple daily baths with hexachlorophene for 2 weeks and developed seizures, irrational behavior and coma; he died after attaining a blood concentration of 2.2 mg/L (Plueckhahn, 1973). Levels of 24 - 74 mg/L have been observed in the serum of 5 adult burn patients whose wounds were washed with 3% hexachlorophene; 3 of these patients exhibited symptoms of toxicity such as diplopia, irritability, vomiting and seizures, and 2 were asymptomatic (Larson, 1968). A number of fatalities have occurred after accidental ingestion of this chemical, with a blood hexachlorophene concentration of 35 mg/L being observed in one adult at autopsy; two infants who survived the ingestion of large amounts of the chemical developed maximal plasma concentrations of 40 and 88 mg/L (Boehm and Czaja, 1979; DiMaio et al., 1973; Herskowitz and Rosman, 1979; Lustig, 1963; Pilapil, 1966; Wear et al., 1962). The acutely lethal dose in humans has been estimated at 250 mg/kg (17.5 g/70 kg) (Kimbrough, 1971).

An increased incidence of congenital malformations has been observed in neonates born to mothers who used hexachlorophene-containing soaps (Halling, 1979).

Biological Monitoring. Whole blood hexachlorophene concentrations in workers exposed to hexachlorophene which exceed a baseline level of 0.03 - 0.08 mg/L are indicative of excessive absorption of the chemical. Women of child-bearing age should be especially protected from exposure due to the known teratogenic effects of hexachlorophene.

Analysis. Hexachlorophene may be analyzed in blood or plasma by electron-capture gas chromatography of an acetyl derivative (Calesnick et al., 1975; Dodson et al., 1977).

References

R. M. Boehm, Jr. and P. A. Czaja. Hexachlorophene poisoning and the ineffectiveness of peritoneal dialysis. Clin. Tox. 14: 257 - 262, 1979.

B. Calesnick, C. H. Costello, J. P. Ryan and C. G. DiGregorio. Percutaneous absorption of hexachlorophene following daily whole body washings. Tox. Appl. Pharm. 32: 204 - 211, 1975.

H. Chung, W. Ts'ao, H. Hsü et al. Hexachlorophene (G-11) as a new specific drug against Clonorchiasis sinensis. Chin. Med. J. 82: 691 - 701, 1963.

A. Curley, R. E. Hawk, R. D. Kimbrough et al. Dermal absorption of hexachlorophene in infants. Lancet 2: 296 - 297, 1971.

V. J. M. DiMaio, F. G. Mullick and L. D. Henry. Hexachlorophene poisoning. J. For. Sci. 18: 303 - 308, 1973.

W. E. Dodson, E. E. Tyrala and R. E. Hillman. Micromethod for measuring hexachlorophene in whole blood by gas-liquid chromatography. Clin. Chem. 23: 944 - 947, 1977.

H. Halling. Suspected link between exposure to hexachlorophene and malformed infants. Ann. N.Y. Acad. Sci. 320: 426 - 435, 1979.

J. Herskowitz and N. P. Rosman. Acute hexachlorophene poisoning by mouth in neonate. J. Pediat. 94: 495 - 496, 1979.

R. D. Kimbrough. Review of the toxicity of hexachlorophene. Arch. Env. Health 23: 119 - 122, 1971.

D. L. Larson. Studies show hexachlorophene causes burn syndrome. Hospitals 42 (Dec.): 63-64, 1968.

F. W. Lustig. A fatal case of hexachlorophane ("pHisoHex") poisoning. Med. J. Aust. 1: 737, 1963.

V. R. Pilapil. Hexachlorophene toxicity in an infant. Am. J. Dis. Child. 111: 333 - 336, 1966.

V. D. Plueckhahn. Infant antiseptic skin care and hexachlorophene. Med. J. Aust. 1: 93 - 100, 1973.

R. M. Shuman, R. W. Leech and E. C. Alvord, Jr. Neurotoxicity of hexachlorophene in the human: I. A clinicopathologic study of 248 children. Pediat. 54: 689 - 695, 1974.

A. G. Ulsamer, F. N. Marzulli and R. W. Coen. Hexachlorophene concentrations in blood associated with the use of products containing hexachlorophene. Food Cos. Tox. 11: 625 - 633, 1973.

J. B. Wear, Jr., R. Shanahan and R. K. Ratliff. Toxicity of ingested hexachlorophene. J. Am. Med. Asso. 181: 587 - 589, 1962.

R. W. West, D. J. Wilson and W. Schaffner. Hexachlorophene concentrations in human milk. Bull. Env. Cont. Tox. 13: 167 - 169, 1975.

Blood Hexachlorophene by Electron-Capture Gas Chromatography

Principle:

Hexachlorophene and an internal standard are extracted from blood with an organic solvent and derivatized with acetic anhydride. The acetyl esters are analyzed by electron-capture gas chromatography.

Reagents:

Stock solution — 1 mg/mL hexachlorophene in methanol
Blood standards — 0.05, 0.10, 0.20 and 0.50 mg/L
Internal standard — 4 mg/L dichlorophene (Aldrich Chemical Co.) in methanol
Extraction solvent — ether/ethanol, 3:1 by volume
Hexane
Derivatization mixture — acetic anhydride/pyridine, 1:1 by volume

Instrumental Conditions:

Gas chromatograph with electron-capture detector
0.5 m x 2 mm i.d. glass column containing 3% OV-225 on 80/100 mesh Supelcoport
Injector, 275° C.; column, 235° C.; detector, 300° C.
Nitrogen flow rate, 35 mL/min

Procedure:

1. Transfer 2 mL blood to a 15 mL screw-cap tube. Add 100 μL internal standard and 2 mL water and vortex.
2. Add 10 mL extraction solvent and shake for 3 min. Centrifuge and transfer the upper solvent layer to a 15 mL centrifuge tube.
3. Evaporate the solvent to dryness under a stream of air at 40° C.
4. Add 200 μL hexane and 30 μL derivatization mixture to the residue and heat for 10 min at 60° C.
5. Adjust the volume to approximately 300 μL with hexane, vortex and inject 3 μL into the gas chromatograph.

	Retention time (min)
internal standard	1.8
hexachlorophene diacetate	4.0

Calculation:

Calculation is based on a response factor derived from a standard curve. A quality control specimen containing 0.10 mg/L hexachlorophene is analyzed daily.

Evaluation:

Sensitivity: 0.010 mg/L
Linearity: 0.05 - 0.50 mg/L
C.V.: not established
Relative recovery: not established

Interferences:

Blood from unexposed subjects was shown to be free of interfering substances. Other drugs and chemicals have not been studied for possible interference.

HYDROGEN SULFIDE

Occurrence and Usage. Although organic and inorganic sulfide compounds have many industrial applications, the most common source of sulfide in episodes of human poisoning is gaseous hydrogen sulfide, a product of organic decomposition. The gas is easily detected by its offensive odor in concentrations as low as 0.03 ppm, but in higher concentrations (150 ppm) it produces paralysis of the olfactory nerves and is therefore dangerous. Hydrogen sulfide is similar to hydrogen cyanide in both its acute effects and its apparent lack of chronic toxicity. The current threshold limit value for hydrogen sulfide in industry is 10 ppm (15 mg/m^3).

Blood Concentrations. Inorganic sulfide is not normally present in biological fluids *in vivo* in significant quantities. The sulfide concentration of whole blood from normal subjects is less than 0.05 mg/L (McAnalley et al., 1979).

Metabolism and Excretion. Exogenous sulfide is partially oxidized both by hemoglobin and by liver enzymes to thiosulfate; a portion may also be excreted unchanged by the lungs as hydrogen sulfide (Sörbo, 1960; Evans, 1967). A small but distinct fraction of normal blood exists as sulfhemoglobin, due to the metabolism of endogenous sulfur, but sulfhemoglobin is not produced during acute exposure to hydrogen sulfide (Adelson and Sunshine, 1966).

Toxicity. Sulfide is thought to produce its systemic toxicity by inhibition of cytochrome oxidase, as with cyanide. Air concentrations of hydrogen sulfide of up to 200 ppm cause primarily local tissue irritation, while concentrations of 1000 - 2000 ppm may result in rapid death. Experimental evidence indicates that methemoglobin induction by nitrite administration protects against sulfide poisoning by complexing hydrosulfide as inactive sulfmethemoglobin (Smith et al., 1976). Numerous instances of acute intoxication have been reported, with many fatalities known to have occurred (Freireich, 1946; Breysse, 1961; Milby, 1962; Kleinfeld et al., 1964; Adelson and Sunshine, 1966; Poda, 1966; Thoman, 1969; Simson and Simpson, 1971; Stine et al., 1976). Following the accidental fatal exposure of 6 workers to hydrogen sulfide in industrial situations, postmortem blood sulfide concentrations of 0.9 - 3.8 mg/L (average 2.4) were observed (Winek et al., 1968; McAnalley et al., 1979).

Biological Monitoring. Whole blood sulfide concentrations should not exceed 0.05 mg/L in workers exposed to hydrogen sulfide. Determination of sulfide in blood or plasma is the only known chemical means of confirming exposure to hydrogen sulfide. Due to the acute nature of most hydrogen sulfide incidents, this test will be used primarily in the diagnosis of intoxication.

Analysis. Sulfide may be demonstrated in biological specimens by microdiffusion isolation and ion-specific potentiometric determination (McAnalley et al.,

1979). Several investigators have stressed the need for promptness in analyzing specimens, due to the rapid loss of sulfide from biological materials.

References

L. Adelson and I. Sunshine. Fatal hydrogen sulfide intoxication. Arch. Path. 81: 375 - 380, 1966.

P. A. Breysse. Hydrogen sulfide fatality in a poultry feather fertilizer plant. Am. Ind. Hyg. Asso. J. 22: 220 - 222, 1961.

C. L. Evans. The toxicity of hydrogen sulphide and other sulphides. Quart. J. Exp. Physiol. 52: 231 - 248, 1967.

A. W. Freireich. Hydrogen sulfide poisoning. Report of two cases, one with fatal outcome, from associated mechanical asphyxia. Am. J. Path. 22: 147 - 150, 1946.

M. Kleinfeld, C. Giel and A. Rosso. Acute hydrogen sulfide intoxication; an unusual source of exposure. Ind. Med. Surg. 33: 656 - 660, 1964.

B. H. McAnalley, W. T. Lowry, R. D. Oliver and J. C. Garriott. Determination of inorganic sulfide and cyanide in blood using specific ion electrodes: application to the investigation of hydrogen sulfide and cyanide poisoning. J. Anal. Tox. 3: 111 - 114, 1979.

T. H. Milby. Hydrogen sulfide intoxication. J. Occ. Med. 4: 431 - 437, 1962.

G. A. Poda. Hydrogen sulfide can be handled safely. Arch. Env. Health 12: 795 - 800, 1966.

R. E. Simson and G. R. Simpson. Fatal hydrogen sulphide poisoning associated with industrial waste exposure. Med. J. Aust. 1: 331 - 334, 1971.

R. P. Smith, R. Kruszyna and H. Kruszyna. Management of acute sulfide poisoning. Arch. Env. Health 22: 166 - 169, 1976.

B. Sörbo. On the mechanism of sulfide oxidation in biological systems. Biochim. Biophys. Acta 38: 349 - 351, 1960.

R. J. Stine, B. Slosberg and B. E. Beacham. Hydrogen sulfide intoxication. Ann. Int. Med. 85: 756 - 758, 1976.

M. Thoman. Sewer gas: hydrogen sulfide intoxication. Clin. Tox. 2: 383 - 386, 1969.

C. L. Winek, W. D. Collom and C. H. Wecht. Death from hydrogen-sulphide fumes. Lancet 1: 1096, 1968.

Blood Sulfide by Ion-Specific Potentiometry

Principle:

Sulfide is isolated from blood by microdiffusion according to the previous procedure. The concentration of the ion is determined by direct potentiometric measurement with a cyanide-specific electrode.

Reagents:

Stock solution — 1 mg/mL sulfide ion in water
Blood standards — 0.1, 0.5 and 1.0 mg/L (prepare fresh)
0.5 mol/L Sulfuric acid
0.1 mol/L Sodium hydroxide
10% Lead acetate solution — 1 g $Pb(C_2H_3O_2)_2$ in 10 mL 0.1 mol/L NaOH

Instrumental Conditions:

pH Meter equipped with cyanide-specific electrode (Orion Research)

Procedure:

1. Process the blood specimen by Conway microdiffusion according to the previous procedure.
2. Stabilize the cyanide electrode by placing in 0.1 mol/L NaOH for 30 minutes or until a constant voltage reading is attained.
3. Determine the electrode response to the NaOH solution from the center well of the Conway cell and compare it to blood standards and a negative control blood processed in the same manner.
4. Add 1 drop 10% lead acetate solution to each NaOH solution after recording the initial reading. A significant change in electrode potential is confirmation of the presence of sulfide in the solution. An initial positive reading which is unaffected by lead acetate addition is indicative of the presence of cyanide.

Calculation:

Calculation is based on a standard curve prepared each time an assay is performed. This procedure cannot be controlled by the usual methods due to the instability of sulfide in biological fluids.

Evaluation:

Sensitivity: 0.01 mg/L
Linearity: 0.1 - 1.0 mg/L
C.V.: not established
Relative recovery: not established

Interferences:

Although cyanide is known to interfere in this procedure, the addition of lead acetate to the final solution will determine its presence or absence. Although fresh whole blood contains less than 0.05 mg/L inorganic sulfide, decomposed specimens may contain up to 0.4 mg/L of the ion.

ISOPROPANOL

Occurrence and Usage. Isopropanol (isopropyl alcohol) is a common industrial and laboratory chemical which is also readily available to the public in a 70% aqueous solution for use as rubbing alcohol. It has about twice the central nervous system depressant potency of ethanol, but is less toxic than methanol. The current threshold limit value in industrial situations is 400 ppm (980 mg/m^3) and the estimated anesthetic concentration is 10,000 ppm. Exposure is by both inhalation and dermal absorption.

Blood Concentrations. Isopropanol has not been measured in the blood of subjects exposed to the chemical under controlled industrial conditions. After a sponge bath with isopropanol, one adult subject was noted to have a blood isopropanol level of 100 mg/L (Wise, 1969).

Metabolism and Excretion. Isopropanol is slowly metabolized in man, probably by alcohol dehydrogenase, to acetone, which contributes to the depressant effects of the alcohol. Both compounds are eliminated to a small degree in the breath and urine, and acetone is probably further metabolized to acetate, formate and carbon dioxide (Kemal, 1927).

Toxicity. Exposure to isopropanol at air concentrations of 400 - 800 ppm produces primarily irritation of the eyes, nose and throat. Higher concentrations may cause nausea, headache, dizziness and coma. Chronic toxicity from isopropanol has not been reported.

An acute lethal dose of isopropanol by ingestion has been estimated at 240 mL for an adult. Several poisoning episodes in children have been reported following excessive use of the alcohol for sponging; blood isopropanol concentrations of 400, 1280 and 1300 mg/L were noted in 3 comatose children (Garrison, 1953; Senz and Goldfarb, 1958; McFadden and Haddow, 1969). Each of these children survived the intoxication, which probably resulted from inhalation of the alcohol vapors. Hemodialysis has been used successfully in the treatment of 2 comatose adults who each ingested about 1 liter of 70% isopropanol. In the first case, blood concentrations were initially 3460 and 1170 mg/L of isopropanol and acetone, respectively, and were 600 and 1500 mg/L, respectively, when the patient awoke. Urine concentrations of isopropanol and acetone over the 2 day period of observation were 7 - 9% higher than the respective blood concentrations (Freireich et al., 1967). In the second case, the blood concentrations of isopropanol and acetone when hemodialysis was begun were 4400 and 400 mg/L, respectively, and converged to 1000 mg/L for each substance when the subject revived, after 5 hours of dialysis (King et al., 1970).

Adelson (1962) has presented clinical and laboratory data in 5 cases of fatal isopropanol intoxication; the victims, all adults, died within 3.5 hours to 15 days of ingesting an estimated 1 pint of 70% isopropanol in most cases. Two men who died within 6 hours of ingestion were both found to have blood isopropanol concentrations of 1500 mg/L at autopsy. The tissues of the persons who survived for longer periods were observed to contain only acetone.

Biological Monitoring. Exposure to isopropanol may be monitored by determination of isopropanol or acetone in blood or urine. While the relationship between these concentrations and environmental isopropanol levels has not been established, blood or urine levels of 100 mg/L for isopropanol and acetone may be proposed as the upper limit for acceptable exposure based on the known toxicity of the two substances.

Analysis. Isopropanol and its metabolite acetone are easily determined in body fluids using the gas chromatographic technique described in the section on acetone (p. 9).

References

L. Adelson. Fatal intoxication with isopropyl alcohol (rubbing alcohol). Am. J. Clin. Path. 38: 144-151, 1962.

R. H. Cravey. Personal communication, 1978.

A. W. Freireich, T. J. Cinque, G. Xanthaky and D. Landau. Hemodialysis for isopropanol poisoning. New Eng. J. Med. 277: 699-700, 1967.

R. F. Garrison. Acute poisoning from use of isopropanol alcohol in tepid sponging. J. Am. Med. Asso. 152: 317-318, 1953.

H. Kemal. Beitrag zur Kenntnis der Schicksale des Isopropylalkohols in menschlichen Organismus. Biochem. Z. 187: 461-466, 1927.

L. H. King, Jr., K. P. Bradley and D. L. Shires, Jr. Hemodialysis for isopropyl alcohol poisoning. J. Am. Med. Asso. 211: 1855, 1970.

S. W. McFadden and J. E. Haddow. Coma produced by topical application of isopropanol. Pediat. 43: 622-623, 1969.

E. H. Senz and D. L. Goldfarb. Coma in a child following use of isopropyl alcohol in sponging. J. Pediat. 53: 322-323, 1958.

J. R. Wise, Jr. Alcohol sponge baths. New Eng. J. Med. 280: 840, 1969.

LEAD

Occurrence and Usage. Lead and inorganic lead compounds are found in a variety of commercial products and industrial materials, including paints, plastics, storage batteries, bearing alloys, insecticides and ceramics. Tetraethyllead is a volatile organic liquid which is covered in a separate section. The average urban adult inhales 20 - 40 μg of inorganic lead daily as atmospheric pollution primarily from automobile exhaust, retaining 30 - 45%, and ingests about 300 μg in the diet, absorbing only 5 - 10%. The threshold limit value for inorganic lead fumes and dusts in industrial situations is 0.15 mg/m^3.

Blood Concentrations. Blood lead concentrations in healthy children gradually increase from a mean of 0.03 mg/L in those less than 1 year old to an average of 0.11 mg/L in 5 year olds (Haas et al., 1972). In healthy suburban adults, a range of 0.07 - 0.22 mg/L was observed for blood lead, 7 - 14% of which was derived from atmospheric sources (Manton, 1977). A group of 50 London taxi drivers was found to have a mean blood lead level of 0.29 mg/L, with a range of 0.16 - 0.49 mg/L (Jones et al., 1972). Generally, 0.40 mg/L is considered the normal upper limit for blood lead, 96% of which is contained within erythrocytes. Lead workers exposed at the current TLV may be expected to develop blood lead concentrations averaging 0.60 mg/L (Williams et al., 1969).

Metabolism and Excretion. Humans are in a state of positive lead balance from the day of birth, such that a slow accumulation occurs until a total body burden of 50 - 350 mg of lead exists by age 60. Over 90% of absorbed lead is deposited in bone, primarily in dense bone, with only minor amounts excreted in hair, nails or urine. Men have higher concentrations in nearly all tissues than women. The following tissue distribution of lead was determined in 60 urban adult males from northwestern England (Barry, 1975):

Lead Concentrations in Normal Subjects (mg/L or mg/kg)

	Brain	Liver	Kidney	Hair	Nails	Urine
Average	0.10	1.0	0.78	6.6	4.7	0.04
(Range)	(0.02 - 0.78)	(0.18 - 3.1)	(0.15 - 1.9)	(1.0 - 20)	(0.65 - 15)	(0.01 - 0.19)

Urine lead concentrations in lead workers average 0.12 mg/L during exposure to 0.15 mg/m^3 lead in air, and 0.14 mg/L during exposure to 0.20 mg/m^3 (Williams et al., 1969).

Toxicity. Lead adversely affects many enzyme systems, but most noteworthy in regard to clinical indices of lead poisoning are the effects on heme synthesis. Many diagnostic tests are based on the abnormalities which result, including increases in erythrocyte zinc protoporphyrin, urinary coproporphyrin and urinary δ-aminolevulinic acid (ALA), and inhibition of erythrocyte ALA dehydrase. These parameters, together with blood lead determinations, are most frequently used in the assessment of lead poisoning (Beattie, 1974; Haeger-Aronsen, 1971).

The symptoms of chronic lead poisoning include gastrointestinal disturbances, anemia, insomnia, weight loss, motor weakness, muscle paralysis and nephropathy. Current sources of exposure to toxic quantities of lead include paint and plumbing in older houses, industrial processes, glazed ceramic vessels, and, rarely, the intentional self-administration of organic or inorganic lead compounds. Chelation therapy with BAL, EDTA or penicillamine, or a combination of these, is usually indicated when the blood lead concentration is found to exceed 0.80 mg/L; above this level, encephalopathy can develop with the possibility of permanent brain damage (Green et al., 1976).

A study of blood lead levels in children of industrially-exposed fathers revealed that 42% were in excess of 0.30 mg/L and 11% exceeded 0.80 mg/L, a result of lead dust carried home on clothing (Baker et al., 1977). Three young children who died of lead poisoning had histories of pica and blood lead concentrations of 1.11 - 3.50 mg/L (Alexander and Delves, 1972). Three persons have been reported poisoned following treatment with Chinese herbal pills, which may contain up to 7.5 mg of lead per dosage unit: a 4 year old child died 7 days after treatment by an herbalist, with lead concentrations of 3 mg/kg in brain and 17 mg/kg in liver (Leung, 1975); a 4 month old child developed a blood lead concentration of 1.37 mg/L and became comatose, but survived with treatment (Chan et al., 1977); and a 59 year old woman with joint pain, insomnia and irritability was found to have a blood lead level of 0.90 mg/L (Kalman, 1977). Several instructors exposed to lead fumes at an indoor pistol range who complained of abdominal pain were found to have blood lead concentrations of 1.09 - 1.39 mg/L (Landrigan et al., 1975).

Although acute lead poisoning is a rare event, death may occur in 1 - 2 days after the ingestion of 10 - 30 g of a lead salt by an adult; one woman survived the ingestion of 7 g of lead acetate after achieving a blood lead level of 2.28 mg/L (Karpatkin, 1961).

Biological Monitoring. There exist numerous tests for the determination of the body burden of lead or of its biologic effect in exposed individuals. For the purposes of monitoring occupationally exposed subjects, Lauwerys (1975) recommends the measurement of ALA in urine for its simplicity and freedom from error, as well as for the fact that the degree of excretion of ALA is related to the deleterious effects of absorbed lead and the lead burden. Urinary ALA does not exceed 4.5 mg/g creatinine in healthy subjects, and a level in excess of 15 mg/g is an indication of overexposure to lead. Williams et al. (1969) found that urine ALA levels average 14 mg/L in workers exposed to lead at an atmospheric concentration of 0.15 mg/m^3, and 18 mg/L at a concentration of 0.20 mg/m^3.

As a second choice, since it requires more sophisticated equipment and skills, lead may be assayed in whole blood. It is generally accepted that the whole blood lead concentration should not exceed 0.7 - 0.8 mg/L in exposed workers. However, the blood lead level alone may not be a sufficiently sensitive index of lead toxicity in some individuals (Joselow, 1976).

Urine lead concentrations are not considered by many authorities to be an accurate index of exposure to inorganic lead due to the slow change in the urine levels in response to an acute elevation in the body burden of lead.

Analysis. ALA in urine is conveniently measured by colorimetry after column chromatography (Davis and Andelman, 1967). Two procedures for the determination of blood lead are presented, the first involving chelation and solvent extraction of the lead followed by flame atomic absorption spectrometry (Berman et al., 1968) and the second, direct introduction of the specimen into the graphite furnace of an atomic absorption spectrometer (Fernandez, 1975). These procedures are also applicable to the determination of lead in urine.

Precautions must be taken when storing specimens for lead analysis and when preparing standards, due to the loss of lead from solutions by adsorption to containers (Unger and Green, 1977).

References

F. W. Alexander and H. T. Delves. Deaths from acute lead poisoning. Arch. Dis. Child. 47: 446-448, 1972.

E. L. Baker, Jr., D. S. Folland, T. A. Taylor et al. Lead poisoning in children of lead workers. New Eng. J. Med. 296: 260-261, 1977.

P. S. I. Barry. A comparison of concentrations of lead in human tissues. Brit. J. Ind. Med. 32: 119-139, 1975.

A. D. Beattie. Clinical and biochemical effects of lead. In *Forensic Toxicology* (B. Ballantyne, ed.), John Wright & Sons, England, 1974, pp. 121-134.

E. Berman, V. Valavanis and A. Dubin. A micromethod for determination of lead in blood. Clin. Chem. 14: 239-242, 1968.

H. Chan, Y. Yeh, G. J. Billmeier, Jr., and W. E. Evans. Lead poisoning from ingestion of Chinese herbal medicine. Clin. Tox. 10: 273-281, 1977.

J. R. Davis and S. L. Andelman. Urinary delta-aminolevulinic acid (ALA) levels in lead poisoning. Arch. Env. Health 15: 53-59, 1967.

F. J. Fernandez. Micromethod for lead determination of whole blood by atomic absorption, with use of the graphite furnace. Clin. Chem. 21: 558-561, 1975.

V. A. Green, G. W. Wise and J. Callenbach. Lead poisoning. Clin. Tox. 9: 33-51, 1976.

T. Haas, K. Mache, K. H. Schaller et al. Investigations into ecological lead levels in children. Zbl. Bakt. Hyg., I. Abt. Orig. B. 156: 353-360, 1972.

B. Haeger-Aronsen. An assessment of the laboratory tests used to monitor the exposure of lead workers. Brit. J. Ind. Med. 28: 52-58, 1971.

D. W. Jones, B. T. Commins and A. A. Cernik. Blood lead and carboxyhaemoglobin levels in London taxi drivers. Lancet 2: 302-303, 1972.

M. M. Joselow. Biological monitoring problems of blood lead levels. In *Health Effects of Occupational Lead and Arsenic Exposure* (B. W. Carnow, ed.), National Institute for Occupational Safety and Health, Cincinnati, Ohio, 1976, pp. 27-37.

S. M. Kalman. The pathophysiology of lead poisoning: a review and a case report. J. Anal. Tox. 1: 277-281, 1977.

S. Karpatkin. Lead poisoning after taking Pb acetate with suicidal intent. Arch. Env. Health 2: 679-684, 1961.

P. J. Landrigan, A. S. McKinney, L. C. Hopkins et al. Chronic lead absorption. J. Am. Med. Asso. 234: 394-397, 1975.

R. Lauwerys. Biological criteria for selected industrial toxic chemicals: a review. Scand. J. Work Env. Health 1: 139 - 172, 1975.

S. C. Leung. Personal communication, 1975.

W. I. Manton. Sources of lead in blood. Arch. Env. Health 32: 149 - 159, 1977.

B. C. Unger and V. A. Green. Blood lead analysis — lead loss to storage containers. Clin. Tox. 11: 237 - 243, 1977.

M. E. Williams, E. King and J. Walford. An investigation of lead absorption in an electric accumulator factory with the use of personal samplers. Brit. J. Ind. Med. 26: 202 - 216, 1969.

Urine δ-Aminolevulinic Acid by Colorimetry

Principle:

Urine is passed through an anion-exchange resin to remove porphobilinogen, and then through a cation-exchange column which retains ALA but allows urea to pass through. ALA is eluted with pH 4.6 acetate buffer and determined colorimetrically after reaction with acetylacetone and Ehrlich's reagent.

Reagents:

Stock solution — 0.1 mg/mL ALA in pH 4.5 1 mol/L acetate buffer (stable for 1 month at 4° C. in the dark)

Aqueous standards — 2.5, 5, 10, 20 and 50 mg/L ALA in pH 4.5 1 mol/L acetate buffer (prepare fresh)

Disposable ion-exchange columns containing AG-1 or AG-50 W resin (both required; Bio-Rad Labs, Richmond, Calif.)

pH 4.5 1 mol/L Acetate buffer — 57 mL glacial acetic acid and 136 g $NaC_2H_3O_2 \cdot 3H_2O$ in 1 liter of water

Acetylacetone

Chromogenic reagent — 3 g p-dimethylaminobenzaldehyde in 90 mL glacial acetic acid and 24 mL 70% perchloric acid; dilute to 150 mL with glacial acetic acid (prepare fresh)

Instrumental Conditions:

Visible spectrophotometer set to 553 nm

Procedure:

1. Piggyback the two ion-exchange columns such that the AG-1 resin is on top. Add 8 mL water to the columns and allow to drain.
2. Add 1 mL urine to the columns and allow to drain. Add three 8 mL portions of water and allow each to drain.
3. Remove the top column. Add 7 mL acetate buffer to the lower column and collect the eluate in a 15 mL graduated centrifuge tube.

4. Add 0.2 mL acetylacetone to the eluate and dilute to 10 mL with acetate buffer. Place the tube in a boiling water bath for 10 min and then cool to room temperature.
5. Transfer 2 mL of this solution to a clean tube and add 2 mL of the chromogenic reagent. After 15 minutes determine the optical density at 553 nm in a spectrophotometer against a reagent blank.

Calculation:

Calculation is based on a standard curve prepared each time an analysis is performed. This procedure cannot be controlled by the usual methods due to the instability of dilute ALA solutions.

Evaluation:

Sensitivity: 0.5 mg/L
Linearity: 1 - 60 mg/L
C.V.: 9%
Relative recovery: not established

Interferences:

Urine ALA is stable for one month when specimens are stored at 4° C. in the dark; if refrigeration is not possible, acidify specimens by adding 1 mL acetic acid per 100 mL. Urine of pH greater than 7 may give falsely low results by this method, and should be treated with acetic acid before analysis.

Blood Lead by Atomic Absorption Spectrometry

Principle:

Lead is extracted from hemolyzed whole blood by chelation with diethyldithiocarbamate. The chelate is partitioned into methylisobutyl ketone and assayed by flame atomic absorption spectrometry.

Reagents:

Stock solution — 1 mg/mL lead (Fisher reference standard)
Aqueous standards — 0.10, 0.20, 0.40 and 0.80 mg/L (prepare fresh)
10% Trichloroacetic acid
5% Trichloroacetic acid
Bromphenol blue solution — 0.1% bromphenol blue in 95% ethanol
2.5 mol/L Sodium hydroxide

DDC solution — 1% sodium diethyldithiocarbamate in water
MIBK — methylisobutyl ketone

All glassware used in this procedure should be soaked overnight in 50% nitric acid and rinsed in distilled-deionized water

Instrumental Conditions:

Atomic absorption spectrometer with an oxidizing air-acetylene flame
Lead hollow cathode lamp
Measure absorption at 283.3 nm

Procedure:

1. Transfer 250 μL of heparinized whole blood to a 10 x 75 mm tube containing 1 mL water. Add 1 mL 10% trichloroacetic acid, vortex and let stand 45 - 60 min.
2. Centrifuge and decant into a 13 x 100 mm tube. Wash precipitate with 1 mL 5% trichloroacetic acid containing 1 drop bromphenol blue solution, centrifuge and add supernatant to the 13 x 100 mm tube.
3. Adjust pH of supernatant to 6.5 - 7.0 with approximately 0.2 mL 2.5 mol/L NaOH.
4. Add 0.2 mL DDC solution and 1 mL MIBK and vortex for 30 seconds. Centrifuge and aspirate upper MIBK layer into the flame of the spectrometer.

Calculation:

Calculation is based on a standard curve prepared each time a specimen is analyzed. This procedure cannot be controlled by the usual methods due to the difficulty in storage of whole blood lead solutions.

Evaluation:

Sensitivity: 0.05 mg/L
Linearity: 0.10 - 3.00 mg/L
C.V.: 1.9 - 9.5%
Relative recovery: 95 - 105%

Interferences:

Glassware and reagents should be carefully checked for lead contamination by analyzing reagent blanks. Addition of anticoagulants or preservatives other than heparin to blood specimens may cause reduced recoveries. Storage of whole blood specimens beyond several days usually results in poor recovery of lead.

Blood Lead by Graphite Furnace Atomic Absorption Spectrometry

Principle:

Whole blood is diluted with a surfactant and injected directly into the graphite furnace of an atomic absorption spectrometer.

Reagents:

Stock solution — 1 mg/mL lead (Fisher reference standard)
Aqueous standards — 0.10, 0.20, 0.40 and 0.80 mg/L (prepare fresh)
Surfactant solution — 0.1% Triton X-100 in water

All glassware used in this procedure should be soaked overnight in 50% nitric acid and rinsed in distilled-deionized water.

Instrumental Conditions:

Atomic absorption spectrometer with graphite furnace and deuterium background corrector
Lead hollow cathode lamp (or electrodeless discharge lamp)
Furnace program:

dry 30 sec at 125° C.
char 40 sec at 525° C.
atomize 13 sec at 2000° C.

Nitrogen purge gas, 15 mL/min
Measure absorption at 283.3 nm

Procedure:

1. Transfer 50 μL heparinized whole blood to a 12 x 75 mm tube containing 200 μL surfactant solution. Rinse the pipet tip several times in the solution. Vortex.
2. Inject 15 μL of the solution into the graphite furnace and begin analysis program.

Calculation:

Calculation is based on a standard curve prepared each time a specimen is analyzed. This procedure cannot be controlled by the usual methods due to the difficulty in storage of whole blood lead solutions.

Evaluation:

Sensitivity: 0.05 mg/L
Linearity: 0.10 - 0.80 mg/L
C.V.: 2.4 - 4.% within run
Relative recovery: 94 - 104%

Interferences:

Glassware and reagents should be carefully checked for lead contamination by analyzing reagent blanks. Anticoagulants other than oxalate do not interfere. Storage of whole blood specimens beyond several days usually results in poor recovery of lead.

LINDANE

Occurrence and Usage. Lindane, an organochlorine insecticide, is the γ-isomer of hexachlorocyclohexane (benzene hexachloride, BHC), one of 8 such isomers isolated and the most toxic. Technical BHC contains 12 - 15% lindane, 65 - 70% α-BHC, 6 - 8% β-BHC and 2 - 5% δ-BHC. The mixture has been extensively used since 1950 for agricultural and domestic purposes (as a fumigant and for the control of body lice) but, as with other organochlorine derivatives, it has recently come under governmental restrictions due to its accumulation in soil, plants and animals. The current threshold limit value for lindane in the industrial atmosphere is 0.5 mg/m^3. Exposure may be via inhalation, dermal absorption or ingestion.

Blood Concentrations. Although lindane itself is not found in the blood or plasma of most members of the general population, blood concentrations of β-BHC in United States residents were found to average 0.0015 and 0.0031 mg/L in two separate studies (Radomski et al., 1971; Dale et al., 1966). Blood lindane concentrations in lindane plant workers averaged 0.004 mg/L (range 0.001 - 0.009) in those with low exposure and 0.031 mg/L (range 0.006 - 0.093) in those with high dermal exposure. The blood concentrations did not appear to increase with continued low-level exposure, but were primarily an index of recent exposure (Milby et al., 1968).

Metabolism and Excretion. Lindane is metabolized in man by oxidation and dehydrohalogenation to a series of chlorinated phenols which are excreted primarily in urine in both free and conjugated form (Starr and Clifford, 1972). Lindane concentrations in the urine of unexposed subjects were less than 0.001 mg/L (Cueto and Biros, 1967) and averaged 0.48 mg/kg (range 0 - 12.3) in adipose tissue obtained randomly at 994 autopsies (Hoffman et al., 1967).

Toxicity. Blood lindane concentrations exceeding 0.02 mg/L were associated with neurological abnormalities, including EEG changes, muscular jerking and emotional changes, in workers exposed to lindane (Czegledi-Janko and Avar, 1970). Chronic exposure to lindane through the use of home vaporizers has been presumptively implicated in seven fatal cases of aplastic anemia (Loge, 1965; West, 1967). Lindane which was probably absorbed dermally was responsible for a mass poisoning episode, producing weakness, mental confusion, anemia, convulsions and the death of 6 persons (Danopoulos et al., 1953).

The mean fatal dose of technical lindane in adults is believed to be 28 g. A young boy who ingested lindane developed a plasma concentration of 0.29 mg/L after 6 hours, 3 hours after the last convulsion; after 7 days the patient was asymptomatic and the plasma level had declined to 0.02 mg/L (Dale et al., 1966). A young girl who ingested 1.6 g of lindane achieved a serum concentration of 0.84 mg/L after 2 hours, just following grand mal seizures; by 4 hours the concentration decreased to 0.49 mg/L. Concentrations of individual free phenolic metabolites in urine collected 5.5 hours after ingestion ranged from 0.04 - 0.74 mg/L (Starr and Clifford, 1972). A fat concentration of 343 mg/kg was observed in a fatality due to lindane (Hayes and Vaughn, 1977).

Biological Monitoring. The blood lindane concentration has been found to be a useful index to lindane exposure and biologic effect. Levels exceeding 0.02 mg/L are associated with a high degree of mild toxicity in exposed workers. The blood concentration produced during exposure at the current TLV has not been determined.

Analysis. Lindane is measurable in body fluids and tissues using the electron-capture gas chromatographic procedure designed for organochlorine insecticides which is presented in the section on aldrin (p. 16).

References

C. Czegledi-Janko and P. Avar. Occupational exposure to lindane: clinical laboratory findings. Brit. J. Ind. Med. 27: 283 - 286, 1970.

C. Cueto, Jr. and F. J. Biros. Chlorinated insecticides and related materials in human urine. Tox. Appl. Pharm. 10: 261 - 269, 1967.

W. E. Dale, A. Curley and C. Cueto, Jr. Hexane extractable chlorinated insecticides in human blood. Life Sci. 5: 47 - 54, 1966.

E. Danopoulos, K. Mellissinos and G. Katsas. Serious poisoning by hexachlorocyclohexane. Arch. Ind. Hyg. Occ. Med. 8: 582 - 587, 1953.

W. J. Hayes, Jr. and W. K. Vaughn. Mortality from pesticides in the United States in 1973 and 1974. Tox. Appl. Pharm. 42: 235 - 252, 1977.

W. S. Hoffman, H. Adler, W. I. Fishbein and F. C. Bauer. Relation of pesticide concentrations in fat to pathological changes in tissues. Arch. Env. Health 15: 758 - 765, 1967.

J. P. Loge. Aplastic anemia following exposure to benzene hexachloride (lindane). J. Am. Med. Asso. 193: 110 - 114, 1965.

T. H. Milby, A. J. Samuels and F. Ottoboni. Human exposure to lindane: blood lindane levels as a function of exposure. J. Occ. Med. 10: 584 - 587, 1968.

J. L. Radomski, W. B. Deichmann, A. A. Rey and T. Merkin. Human pesticide blood levels as a measure of body burden and pesticide exposure. Tox. Appl Pharm. 20: 175 - 185, 1971.

H. G. Starr, Jr. and N. J. Clifford. Acute lindane intoxication. Arch. Env. Health 25: 374 - 375, 1972.

I. West. Lindane and hematologic reactions. Arch. Env. Health. 15: 97 - 101, 1967.

LITHIUM

Occurrence and Usage. Lithium hydride, which is used in metallurgy and in chemical synthesis, is the most toxic of the lithium compounds encountered industrially. Exposure is usually by inhalation; the current threshold limit value for lithium hydride in the industrial atmosphere is 0.025 mg/m^3. The metal is administered therapeutically as the carbonate salt in daily oral doses of 900 - 2400 mg for the treatment of mania and endogenous depression. The optimum maintenance dosage is often determined by monitoring the serum concentration.

Blood Concentrations. In unexposed persons, the physiological serum lithium concentration ranges from 0.0001 to 0.0003 mmol/L. Following a single oral dosage of 1500 mg of the carbonate to 3 adult subjects, an average peak plasma concentration of 1.66 mmol/L was observed at 1 hour. Plasma concentrations declined rapidly during the first 20 hours, with a half-life of 5.2 hours, and then more slowly over the next 6 days, with an elimination half-life of 17 - 24 hours (Groth et al., 1974). Optimum serum lithium concentrations for most patients have been found to range from 0.5 - 1.3 mmol/L in early morning specimens drawn 12 hours after the last dose (Amidsen, 1975). In patients receiving average daily doses of 1500 - 1700 mg of lithium carbonate, serum concentrations were in the range of 0.7 - 0.9 mmol/L (Marini and Sheard, 1976).

Metabolism and Excretion. In normal subjects lithium is excreted essentially quantitatively in the urine, an average of 97% of a single dose being eliminated within 10 days (Groth et al., 1974). Hyponatremia causes lithium retention, and conversely, the administration of large doses of sodium chloride hastens the renal excretion of the metal.

Toxicity. Lithium hydride is a severe irritant when applied to the skin or mucous membranes. The absorption of inhaled or ingested lithium, on either an acute or chronic basis, can cause symptoms of toxicity. Lithium toxicity, which results in nausea, vomiting, tremor, confusion and coma, is often manifested at serum concentrations exceeding 2 mmol/L. In one subject who ingested 60 g of lithium carbonate, a peak serum concentration of 14 mmol/L was recorded after 50 hours, when the patient was comatose; the level dropped to 5 mmol/L by 64 hours and death occurred at 92 hours (Achong et al., 1975). Another person who ingested an unknown amount of lithium carbonate was found to have a serum concentration of 6.8 mmol/L 48 hours later; death occurred after 21 days, at which time a serum lithium concentration of 0.4 mmol/L was observed (Amdisen et al., 1974).

Biological Monitoring. Serum and urine lithium concentrations have not been correlated with controlled industrial exposure to lithium. The determination of these levels is currently limited to the diagnosis of lithium toxicity.

Analysis. Lithium may be conveniently determined in serum or urine by atomic absorption spectrophotometry (Hansen, 1968).

References

M. R. Achong, P. G. Fernandez and P. J. McLeod. Fatal self-poisoning with lithium carbonate. Can. Med. Asso. J. 112: 868 - 870, 1975.

A. Amdisen. Monitoring of lithium treatment through determination of lithium concentration. Dan. Med. Bull. 22: 277 - 291, 1975.

A. Amdisen, C. G. Gottsfries, L. Jacobsson and B. Winblad. Grave lithium intoxication with fatal outcome. Acta Psych. Scand. Supp. 4: 25 - 33, 1974.

U. Groth, W. Prellwitz and E. Jahnchen. Estimation of pharmacokinetic parameters of lithium from saliva and urine. Clin. Pharm. Ther. 16: 490 - 498, 1974.

J. L. Hansen. The measurement of serum and urine lithium by atomic absorption spectrophotometry. Am. J. Med. Tech. 34: 1 - 9, 1968.

J. L. Marini and M. H. Sheard. Sustained-release lithium carbonate in a double-blind study: serum lithium levels, side effects, and placebo response. J. Clin. Pharm. 16: 276 - 283, 1976.

Serum and Urine Lithium by Atomic Absorption Spectrometry

Principle:

Serum and urine are diluted with water and directly analyzed by flame atomic absorption spectrometry.

Reagents:

Stock solution — 1 mg/mL lithium ion (Fisher reference standard)
Serum standards — 0.2, 0.5, 1.0 and 2.0 mmol/L
Urine standards — 1.0, 2.5, 5.0 and 10.0 mmol/L (in pooled urine or in water)

Instrumental Conditions:

Atomic absorption spectrometer with air-acetylene oxidizing flame and three slot burner head
Lithium hollow cathode lamp
Measure absorption at 670.8 nm

Procedure:

1. Serum: dilute 0.2 mL to 5.0 mL with water.
   Urine: dilute 0.2 ml to 25.0 mL with water.
2. Aspirate diluted specimen into flame of atomic absorption spectrometer.

Calculation:

Calculation is based on a response factor derived from a standard curve. A quality control specimen containing 1.0 mmol/L lithium (serum) or 5.0 mmol/L lithium (urine) is analyzed daily.

Evaluation:

Sensitivity: 0.1 mmol/L for serum and 0.5 mmol/L for urine
Linearity: 0.2 - 4.0 mmol/L for serum and 1 - 20 mmol/L for urine
C.V.: 5.3% within-run
Relative recovery: 89 - 112%

Interferences:

Sodium and potassium at concentrations of up to 180 and 8.0 mmol/L, respectively, did not interfere in this procedure. Clogging of the burner head by serum protein does not occur if a three slot burner head is used.

MALATHION

Occurrence and Usage. Malathion is one of the least toxic of the commercially available organophosphate insecticides, and therefore one of the safest for domestic usage. It is commonly employed as a dusting powder in concentrations of 1 - 5% and in solutions of up to 50% strength for spraying. The pure compound is an oily liquid which decomposes when heated or moistened; it is biologically degradable and so does not present an environmental threat. Occupational exposure is commonly by inhalation or dermal absorption. The current threshold limit value is 10 mg/m^3.

Blood Concentrations. Persons occupationally exposed to malathion were found to have dimethyldithiophosphate serum concentrations ranging from 0 - 3.50 mg/L, the level being directly proportional to the degree of exposure (Shafik and Enos, 1969). Subjects who were exposed to controlled amounts of 5% and 20% malathion sprays at atmospheric concentrations of 5 - 85 mg/m^3 for one hour periods over six consecutive weeks exhibited erythrocyte and plasma cholinesterase values of 90% or greater on all but a few sampling occasions (Golz, 1959). In another study, volunteers ingested 16 mg of malathion daily for 47 days without effect on plasma or erythrocyte cholinesterase activity. Doses of 24 mg, however, when administered for 56 days caused 25% depression of cholinesterase activity, with maximal effects occurring 3 weeks after cessation of administration; no toxic effects were apparent in spite of depression of both plasma and erythrocyte cholinesterase (Moeller and Rider, 1962).

Metabolism and Excretion. In man, malathion is believed to be activated by conversion to malaoxon, an oxygen analogue, with hydrolysis and inactivation of both malathion and malaoxon to dimethyldithiophosphoric acid (DMDTP) and dimethylthiophosphoric acid (DMTP), respectively. DMDTP and DMTP have been identified in the urine of exposed workers in concentrations of 0.20 - 1.86 mg/L and 0 - 0.11 mg/L, respectively, with the levels correlating to the severity of exposure (Shafik and Enos, 1969). Up to 23% of a single oral dose of malathion is excreted in the 16 hour urine as ether-extractable phosphates (Mattson and Sedlak, 1960). In animals and probably in man the compound is also detoxified by hydrolysis of either or both of its carboxyester functions (Matsumura, 1975).

Toxicity. Malathion has resulted in fewer episodes of poisoning than most other organophosphate derivatives due to its lower toxicity; the mean fatal dose in man is estimated at 60 g. However, several hundred fatalities have been reported, usually after ingestion of large amounts of the chemical (Nalin, 1973). One such case involved an adult who died 6 days after ingestion of 60 - 90 g of malathion; the following cholinesterase levels were determined at autopsy (Namba et al., 1970):

Cholinesterase Activity in a Malathion Fatality (% of normal)

Plasma	Cerebrum	Cerebellum	Muscle	Liver	Kidney
4%	32%	3%	1%	19%	13%

Cholinesterase activity was reduced to 22% and 10% of normal in the serum and erythrocytes, respectively, of a woman who survived the ingestion of 60 g of malathion due to treatment with atropine and PAM; the levels gradually returned to normal after a period of 31 days for plasma and 130 days for erythrocytes (Goldin et al., 1964). Malathion blood concentrations of 100 - 1880 mg/L (average 815) were measured by colorimetry (palladium chloride complex) after thin-layer chromatography in four instances of fatal suicidal poisoning; these involved the ingestion of 25 - 70 g of malathion and in 2 cases death occurred after 2 - 14 hours (Farago, 1967).

Biological Monitoring. Blood cholinesterase determinations are the best index for monitoring exposure to malathion and other cholinesterase inhibitors; a blood cholinesterase level which is less than 70% of the pre-exposure level is indicative of excessive exposure to malathion. The measurement of organic phosphates in urine is a useful adjunct to cholinesterase determination in malathion-exposed workers. Total urinary organic phosphate levels in excess of 0.2 mg/L represent significant exposure to organophosphate insecticides.

Analysis. A method for blood cholinesterase determination was presented in the section on carbaryl (p. 60). The phosphoric acid metabolites of malathion may be assayed in urine by the colorimetric procedure described in the section on diazinon (p. 106).

References

A. Farago. Fatal, suicidal malathion poisonings. Arch. Tox. 23: 11 - 16, 1967.

A. R. Goldin, A. H. Rubenstein, B. A. Bradlow and G. A. Elliott. Malathion poisoning with special reference to the effect of cholinesterase inhibition on erythrocyte survival. New Eng. J. Med. 271: 1289 - 1293, 1964.

H. H. Golz. Controlled human exposures to malathion aerosols. Arch. Ind. Health 19: 516-523, 1959.

F. Matsumura. *Toxicology of Insecticides*, Plenum Press, New York, 1975, pp. 224 - 226.

A. M. Mattson and V. A. Sedlak. Ether-extractable urinary phosphates in man and rats derived from malathion and similar compounds. J. Agr. Food Chem. 8: 107 - 110, 1960.

H. C. Moeller and J. A. Rider. Plasma and red blood cell cholinesterase activity as indications of the threshold of incipient toxicity of ethyl-p-nitrophenyl thionobenzenephosphonate (EPN) and malathion in human beings. Tox. Appl. Pharm. 4: 123 - 130, 1962.

D. R. Nalin. Epidemic of suicide by malathion poisoning in Guyana. Trop. Geogr. Med. 25: 8 - 14, 1973.

T. Namba, M. Greenfield and D. Grob. Malathion poisoning. A fatal case with cardiac manifestation. Arch. Env. Health 21: 533 - 541, 1970.

M. T. Shafik and H. F. Enos. Determination of metabolic and hydrolytic products of organophosphorus pesticide chemicals in human blood and urine. J. Agr. Food Chem. 17: 1186 - 1189, 1969.

MANGANESE

Occurrence and Usage. Manganese is widely used industrially in the manufacture of steel, welding rods, batteries, ceramics and refractory materials. It is also an essential trace element and is supplied in daily amounts of 3 - 7 mg by dietary intake. Occupational exposure usually occurs by inhalation or ingestion of fumes and dusts produced during the refining of manganese ores or the treatment of manganese alloys. The current threshold limit value for manganese fume is 1 mg/m^3 and for manganese and its compounds, 5 mg/m^3 (both expressed as Mn).

Blood Concentrations. Whole blood manganese, most of which is bound to hemoglobin in the erythrocytes, averages 9 $\mu g/L$ (range 3.9 - 15) in normal adults when measured by atomic absorption spectrometry. Serum manganese in normal adults averages 1.8 $\mu g/L$, ranging from 0.9 - 2.9 $\mu g/L$ (Pleban and Pearson, 1979). Other authors, using either similar techniques, colorimetry or neutron activation analysis, are in general agreement with this data (Cotzias et al., 1966; Cotzias et al., 1968; Weissman and Pileggi, 1974; Buchet et al., 1976). However, many discrepancies exist in the literature on endogenous manganese concentrations, probably as a result of methodological difficulties and problems with contamination, with some authors claiming normal blood or serum levels 5 to 40 times higher than those cited above (Nilubol et al., 1968; Mahoney et al., 1969; Jonderko et al., 1971).

Metabolism and Excretion. Most inhaled manganese is mobilized up the trachea and is swallowed. The efficiency of gastrointestinal absorption of the element is low, usually less than 10%, but is quite variable and appears to correlate inversely to the amount available for absorption (Mena et al., 1969). The absorbed manganese leaves the blood quickly and is stored in parenchymatous tissues; the half-time for excretion of manganese from the body in normal subjects is about 40 days. Elimination of injected manganese is largely via the feces, which contain from 14 - 54% of a single dose after 15 days, and to a very minor extent in urine (Mena et al., 1967; Mahoney and Small, 1968).

Urinary manganese concentrations in normal persons have been reported to range from less than 1 to 10 $\mu g/L$ (Cholak and Hubbard, 1960; Nilubol et al., 1968; Ajemian and Whitman, 1969; Weissman and Pileggi, 1974; Buchet et al., 1976). These concentrations in asymptomatic manganese workers have ranged from 25 - 124 $\mu g/L$ (Nilubol et al., 1968), although it has been found that urine concentrations do not usually exceed 8 $\mu g/L$ when occupational manganese exposure is limited to 5 mg/m^3 (Tanaka and Lieben, 1969).

Toxicity. Typical metal fume fever may develop after acute exposure to manganese oxide fumes, with symptoms of fever, muscle pains, chills and dryness of the mouth and throat. However, chronic overexposure to manganese is more frequently encountered in occupational medicine. This may require a year or more of exposure prior to the manifestation of CNS symptoms such as headache, restlessness, irritability, personality change, hallucinations and hearing impairment. Severe toxicity results in muscle weakness and rigidity, tremor and other extrapyramidal symptoms. Administration of levodopa has been successfully employed in the treatment of manganism (Hine and Pasi, 1975).

Manganese concentrations in a patient with chronic poisoning were elevated in blood (75μg/L) but normal in urine (Rosenstock et al., 1971); another patient demonstrated blood concentration of 20 μg/L and urine concentrations of 100 - 150 μg/L (Hine and Pasi, 1975). Urine manganese concentrations in other manganism patients have ranged from less than 10 μg/L to as high as 260 μg/L (Nilubol et al, 1967; Tanaka and Lieben, 1969; Smyth et al., 1973).

Biological Monitoring. The lack of agreement of literature studies on the usefulness of manganese levels in biologic specimens can be at least partially attributed to technical problems with manganese analysis, the rapid clearance of manganese from blood and the unimportance of urine as an elimination route for the element. It is possible that, using more sophisticated techniques, measurement of blood manganese will prove to be a useful tool in monitoring worker exposure. At present it is only of secondary importance in the confirmation of manganism.

On the other hand, urinary manganese concentrations in exposed workers have been found to be positively correlated with atmospheric manganese levels, although not necessarily with clinical signs of poisoning (Tanaka and Lieben, 1969). Administration of EDTA to mobilize the metal followed by determination of manganese in urine has been used to diagnose manganese intoxication.

Analysis. A procedure is presented for the analysis of manganese in urine which utilizes the method of standard additions and flameless atomic absorption spectrometry (Buchet et al., 1976).

References

R. S. Ajemian and N. E. Whitman. Determination of manganese in urine by atomic absorption spectrometry. Am. Ind. Hyg. Asso. J. 30: 52 - 56, 1969.

J. P. Buchet, R. Lauwerys and H. Roels. Determination of manganese in blood and urine by flameless atomic absorption spectrophotometry. Clin. Chim. Acta 73: 481 - 486, 1976.

J. Cholak and D. M. Hubbard. Determination of manganese in air and biological material. Am. Ind. Hyg. Asso. J. 21: 356 - 360, 1960.

G. C. Cotzias, S. T. Miller and J. Edwards. Neutron activation analysis: the stability of manganese concentrations in human blood and serum. J. Lab. Clin. Med. 67: 836 - 849, 1966.

G. C. Cotzias, P. S. Papavasiliou, E. R. Hughes et al. Slow turnover of manganese in active rheumatoid arthritis accelerated by prednisone. J. Clin. Invest. 47: 992 - 1001, 1968.

C. H. Hine and A. Pasi. Manganese intoxication. West. J. Med. 123: 101 - 107, 1975.

G. Jonderko, A. Kujawska and H. Langauer-Lewowicka. Problems of chronic manganese poisoning on the basis of investigations of workers at a manganese alloy foundry. Int. Arch. Arbeitsmed. 28: 250 - 264, 1971.

J. P. Mahoney and W. J. Small. Studies on manganese. III. The biological half-life of radiomanganese in man and factors which affect this half-life. J. Clin. Invest. 47: 643 - 653, 1968.

J. P. Mahoney, K. Sargent, M. Greland, and W. Small. Studies on manganese. I. Determination in serum by atomic absorption spectrophotometry. Clin. Chem. 15: 312 - 322, 1969.

I. Mena, O. Marin, S. Fuenzalida nd G. C. Cotzias. Chronic manganese poisoning. Clinical picture and manganese turnover. Neurology 17: 128 - 136, 1967.

I. Mena, K. Horiuchi, K. Burke and G. C. Cotzias. Chronic manganese poisoning. Individual susceptibility and absorption of iron. Neurology 19: 1000 - 1006, 1969.

M. L. A. Nilubol, K. Chayawatanangkur and S. Kritalugsana. Manganese toxication in the human body determined by activation analysis. J. Nucl. Med. 9: 178 - 180, 1968.

P. A. Pleban and K. H. Pearson. Determination of manganese in whole blood and serum. Clin. Chem. 25: 1915 - 1918, 1979.

H. A. Rosenstock. D. G. Simons and J. S. Meyer. Chronic manganism. Neurologic and laboratory studies during treatment with levodopa. J. Am. Med. Asso. 217: 1354 - 1358, 1971.

L. T. Smyth, R. C. Ruhf, N. E. Whitman and T. Dugan. Clinical manganism and exposure to manganese in the production and processing of ferromanganese alloy. J. Occ. Med. 15: 101 - 109, 1973.

S. Tanaka and J. Lieben. Manganese poisoning and exposure in Pennsylvania. Arch. Env. Health 19: 674 - 684, 1969.

N. Weissman and W. J. Pileggi. Inorganic ions. In *Clinical Chemistry, Principles and Techniques* (R. J. Henry, D. C. Cannon and J. W. Winkelman, eds.), Harper and Row, New York, 2nd ed., 1974, pp. 707 - 712.

Urine Manganese by Graphite-Furnace Atomic Absorption Spectrometry

Principle:

Manganese is extracted from urine as the cupferron chelate with methylisobutylketone. The organic extract is analyzed by atomic absorption spectrometry, utilizing the method of standard additions.

Reagents:

Stock solution — 1 mg/mL manganese ion (Fisher reference standard)
Aqueous standards — 0.5 and 1.0 mg/L (prepare fresh)
Cupferron solution — 10% cupferron in 0.1 M pH 7.1 imidazole-HCl buffer
Methylisobutylketone

Instrumental Conditions:

Atomic absorption spectrometer with graphite furnace
Manganese hollow cathode lamp
Furnace program:
- dry at 85° C. for 5 sec
- ash at 600° C. for 10 sec
- atomize at 2600° C. for 7 sec

Nitrogen purge gas on interrupt mode
Measure absorption at 279.5 nm

Procedure:

1. Adjust about 20 mL of urine to pH 7.1 ± 0.1. Transfer three 5 mL portions of this solution to separate 12 mL polyethylene tubes marked 0, 5 and 10.
2. Add 50 μL of the 0.5 mg/L standard to the tube marked 5 and 50 μL of the 1.0 mg/L standard to the tube marked 10.
3. To all tubes add 0.5 mL cupferron solution and vortex. Let stand for 10 minutes.
4. Add 2 mL methylisobutylketone to each tube, stopper and shake vigorously for 2 minutes. Centrifuge to separate layers.
5. Inject 20 μL of the organic phase into the graphite furnace and begin the temperature program.

Calculation:

Calculation is based on a standard curve of signal peak height versus concentration of the added standard (0, 5 or 10 μg/L). The negative intercept of the line drawn through the three points represents the concentration of the unknown urine specimen. This procedure cannot be controlled by the usual methods due to the instability of dilute manganese solutions.

Evaluation:

Sensitivity: 1 μg/L
Linearity: 1 - 25 μg/L
C.V.: 3 - 5%
Relative recovery: not established

Interferences:

Specimens with manganese concentrations of 25 - 50 μg/L may be determined by diluting the organic extract with additional methylisobutylketone; specimens with higher concentrations should be diluted with water prior to the analysis. Other metal ions were not found to interfere in the procedure.

MERCURY

Occurrence and Usage. Mercury is a nonessential trace element, the presence of which in human tissues represents uptake from both natural and man-made sources. Inorganic mercury released by industries into waterways can be converted to methylmercury by microflora; this lipid-soluble organic form of the element is efficiently concentrated by fish and other aquatic organisms. In the United States, a total mercury limit of 0.5 mg/kg has been established for commercial fish; mercury levels in marine fish have ranged from undetectable to 5.0 mg/kg, averaging 0.2 - 0.5 mg/kg in some species, while freshwater fish in contaminated areas have accumulated concentrations up to 40 mg/kg (80 - 90% of which is methylmercury). Organic mercury compounds are used as preservatives in paints and for agricultural purposes, and as diuretics in clinical medicine. Mercury is widely used industrially, especially in electrical components, and also in dentistry. The daily dietary intake of mercury ranges from 1 - 30 μg for most persons. The current threshold limit value for mercury and its inorganic compounds is 0.05 mg/m^3, while for alkyl mercury compounds it is 0.01 mg/m^3 (as Hg). Industrial exposure is usually by inhalation or dermal absorption.

Blood Concentrations. Total blood mercury ranges up to 0.006 mg/L in persons having low fish consumption, up to 0.050 mg/L in dieters eating moderate quantities of tunafish and up to 0.200 mg/L or higher in those consuming large amounts of predatory marine fish. About 95% of the mercury in whole blood is contained in red cells, largely as methylmercury (Clarkson, 1977). A concentration of 0.020 mg/L is considered an acceptable level of mercury in whole human blood (Panel on Mercury, 1978).

Metabolism and Excretion. Methylmercury is well absorbed from dietary sources and has a biological half-life of about 70 days in man. It is slowly converted in man, possibly by the intestinal flora, to inorganic divalent mercury at the rate of about 1% of the body burden daily. Individuals in mercury equilibrium have a body burden of approximately 100 times the daily intake, and about 1% of the daily intake is found in 1 liter of blood. Metallic mercury vapor, in contrast, is very rapidly oxidized to divalent mercury. Mercury is eliminated in all body secretions but primarily in feces after biliary excretion; urine concentrations in normal persons are nearly always less than 0.010 mg/L. Hair concentrations correlate well with blood concentrations during exposure to methylmercury, but not to mercury vapor; urine levels are the best guide to blood levels during exposure to inorganic or metallic mercury (Clarkson, 1977). In Japanese workers, urine mercury concentrations averaged 0.119 mg/L in an unexposed group and 0.403 mg/L in an asymptomatic group exposed to mercury vapor (Nakayama et al., 1977). Urine mercury levels in exposed workers may remain elevated for some years following cessation of the exposure (Goldwater et al., 1966).

Toxicity. The average lethal dose of mercury is about 100 mg for organic mercury and 1 g for inorganic mercuric salts. The organic mercury compounds can produce severe and often irreversible central nervous system toxicity in overdosage, while inorganic compounds result in primarily peripheral effects, including gastroenteritis and tubular nephritis leading to renal failure. Elemental mercury by inhalation produces central effects initially, progressing to renal toxicity after its oxidation to mercuric ion. Several mass poisonings, involving over 8000 people, have been caused by accidental ingestion of organic mercury in contaminated seafood (Minimata disease) or of mercury-treated seed grain. A daily intake of methylmercury exceeding 300 μg will produce chronic mercury poisoning in the average 70 kg adult; this level of intake is associated with steady-state concentrations of 0.200 mg/L in blood, 60 mg/kg in hair and a body burden of 20 - 30 mg of mercury (Panel on Mercury, 1978). Hair concentrations of methylmercury have ranged from 200 - 800 mg/kg during moderate intoxication (Gerstner and Huff, 1977). Postmortem blood mercury levels of 0.6 - 6.0 mg/L (average 2.6) were established in 8 victims of accidental methylmercury poisoning due to ingestion of treated seed wheat (Al-Saleem, 1976).

Poisoning from inorganic mercury has been described after both ingestion and external application of soluble mercuric salts. Urine mercury concentrations of 0.09 - 0.25 mg/L were reported in nephrotic patients who had developed chronic intoxication through the use of a skin-lightening cream (Gerstner and Huff, 1977). Postmortem blood mercury concentrations of 1.7 and 2.1 mg/L were observed in 2 adults who received peritoneal lavage with mercuric chloride during surgery and who absorbed lethal amounts of the metal (Cross et al., 1979).

Mercury concentrations in three patients, two of whom died, suffering from acute mercury vapor poisoning, were 0.4 - 0.9 mg/L in blood and 0.5 - 1.6 mg/L in urine (Jaeger et al., 1979). In five victims of chronic mercury vapor poisoning, who suffered symptoms of nervousness, lassitude, tremor, burning eyes and bleeding gums, blood mercury concentrations ranged from 0.18 - 0.62 mg/L and urine concentrations, from 2.4 - 8.3 mg/L (Sexton et al., 1978). Exposure to metallic mercury vapor has produced elevated body burdens in many dental personnel and toxicity in some (Joselow et al., 1968; Cook and Yates, 1969; Buchwald, 1972; Gutenmann et al., 1973; Battistone et al., 1977; Kelman, 1978).

Biological Monitoring. Exposure to inorganic mercury may be evaluated by determination of mercury in blood or urine. Workers exposed to the TLV of 0.05 mg/m^3 develop blood mercury levels of about 0.03 mg/L and urine levels of 0.05 - 0.10 mg/L (Smith et al., 1970; Bell et al., 1973).

Organic mercury exposure is best monitored by the measurement of total mercury (or the specific derivative) in whole blood. It has been recommended that the blood mercury level not be allowed to exceed 0.10 mg/L in workers exposed to organomercury compounds (Berlin et al., 1969).

Analysis. Extensive losses of mercury from solutions during several days' storage have been noted, and it has been suggested that acidification with nitric acid and prompt analysis be performed to reduce mercury loss (Rosain and Wai, 1973). A method based on atomic absorption spectrometry with the cold vapor technique is presented for the determination of total mercury in blood or urine (Sharma and Davis, 1979; Clarkson et al., 1977). An alternative method which is specific for methylmercury in blood relies on electron-capture gas chromatography (Von Burg et al., 1974; Cappon and Smith, 1978).

References

T. Al-Saleem. Levels of mercury and pathological changes in patients with organomercury poisoning. Bull. WHO 53 (Suppl.): 99 - 104, 1976.

G. C. Battistone, J. J. Hefferren, R. A. Miller and D. E. Cutright. Mercury as an occupational hazard in the practice of dentistry. In *Clinical Chemistry and Chemical Toxicology of Metals*, (S. S. Brown, ed.), Elsevier/North Holland, New York, 1977, pp. 205 - 208.

Z. G. Bell, Jr., H. B. Lovejoy and T. R. Vizena. Mercury exposure evaluations and their correlations with urine mercury excretions. J. Occ. Med. 15: 501 - 508, 1973.

M. H. Berlin, T. W. Clarkson, L. T. Friberg et al. Maximum allowable concentrations of mercury compounds. Arch. Env. Health 19: 891 - 905, 1969.

H. Buchwald. Exposure of dental workers to mercury. Am. Ind. Hyg. Asso. J. 33: 492 - 502, 1972.

C. J. Cappon and J. C. Smith. A simple and rapid procedure for the gas-chromatographic determination of methylmercury in biological specimens. Bull. Env. Cont. Tox. 19: 600 - 607, 1978.

T. W. Clarkson. Mercury poisoning. In *Clinical Chemistry and Chemical Toxicology of Metals* (S. S. Brown, ed.), Elsevier/North Holland, New York. 1977, pp. 189 - 200.

T. W. Clarkson, M. R. Greenwood and L. Magos. Atomic absorption determination of total, inorganic, and organic mercury in biological fluids. In *Clinical Chemistry and Chemical Toxicology of Metals* (S. S. Brown, ed.), Elsevier/North Holland, New York, 1977, pp. 201 - 208.

T. A. Cook and P. O. Yates. Fatal mercury intoxication in a dental surgery assistant. Brit. Dent. J. 127: 553 - 555, 1969.

J. D. Cross, I. M. Dale, H. L. Elliott and H. Smith. Postoperative mercury poisoning. Med. Sci. Law 19: 202 - 204, 1979.

H. G. Gerstner and J. E. Huff. Selected case histories and epidemiologic examples of human mercury poisoning. Clin. Tox. 11: 131 - 150, 1977.

L. J. Goldwater and A. Nicolau. Absorption and excretion of mercury in man. Arch. Env. Health 12: 196 - 198, 1966.

W. H. Gutenmann, J. J. Silvin and D. J. Lisk. Elevated concentrations of mercury in dentists' hair. Bull. Env. Cont. Tox. 9: 318 - 320, 1973.

A. Jaeger, J. D. Tempe, J. M. Haegy et al. Accidental acute mercury vapor poisoning. Vet. Hum. Tox. 21: 62 - 63, 1979.

M. M. Joselow, L. J. Goldwater, A. Alvarez and J. Herndon. Absorption and excretion of mercury in man. XV. Occupational exposure among dentists. Arch. Env. Health 17: 39 - 43, 1968.

G. R. Kelman. Urinary mercury excretion in dental personnel. Brit. J. Ind. Med. 35: 262 - 265, 1978.

E. Nakayama, H. Momotani and S. Ishizu. A pattern of urinary mercury excretion in workers exposed to mercury vapor of relatively low and constant concentration. In *Clinical Chemistry and Chemical Toxicology of Metals* (S. S. Brown, ed.), Elsevier/North Holland, New York. 1977, pp. 209 - 212.

Panel on Mercury. *An Assessment of Mercury in the Environment*, National Academy of Sciences, Washington, D.C., 1978.

R. M. Rosain and C. M. Wai. The rate of loss of mercury from aqueous solution when stored in various containers. Anal. Chim. Acta 65: 279 - 284, 1973.

D. J. Sexton, K. E. Powell, J. Liddle et al. A nonoccupational outbreak of inorganic mercury vapor poisoning. Arch. Env. Health 33: 186 - 191, 1978.
D. C. Sharma and P. S. Davis. Direct determination of mercury in blood by use of sodium borohydride reduction and atomic absorption spectrophotometry. Clin. Chem. 25: 769 - 772, 1979.
R. G. Smith, A. J. Vorwald, L. S. Patil and T. F. Mooney. Effects of exposure to mercury in the manufacture of chlorine. Am. Ind. Hyg. Asso. J. 31: 687 - 700, 1970.
R. Von Burg, F. Farris and J. C. Smith. Determination of methylmercury in blood by gas chromatography. J. Chrom. 97: 65 - 70, 1974.

Blood and Urine Mercury by Atomic Absorption Spectrometry

Principle:

Inorganic and organic mercury in blood or urine is reduced to elemental mercury by reaction with sodium borohydride in a sealed vessel. The released mercury vapor is flushed through the absorption cell of an atomic absorption spectrometer.

Reagents:

Stock solution — 1 mg/mL mercury ion (Fisher reference standard)
Aqueous standards — 0.01, 0.05, 0.10 and 0.20 mg/L (prepare fresh)
Antifoam — tri-n-butyl phosphate
Borohydride reagent — 50 g/L sodium borohydride in 1 mol/L NaOH (prepare fresh)
Apparatus — a reaction vessel and washing vessel are connected in series to the spectrometer absorption cell by means of polyvinyl chloride tubing; the vessels are made of 15 x 2.5 cm test tubes and each inlet tube comes to within 0.5 cm of the bottom of the vessel and ends in a fine tip; the first vessel is initially empty and the second contains 10 mL water and 3 drops antifoam and is immersed in ice water; an air source capable of delivering a constant 3 L/min flow is connected to the inlet of the reaction vessel

Instrumental Conditions:

Atomic absorption spectrometer with flow-through quartz absorption cell
Mercury hollow cathode lamp
Measure absorption at 253.7 nm

Procedure:

1. With the air flow off, transfer 2 mL blood or urine to the reaction vessel. Add 3 mL water and 1 drop of antifoam and close the vessel with the stopper containing the inlet and outlet tubes.

2. Inject 1 mL borohydride reagent through the rubber stopper of the reaction vessel using a hypodermic syringe. Vortex the vessel for 2 min.
3. Turn on the air supply and read the absorbance peak of the mercury vapor as it passes through the absorption cell of the spectrometer. Clean the reaction vessel and flush the system with air before analyzing the next sample.

Calculation:

Calculation is based on a standard curve prepared each time an analysis is performed. Quality control urine specimens containing known amounts of mercury are available commercially and should be analyzed with each specimen.

Evaluation:

Sensitivity: <0.001 mg/L
Linearity: 0.01 - 0.05 mg/L
C.V.: 5 - 7%
Relative recovery: 97 - 124% for inorganic mercury, 89 - 117% for methylmercury

Interferences:

Reagent blanks should be analyzed frequently to monitor contamination from reagents, glassware and residual mercury in the analytical apparatus. The method is highly specific for mercury.

Blood Methylmercury by Electron-Capture Gas Chromatography

Principle:

Methylmercury is extracted from blood as the iodide into benzene. Following several clean-up steps, the extract is analyzed by electron-capture gas chromatography. The procedure is also applicable to the determination of ethylmercury.

Reagents:

Stock solution — 1 mg/mL methylmercury in methanol (as the chloride salt)
Aqueous standards - 0.01, 0.02, 0.05 and 0.10 mg/L (prepare fresh)
8 mol/L Urea
1 mol/L Oxalic acid
1 mol/L Potassium iodide
Benzene

0.1 mol/L Sodium hydroxide
Cysteine solution — 1.5% cysteine in water, adjust to pH 10 with ammonium hydroxide

Instrumental Conditions:

Gas chromatograph with electron-capture detector
1.2 m x 4 mm i.d. glass column containing 2% ethylene glycol succinate on 60/80 mesh Chromosorb G
Injector, 180° C.; column, 150° C.; detector, 180° C.
Nitrogen flow rate, 120 mL/min

Procedure:

1. Transfer 1 mL heparinized whole blood to a 50 mL polypropylene tube. Add 8 mL 8 mol/L urea, 2 mL 1 mol/L oxalic acid and 1 mL 1 mol/L KI and vortex.
2. Add 15 mL benzene and shake to extract. Centrifuge and transfer the benzene to a clean tube. Repeat the extraction with a second 15 mL aliquot of benzene and combine this extract with the first.
3. Add 1 mL 0.1 mol/L NaOH to the benzene. Shake, centrifuge and discard the lower aqueous layer.
4. Add 1 mL cysteine solution to the benzene and extract. Centrifuge and transfer the cysteine solution to a 15 mL screw-cap tube.
5. Add 1 mL 1 mol/L oxalic acid, 1 mL 1 mol/L KI and 1 mL benzene to the cysteine solution. Vortex for several minutes and centrifuge.
6. Transfer the benzene layer to a clean tube. Inject 10 μL into the gas chromatograph.

	Retention time (min)
methylmercuric iodide	0.6
ethylmercuric iodide	1.6

Calculation:

Calculation is based on a standard curve prepared each time a specimen is analyzed. This procedure cannot be controlled by the usual methods due to the instability of dilute methyl mercury solutions.

Evaluation:

Sensitivity: 0.001 mg/L
Linearity: 0.01 - 0.10 mg/L
C.V.: not established
Relative recovery: not established

Interferences:

Recovery of methylmercury from blood averages only 60 - 70% and so it is preferable, if sample volume allows, to use the method of standard additions for accurate calibration rather than to rely on aqueous standards. The original methods required addition to each specimen of radioactive methylmercury as an internal standard to calculate absolute recovery. Reagents and glassware should be checked for interfering peaks on the gas chromatogram by analyzing reagent blanks.

METHANOL

Occurrence and Usage. Methanol finds widespread commercial use as a solvent, especially in paints and varnishes. It is also a constituent of some antifreeze solutions, is used to denature ethanol and is being considered as an alternative energy source. The current threshold limit value for methanol in industry is 200 ppm (260 mg/m^3). The methanol content of 20 commercial wines was found to range from 50 - 325 mg/L (Lee et al., 1975) and of 24 distilled liquors, from 13 - 106 mg/L (Carroll, 1970). Occupational exposure may be via inhalation, dermal absorption or ingestion.

Blood Concentrations. Normal blood methanol concentrations, derived from endogenous production and dietary sources, are on the order of 1.5 mg/L or less (Eriksen and Kulkarni, 1963). During a 10 - 15 day period of chronic bourbon consumption by volunteers, blood methanol concentrations rose steadily to an average peak of 27 mg/L, and did not decline until blood ethanol concentrations fell to less than 0.2 - 0.7 g/L. This accumulation was believed due to the inhibition of metabolism of endogenous and exogenous methanol by ethanol (Majchrowicz and Mendelson, 1971). A peak blood concentration of 117 mg/L was attained at 1 hour after the ingestion of 7 mL of methanol by a 78.5 kg adult male volunteer (Leaf and Zatman, 1952).

Blood formic acid concentrations in normal subjects average about 5 mg/L. In workers exposed to 85 - 134 ppm of methanol vapor, blood formic acid increased from an average of 3.2 mg/L in pre-exposed specimens to 7.9 mg/L by the late afternoon (Baumann and Angerer, 1979).

Metabolism and Excretion. Methanol has a half-life of about 24 hours in man, being oxidized by liver alcohol dehydrogenase at about one-tenth the rate of ethanol (Kane et al., 1968; Mani et al., 1970). The highly toxic formaldehyde which is formed has not been found to accumulate, but is oxidized to formic acid, which is 6 times more toxic than methanol and which probably accounts for the insidious toxicity of its parent. Formic acid is further oxidized to carbon dioxide by a folate-dependent pathway in the rat (Palese and Tephly, 1975). From 10 - 20% of a dose of methanol is eliminated unchanged through the lungs and about 3% by the kidneys; up to 60% is oxidized and, although formaldehyde is not found in urine, urinary formic acid may account for 2 - 5% over a 4 - 10 day period (Lund, 1948; Keeney and Mellinkoff, 1951). The average urine/blood concentration ratio for methanol in man is 1.30, identical to that for ethanol (Leaf and Zatman, 1952).

Methanol breath concentrations in workers exposed to 85 - 134 ppm of methanol vapor averaged 0.8 ppm before work and 2.5 ppm by late afternoon (Baumann and Angerer, 1979).

Urine formic acid concentrations average from 12 to 17 mg/L in unexposed subjects as a result of normal metabolism (Triebig et al., 1978; Baumann and Angerer, 1979). After oral ingestion of 4 mL of methanol by volunteers, urinary formic acid levels reached a maximum of about 56 mg/L within 2 hours and declined rapidly thereafter (Kendal and Ramanathan, 1953). In workers exposed to methanol at vapor concentrations of 85 - 134 ppm, urine formic acid concentrations increased from an average of 13 mg/L in the morning to 20 mg/L by late afternoon (Baumann and Angerer, 1979).

Toxicity. The accumulation of formic acid has been held primarily responsible for the severe metabolic acidosis and ocular toxicity of methanol (Makar and Tephly, 1977). The initial narcotic effects of methanol are much milder than those of ethanol, and the characteristic toxic syndrome may not appear until 6 - 30 hours after ingestion; treatment may include administration of ethanol to inhibit methanol metabolism, administration of folate to induce formic acid detoxification and hemodialysis for the removal of methanol and formic acid (Gosselin et al., 1976; Manoguerra et al., 1977).

Chronic exposure to air concentrations of 3000 ppm or greater is believed to cause accumulation of methanol in the body, with resulting toxicity (Leaf and Zatman, 1952). However, exposure for long periods of time to levels of only 800 - 1000 ppm may be sufficient to produce serious eye damage in some persons (ACGIH, 1971).

The acute ingestion of as little as 10 mL of methanol has caused permanent blindness and 100 - 200 mL is fatal to most adults. Of 725 cases of methanol poisoning by ingestion which occurred prior to 1939, 54% resulted in death, 12% in total blindness and 12% in visual impairment (Keeney and Mellinkoff, 1951). Blood methanol concentrations are not necessarily a good prognostic index. Bennett et al. (1953) reported blood concentrations ranging from 0 - 3.9 g/L (average 1.3) in 11 patients who survived, and concentrations of 0 - 4.0 g/L (average 1.6) in 7 who died during treatment. In 9 hospitalized patients, Lund (1948) found blood methanol concentrations of 0 - 1.2 g/L (average 0.6) and blood formic acid levels of 8 - 134 mg/L (average 56). Blood methanol concentrations in 20 fatal cases averaged 1.9 g/L with a range of 0.2 - 6.3 g/L (Kane et al., 1968; Tonkabony, 1975). The body distribution of methanol in man has been found to be very similar to that of ethanol (Harger et al., 1938).

Biological Monitoring. Exposure to methanol may be evaluated by measuring methanol or its formic acid metabolite. Urine methanol should not exceed 50 mg/L in workers exposed at the 200 ppm (260 mg/m^3) TLV. The air methanol concentration in mg/m^3 may be estimated by multiplying the urinary methanol concentration in mg/L by a factor of 3 (Lauwerys, 1975; Piotrowski, 1977). The determination of methanol in expired breath has also been recommended for monitoring exposure to methanol, although breath concentrations have not been correlated with atmospheric concentrations (Dutkiewicz, 1979).

Urinary formic acid concentrations in workers exposed to 200 ppm of methanol should probably not exceed 50 - 100 mg/L when measured by a specific method such as gas chromatography. Baumann and Angerer (1979) found, however, that urine formic acid levels were too unpredictable and suggested that the blood formic acid level was the most useful parameter for estimating methanol exposure. These authors cautioned that the large interindividual variability in blood formic acid concentration requires pre- and post-exposure determinations for each subject.

Analysis. The gas chromatographic technique presented in the section on acetone (p. 9) is applicable as well to the determination of methanol in biological fluids. A method for the analysis of formic acid in urine was described in the section on formaldehyde (p. 145).

References

ACGIH. *Documentation of the Threshold Limit Values,* American Conference of Governmental Industrial Hygienists, Cincinnati, Ohio, 1971, pp. 155 - 156.

K. Baumann and J. Angerer. Occupational chronic exposure to organic solvents. Int. Arch. Occ. Env. Health 42: 241 - 249, 1979.

I. L. Bennett, Jr., F. H. Cary, G. L. Mitchell, Jr. and M. N. Cooper. Acute methyl alcohol poisoning: a review based on experiences in an outbreak of 323 cases. Medicine 32: 431 - 463, 1953.

R. B. Carroll. Analysis of alcoholic beverages by gas-liquid chromatography. Quart. J. Stud. Alc. Suppl. 5: 6 - 19, 1970.

B. Dutkiewicz. Comparative study on methanol elimination with expired air, after skin and per os administration. In *Industrial and Environmental Xenobiotics* (J. R. Fouts and I. Gut, eds.), Excerpta Medica, Amsterdam, 1978, pp. 106 - 109.

S. P. Eriksen and A. B. Kulkarni. Methanol in normal human breath. Science 141: 639 - 640, 1963.

R. E. Gosselin, H. C. Hodge, R. P. Smith and M. N. Gleason. *Clinical Toxicology of Commercial Products,* 4th ed., Williams and Wilkins, Baltimore, 1976, pp. 229 - 233 (Section III).

R. N. Harger, S. L. Johnson and E. G. Bridwell. Detection and estimation of methanol, with results in human cases of methanol poisoning. J. Biol. Chem. 123: Suppl. 50 - 51, 1938.

R. L. Kane, W. Talbert, J. Harlan et al. A methanol poisoning outbreak in Kentucky. Arch. Env. Health 17: 119 - 129, 1968.

A. H. Keeney and S. M. Mellinkoff. Methyl alcohol poisoning. Ann. Int. Med. 34: 331 - 338, 1951.

L. P. Kendal and A. N. Ramanathan. Excretion of formate after methanol ingestion in man. Biochem. J. 54: 424 - 426, 1953.

R. Lauwerys. Biological criteria for selected industrial toxic chemicals: a review. Scand. J. Work Env. Health 1: 139 - 172, 1975.

G. Leaf and L. J. Zatman. A study of the conditions under which methanol may exert a toxic hazard in industry. Brit. J. Ind. Med. 9: 19 - 31, 1952.

C. Y. Lee, T. E. Acree and R. M. Butts. Determination of methyl alcohol in wine by gas chromatography. Anal. Chem. 47: 747 - 748, 1975.

A. Lund. Excretion of methanol and formic acid in man after methanol consumption. Acta Pharm. Tox. 4: 205 - 212, 1948.

E. Majchrowicz and J. H. Mendelson. Blood methanol concentrations during experimentally induced ethanol intoxication in alcoholics. J. Pharm. Exp. Ther. 179: 293 - 300, 1971.

A. B. Makar and T. R. Tephly. Methanol poisoning VI: role of folic acid in the production of methanol poisoning in the rat. J. Tox. Env. Health 2: 1201 - 1209, 1977.

J. C. Mani, R. Pietruszko and H. Theorell. Methanol activity of alcohol dehydrogenases from human liver, horse liver, and yeast. Arch. Biochem. Biophys. 140: 52 - 59, 1970.

A. S. Manoguerra, R. J. Cipolle, D. E. Zaske and S. M. Ehlers. Serum concentration studies during hemodialysis in a patient with severe methanol intoxication. In *Management of the Poisoned Patient* (B. H. Rumack and A. R. Temple, eds.), Science Press, Princeton, 1977, pp. 103 - 114.

M. Palese and T. R. Tephly. Metabolism of formate in the rat. J. Tox. Env. Health 1: 13 - 24, 1975.

J. K. Piotrowski. *Exposure Tests for Organic Compounds in Industrial Toxicology,* U. S. Government Printing Office, Washington, D.C., 1977, p. 122.

S. E. H. Tonkabony. Post-mortem blood concentration of methanol in 17 cases of fatal poisoning from contraband vodka. For. Sci. 6: 1 - 3, 1975.

G. Triebig, K. H. Schaller and K. Gossler. Ein einfache und zuverlässige gas-chromatographische Bestimmung von Ameisensäure im Urin. Z. Anal. Chem. 290: 114, 1978.

METHYL BROMIDE

Occurrence and Usage. Methyl bromide is a gaseous chemical (b.p. 5° C.) which is frequently employed as a fumigant for large enclosed industrial and agricultural areas. It has also been used as a refrigerant and fire extinguishant. The threshold limit value for industrial usage is 15 ppm (60 mg/m^3) in the atmosphere; at this level the compound has practically no detectable odor, but at higher concentrations the odor resembles that of chloroform. The TLV for methyl bromide is scheduled for possible reduction to 5 ppm. Exposure may be by inhalation or dermal absorption.

Blood Concentrations. Blood concentrations of intact methyl bromide after low-level occupational exposure have not been established. However, inorganic bromide blood concentrations have been measured in 12 asymptomatic methyl bromide workers and found to average 15 mg/L, with a range of 4 - 36 mg/L (Rathus and Landy, 1961). In another study, a range of 0 - 114 mg/L (average 55) was found in workers (Drawneek et al., 1964). By contrast, patients receiving sodium bromide as an anticonvulsant or sedative often develop serum bromide concentrations of at least 75 - 100 mg/L (Maynert, 1965). Baseline blood bromide concentrations in normal subjects average 3 mg/L, with a range of 1 - 5 mg/L (Cross and Smith, 1978). The half-life of bromide in blood is about 12 days (Soremark, 1960).

Metabolism and Excretion. Methyl bromide is known to be partially converted in man to inorganic bromide. The contribution of this metabolite to the toxicity of the parent is not clear, but since inorganic bromide blood concentrations after methyl bromide poisoning are generally much lower than during intoxication by bromide salts, it is felt that methyl bromide itself is the primary toxic agent. Its ability to methylate sulfhydryl groups and thus inactivate enzymes has been postulated to play an important role in methyl bromide poisoning (Gosselin et al., 1976). There is a suggestion that a fraction of a dose (2 - 3%) may be eliminated in the urine as a mercapturic acid conjugate (Drawneek et al., 1964). Undoubtedly, much of the compound is rapidly exhaled unchanged, whereas the inorganic bromide which is formed as a metabolite has a serum half-life of about 15 days and is slowly excreted in the urine (Maynert, 1965).

Toxicity. Methyl bromide toxicity following exposure often develops after a latent period of several hours, and is manifested by confusion, abdominal pain, weakness, nausea, convulsions, coma and occasionally pulmonary edema. Exposure to atmospheric concentrations of 600 ppm for a period of several hours may prove fatal. Persons who survive often require a long period of convalescence and may experience permanent disability due to continued weakness, vertigo and mental and motor impairment (Hine, 1969). The serum inorganic bromide level in poisoned patients can often be correlated with severity of symptoms and has ranged from 24 mg/L in a person experiencing only dizziness to 550 mg/L in a subject who suffered convulsions, with an overall average of 164 mg/L for 17 survivors (Clarke et al., 1945; Benatt and Courtney, 1948; Longley and Jones, 1965; Hine, 1969). In 4 fatal cases of methyl bromide intoxication, blood bromide concentrations of 92 - 400 mg/L (average 206) were noted (Clarke et al., 1945; Hine, 1969). These concentrations of inorganic bromide are only one-eighth those observed in fatalities due to carbromal, a brominated monoureide used as a sedative, and one-tenth those measured in nonfatal intoxications with inorganic bromide salts (Wenk et al., 1976).

Biological Monitoring. The determination of inorganic bromide in serum may be used as an index of exposure to methyl bromide. The long serum half-life of bromide limits the usefulness of this value, but on the basis of past industrial experience the serum bromide level in methyl bromide workers should probably not exceed 15 - 30 mg/L. The possible contribution of inorganic and organic bromide sedatives to the serum level must be considered in the evaluation of the analytical findings.

Analysis. Intact methyl bromide has not been isolated from human tissues following exposure. Inorganic bromide which is released during the metabolism of methyl bromide may be determined by gas chromatography after derivatization (Corina et al., 1979). The usual gold chloride procedure is limited to measurement of bromide concentrations in excess of 50 - 100 mg/L (Sunshine, 1975).

References

A. J. Benatt and T. R. B. Courtney. Uraemia in methyl bromide poisoning: a case report. Brit. J. Ind. Med. 5: 21 - 25, 1948.

C. A. Clarke, C. G. Roworth and H. E. Holling. Methyl bromide poisoning. Brit. J. Ind. Med. 2: 17 - 23, 1945.

D. L. Corina, K. E. Ballard, D. Grice et al. Bromide measurement in serum and urine by an improved gas chromatographic method. J. Chrom. 162: 382-387, 1979.

J. D. Cross and H. Smith. Bromine in human tissue. For. Sci. 11: 147 - 153, 1978.

W. Drawneek, M. J. O'Brien, H. J. Goldsmith, and R. E. Bourdillion. Industrial methyl-bromide poisoning in fumigators. Lancet 2: 855 - 856, 1964.

R. E. Gosselin, H. C. Hodge, R. P. Smith and M. N. Gleason. *Clinical Toxicology of Commercial Products*, 4th ed., Williams and Wilkins, Baltimore, 1976, pp. 233 - 237 (Section III).

C. H. Hine. Methyl bromide poisoning. A review of ten cases. J. Occ. Med. 11: 1 - 10, 1969.

E. O. Longley and A. T. Jones. Methyl bromide poisoning in man. Ind. Med. Surg. 34: 499 - 502, 1965.

E. W. Maynert. Sedatives and hypnotics I: Nonbarbiturates. In *Drill's Pharmacology in Medicine* (J. R. DiPalma, ed.), 3rd ed., McGraw-Hill, New York, 1965, p. 184.

E. M. Rathus and P. J. Landy. Methyl bromide poisoning. Brit. J. Ind. Med. 18: 53 - 57, 1961.

R. Soremark. The biological half-life of bromide ions in human blood. Acta Physiol. Scand. 50: 119 - 123, 1960.

I. Sunshine (ed.). Bromide, type A procedure. In *Methodology for Analytical Toxicology*, CRC Press, Cleveland, 1975, pp. 54-55.

R. E. Wenk, J. A. Lustgarten, N. J. Pappas et al. Serum chloride analysis, bromide detection and the diagnosis of bromism. Am. J. Clin. Path. 64: 49 - 57, 1976.

Serum Bromide by Gas Chromatography

Principle:

A protein-free solution is prepared from serum. Bromide ion is oxidized to bromine with sodium hypochlorite, and the bromine is allowed to react with 2, 4-dimethylphenol. The bromine derivative is extracted into petroleum ether containing an internal standard and the concentrated extract is analyzed by flame-ionization gas chromatography.

Reagents:

Stock solution — 1 mg/mL bromide ion (14.89 mg KBr/10 mL water)
Aqueous standards — 10, 25, 50 and 100 mg/L
30% Trichloroacetic acid
Activated charcoal
Internal standard — 50 mg/L ethanolic solution of 2,3-dibromocyclohexanol (prepare by adding a slight excess of bromine to a solution of 2-cyclohexen-1-ol [Aldrich Chemical Co.] in CCl_4; evaporate to dryness to remove excess bromine and recrystallize product from CCl_4 at −10° C.)
Sodium hypochlorite solution
DMP solution — 200 mg 2,4-dimethylphenol in 20 mL petroleum ether (prepare fresh)
Hexane

Instrumental Conditions:

Gas chromatography with flame-ionization detector
2.1 m x 2 mm i.d. glass column containing 3% OV-17 on Diatomite CQ
Injector, 200° C.; column, 145° C.; detector, 200° C.
Nitrogen flow rate, 15 mL/min

Procedure:

1. Transfer 1 mL serum to a centrifuge tube and add 1 mL 30% trichloroacetic acid. Add 50 mg activated charcoal, vortex and let stand for 5 min.
2. Centrifuge and filter the supernatant through a plug of glass wool in a disposable pipet. Transfer 1 mL of filtrate to a 2 mL capped vial.
3. Add 10 μL internal standard and 30 μL sodium hypochlorite and vortex. Add 0.3 mL DMP solution, cap the vial and shake vigorously for 1 min.
4. Centrifuge if necessary to separate layers and transfer the upper organic layer to a 5 mL conical centrifuge tube. Evaporate to dryness under a stream of nitrogen.
5. Dissolve the residue in 20 μL hexane, vortex and let stand for 10 min. Inject 2 μL into the gas chromatograph.

	Retention time (min)
bromide derivative	2.1
internal standard	5.0

Calculation:

Calculation is based on a response factor derived from a standard curve. A quality control specimen containing 25 mg/L bromide is analyzed daily.

Evaluation:

Sensitivity: 10 mg/L
Linearity: 15 - 150 mg/L
C.V.: 3.9%
Relative recovery: not established

Interferences:

None is known. Normal serum bromide concentrations are generally less than 5 mg/L.

NICKEL

Occurrence and Usage. Nickel is a component of many alloys, being present in amounts of up to 15% in stainless steel. It is used to plate other metals and is widely used in electrical devices. Nickel is an essential trace element and is supplied at the rate of 0.3 - 0.6 mg per day by the diet. The metal or its compounds are absorbed following inhalation or ingestion. The threshold limit values for nickel in the industrial atmosphere range from 0.1 mg/m^3 for soluble compounds of nickel to 1 mg/m^3 for the metal itself. Nickel carbonyl is dealt with in the subsequent section.

Blood Concentrations. Nickel in the plasma of healthy subjects averages 2.1 μg/L, with a range of 1.4 - 3.4 μg/L. In six asymptomatic nickel-exposed workers, plasma concentrations ranged from 3.2 - 11.1 μg/L (Andersen et al., 1978). Plasma concentrations as high as 100 μg/L have been observed in nickel refinery workers (Hogetveit et al., 1978). Whole blood concentrations are approximately twice those of plasma or serum (Sunderman, 1977).

Metabolism and Excrction. Of the nickel which is ingested, over 90% is excreted unabsorbed in the feces (Sunderman, 1977). Absorbed nickel tends to localize in the connective tissue, kidney and lungs (Oskarsson and Tjalve, 1977). Nickel concentrations in parenchymal tissues are generally quite low, usually less than 25 μg/kg in lung and less than 10 μg/kg in liver, and do not appear to increase with age in healthy non-occupationally exposed subjects (Panel on Nickel, 1975). Most of the absorbed nickel is believed to be excreted in urine, with an average of 4.5 μg/L (range 1.9 - 9.6) found in the urine of unexposed persons (Andersen et al., 1978). Urine nickel concentrations in healthy electroplating shop employees have ranged from 4 - 65 μg/L in one study (Bernacki et al., 1978) and 10 - 120 μg/L in another (Tola et al., 1979). Urine levels as high as 1200 μg/L have been observed in nickel refinery workers (Hogetveit and Barton, 1976).

Insoluble nickel compounds which are inhaled tend to accumulate in the nasal mucosa and lungs, and nickel levels in these tissues may remain elevated for years after cessation of exposure (Torjussen and Andersen, 1979).

Toxicity. Nickel is well-known for producing contact dermatitis in sensitized persons which can become quite severe. Acute exposure to nickel fume has occasionally produced typical metal fume fever. Few industrial problems have arisen in regard to acute toxicity from exposure to soluble or insoluble nickel compounds, with the exception of nickel carbonyl (see next section) and the rare instance of accidental ingestion of a soluble salt. Nickel carcinogenicity, especially with exposure to insoluble compounds, is a more serious cause for concern, having been demonstrated experimentally and in a number of epidemiologic studies involving refinery workers.

Biological Monitoring. Both plasma and urine nickel concentrations have been shown to be good indices of exposure to nickel or its soluble salts, and both are generally related to the atmospheric content of nickel as well as to each other (Bernacki et al., 1978). The soluble salts of nickel do not tend to accumulate in the body, so that an end-of-shift specimen is representative of that day's exposure. If substantial overexposure has occurred, however, it may require some days or even weeks for the plasma and urine nickel values to return to baseline (Tola et al., 1979). It has been suggested that a plasma nickel level of 10 μg/L be used as a biological threshold limit for industrial exposure (Hogetveit et al., 1978).

Analysis. An electrothermal atomic absorption spectrometry procedure which requires minimal sample preparation is described for the analysis of nickel in plasma and urine (Andersen et al., 1978).

References

I. Andersen, W. Torjussen and H. Zachariasen. Analysis for nickel in plasma and urine by electrothermal atomic absorption spectrometry, with sample preparation by protein precipitation. Clin. Chem. 24: 1198 - 1202, 1978.

E. J. Bernacki, G. E. Parsons, B. R. Roy et al. Urine nickel concentrations in nickel-exposed workers. Ann. Clin. Lab. Sci. 8: 184 - 189, 1978.

A. C. Hogetveit and R. T. Barton. Preventive health program for nickel workers. J. Occ. Med. 18: 805 - 808, 1976.

A. C. Hogetveit, R. T. Barton and C. O. Kostol. Plasma nickel as a primary index of exposure in nickel refining. Ann. Occ. Hyg. 21: 113 - 120, 1978.

A. Oskarsson and H. Tjalve. Autoradiography of nickel chloride and nickel carbonyl in mice. Acta Pharm. Tox. 41: 158 - 159, 1977.

F. W. Sunderman, Jr. A review of the metabolism and toxicology of nickel. Ann. Clin. Lab. Sci. 7: 377 - 398, 1977.

S. Tola, J. Kilpio and M. Virtamo. Urinary and plasma concentrations of nickel as indicators of exposure to nickel in an electroplating shop. J. Occ. Med. 21: 184 - 188, 1979.

W. Torjussen and I. Andersen. Nickel concentrations in nasal mucosa, plasma, and urine in active and retired nickel workers. Ann. Clin. Lab. Sci. 9: 289 - 298, 1979.

Plasma and Urine Nickel by Graphite-Furnace Atomic Absorption Spectrometry

Principle:

Nickel is extracted from the deproteinized specimen as a chelate into an organic solvent. The extract is analyzed by electrothermal atomic absorption spectrometry.

Reagents:

Stock solution — 1 mg/mL nickel ion (Fisher reference standard)
Aqueous standards — 1, 2, 5, 10 and 20 μg/L (prepare fresh)

3 mol/L Trichloroacetic acid (ultra-pure)
Sulfuric acid — conc. H_2SO_4 (ultra-pure)
APDC solution — 0.12 mol/L ammonium pyrrolidinedithiocarbamate in water (prepare fresh and extract 4 times with MIBK before use)
pH Indicator — 1 g/L m-cresol
Ammonium hydroxide — conc. NH_4OH (ultra-pure)
Methylisobutyl ketone

All glassware is soaked overnight in 50% nitric acid and rinsed before use; all water for reagent preparation and rinsing is deionized-distilled.

Instrumental Conditions:

Atomic absorption spectrometer with graphite furnace
Nickel hollow cathode lamp
Furnace program:
- dry 20 sec at 140° C.
- char 10 sec at 420° C.
- ash 10 sec at 1060° C.
- atomize 15 sec at 2600° C

Argon purge gas in interrupt mode
Measure absorption at 232 nm

Procedure:

1. Transfer 3 mL plasma or urine to a 12 mL centrifuge tube. Add 1 mL 3 mol/L trichloroacetic acid and 1 mL conc. H_2SO_4 and vortex.
2. Centrifuge to separate proteins and decant supernatant to a 12 mL glass-stoppered centrifuge tube. Add 0.3 mL APDC solution and 1 drop pH indicator and vortex.
3. Adjust solution to pH 9 with conc. NH_4OH. Add 1 mL methylisobutyl ketone and shake for 2 min.
4. Centrifuge and transfer a portion of the upper organic layer to a 3 mL test tube. Inject 20 μL into the furnace and begin temperature program. Determine the average peak absorbance of 3 - 5 injections for each specimen.

Calculation:

Calculation is based on a response factor derived from a standard curve. A quality control specimen consisting of pooled plasma or urine is analyzed daily.

Evaluation:

Sensitivity: <1 μg/L
Linearity: 1 - 20 μg/L
C.V.: 12%
Relative recovery: not established

Interferences:

Nickel contamination of reagents and glassware will always be present. Reagent blanks must be run frequently and their average value subtracted from that of the aqueous standards and specimens. A deuterium background corrector is not necessary when the 10 second ashing step at 1060° C. is performed.

NICKEL CARBONYL

Occurrence and Usage. Nickel carbonyl is an especially toxic form of nickel which is produced as an intermediate in the purification of nickel ore and is used in organic synthesis and in electroplating operations. It may be formed inadvertently whenever carbon monoxide comes into contact with active nickel; tobacco smoke has been found to contain an average of approximately 3.5 ppm of nickel carbonyl. The substance is generally encountered in industry as a vapor (b.p. of the liquid is 43° C.) which is rapidly absorbed after inhalation. The current threshold limit value is 0.05 ppm (0.35 mg/m^3); it had been set as low as 0.001 ppm in earlier years due to concern over the carcinogenic potential of the compound.

Blood Concentrations. Due to its rapid metabolism and elimination, intact nickel carbonyl has not been measured in the blood of exposed subjects. Ionic nickel, a metabolite of nickel carbonyl, has been found at concentrations of 4.3 - 4.8 μg/L in the serum of two asymptomatic workers exposed to nickel carbonyl; by comparison, serum nickel concentrations average 2.6 μg/L (range 1.1 - 4.6) in healthy unexposed subjects (Nomoto and Sunderman, 1970).

Metabolism and Excretion. Inhaled nickel carbonyl is rapidly absorbed into the blood and distributed primarily to the lungs, brain, adrenals and kidney. Oxidation to divalent nickel takes place intracellularly within minutes (Oskarsson, 1979). Slightly more than one-third of a dose is exhaled unchanged by rats over a period of 6 hours (Kasprzak and Sunderman, 1969). The divalent nickel which is formed is nearly totally excreted in the urine within six days (Tedeschi and Sunderman, 1957).

Urine nickel concentrations in asymptomatic nickel carbonyl workers have been observed to range from 10 - 50 μg/L (Kincaid et al., 1956), compared to a range of 2 - 10 μg/L in normal unexposed persons (Andersen et al., 1978). Two workers who were exposed to excessive amounts of nickel carbonyl but did not develop symptoms of toxicity were found to have nickel levels of 110 and 180 μg/L in urine collected during the 8 hours following exposure (Sunderman and Kincaid, 1954).

Toxicity. The immediate effects of nickel carbonyl exposure include headache, chest pain and dizziness. These may disappear after a few hours, to be followed within 12 hours to five days by the delayed effects. In severe cases, cough, dyspnea, cyanosis and weakness have been observed. Death usually occurs within 3 - 7 days and is the result of diffuse interstitial pneumonitis and cerebral edema (Sunderman, 1977).

Several hundred instances of acute nickel carbonyl poisoning have occurred, with between 20 and 30 reported deaths (Panel on Nickel, 1975; Sunderman, 1979). In these cases urine specimens taken on the first day of exposure have contained nickel at concentrations of 100 - 2470 μg/L, the concentrations being reasonably well-correlated with the severity of the symptoms. Sunderman and Sunderman (1958) have suggested that if an initial 8-hour urine specimen contains less than 100 μg/L nickel, the exposure should be classified as mild; if it contains from 100 - 500 μg/L, as moderately severe; and if more than 500 μg/L, as severe. Oral administration of sodium diethyldithiocarbamate is often prescribed for treatment of serious cases of nickel carbonyl poisoning.

Biological Monitoring. Preliminary investigations have been made into the measurement of intact nickel carbonyl in the breath of exposed workers. The early results indicated that breath concentrations measured within two hours of exposure show a good correlation to the amount of nickel carbonyl inhaled (Metcalfe et al., 1977).

Currently, measurement of plasma or urine concentrations of divalent nickel provide the best index to nickel carbonyl exposure in workers. Plasma nickel levels should not exceed 10 μg/L in exposed workers (Hogetveit et al., 1978). It has been recommended that a urine nickel concentration of 150 μg/L be considered an action level; at one large refinery, chelation therapy is initiated for employees with urine concentrations exceeding this level (ACGIH, 1977).

Analysis. Plasma and urine nickel concentrations may be determined using the atomic absorption spectrometric method described in the section on nickel (p. 194).

References

ACGIH. *Documentation of Threshold Limit Values for Substances in Workroom Air*, American Conference of Governmental Industrial Hygienists, Cincinnati, Ohio, 1977, pp. 389 - 390.

I. Andersen, W. Torjussen and H. Zachariasen. Analysis for nickel in plasma and urine by electrothermal atomic absorption spectrometry, with sample preparation by protein precipitation. Clin. Chem. 24: 1198 - 1202, 1978.

A. C. Hogetveit and R. T. Barton. Preventive health program for nickel workers. J. Occ. Med. 18: 805 - 808, 1976.

K. S. Kasprzak and F. W. Sunderman, Jr. The metabolism of nickel carbonyl-^{14}C. Tox. App. Pharm. 15: 295 - 303, 1969.

J. F. Kincaid, E. L. Stanley, C. H. Beckworth and F. W. Sunderman. Nickel poisoning. Am. J. Clin. Path. 26: 107 - 119, 1956.

L. P. Metcalfe, L. G. Morgan and G. O. R. Williams. Gas chromatographic detection of nickel carbonyl. Presented at the International Symposium on Clinical Chemistry and Clinical Toxicology of Metals, Monte Carlo, March 2 - 5, 1977.

S. Nomoto and F. W. Sunderman. Atomic absorption spectrometry of nickel in serum, urine, and other biological materials. Clin. Chem. 16: 477 - 485, 1970.

A. Oskarsson. Tissue localization of some nickel compounds. Abstract of Doctoral Dissertation, University of Uppsala, Sweden, 1979.

Panel on Nickel. *Nickel,* National Academy of Sciences, Washington, D. C., 1975.

F. W. Sunderman and J. F. Kinkaid. Nickel poisoning. II. Studies on patients suffering from acute exposure to vapors of nickel carbonyl. J. Am. Med. Asso. 155: 889 - 894, 1954.

F. W. Sunderman and F. W. Sunderman, Jr. Nickel poisoning. VIII. Dithiocarb: a new therapeutic agent for persons exposed to nickel carbonyl. Am. J. Med. Sci. 236: 26 - 31, 1958.

F. W. Sunderman, Jr. A review of the metabolism and toxicology of nickel. Ann. Clin. Lab. Sci. 7: 377 - 398, 1977.

F. W. Sunderman, Sr. Efficacy of sodium diethyldithiocarbamate (dithiocarb) in acute nickel carbonyl poisoning. Ann. Clin. Lab. Sci. 9: 1 - 10, 1979.

R. E. Tedeschi and F. W. Sunderman. Nickel poisoning. V. The metabolism of nickel under normal conditions and after exposure to nickel carbonyl. Arch. Ind. Health 16: 486 - 488, 1957.

NICOTINE

Occurrence and Usage. Nicotine is a highly toxic alkaloid which causes stimulation of autonomic ganglia and the central nervous system. In its free state it is a liquid (b.p. 247° C.) which slowly darkens on exposure to air. The compound was first isolated in 1828 from tobacco, in which it is present in amounts of 0.5 - 8.0% by weight; certain varieties of tobacco contain nornicotine to the extent of 10 - 20% of the nicotine content. The average cigarette in the United States contains 1.5% nicotine; of the amount which survives the combustion process and is presented to the respiratory tract (0.2 - 2.4 mg), 10 - 50% is absorbed during mouth puffing and 80 - 100% during deep lung inhalation. Nicotine is a drug to which virtually every member of a tobacco-smoking society is exposed. The concentrations of nicotine in the air of public places range from 1 - 10 $\mu g/m^3$ (Hinds and First, 1975), and nicotine can be found in the urine of most nonsmokers. Nicotine is used as a horticultural pesticide and is commercially available in a crude 40% solution of the sulfate which is applied as a spray. The threshold limit value for industrial exposure is 0.5 mg/m^3. The compound is absorbed following inhalation, ingestion or dermal contact.

Blood Concentrations. Of a group of 39 urban non-smokers, about half had measurable amounts of nicotine in their plasma, with a concentration range of 0 - 0.006 mg/L (Russell and Feyerabend, 1975). Plasma nicotine concentrations were found to range from 0.012 - 0.044 mg/L 30 minutes after a 6.5 hour *ad libitum* smoking period, during which the total abstracted nicotine dose ranged from 7.8 - 33 mg (Isaac and Rand, 1972). In a study performed with multiple sampling of plasma during the smoking of 7 cigarettes at the rate of 1 per hour, it was found that the plasma nicotine concentration peaked rapidly after each cigarette (peak level range 0.035 - 0.054 mg/L) and declined rapidly, with only moderate accumulation of nicotine over the 7 hour period (Russell et al., 1976). The plasma half-life of nicotine in smokers has been found to range from 24 to 84 min, with an average of 40 minutes (Armitage et al., 1975).

Metabolism and Excretion. The fate of nicotine in man has not been thoroughly elucidated, but it is known to be extensively transformed to largely inactive metabolites. The first step in its biotransformation appears to be oxidation to cotinine, which is further degraded by oxidation to hydroxycotinine and a ring cleavage product. Nicotine-1′-N-oxide and norcotinine have also been identified as metabolites. Only about 5% of a dose of nicotine is excreted unchanged in the 24 hour urine, with 10% as cotinine and about 4% as nicotine-1′-N-oxide; the quantities of the other known metabolites have not been established (Bowman et al., 1959; Bowman and McKennis, 1962; Beckett et al., 1971; Armitage et al., 1975). The excretion of nicotine is enhanced by acidification of the urine (Matsukura et al., 1979a), whereas cotinine excretion is less affected by pH changes (Matsukura et al., 1979b). In urban nonsmokers the average urinary nicotine concentration is 0.010 mg/L (range 0 - 0.064), although after spending 78 minutes in a smoky room this average increased to 0.080 mg/L (range 0.013 - 0.208). By contrast the urine nicotine concentrations in a group of 18 smokers (8 - 70 cigarettes/day) averaged 1.236 mg/L with a range of 0.104 - 2.743 (Russell and Feyerabend, 1975).

Toxicity. Small doses of nicotine produce nausea, vomiting, dizziness, tachycardia, hypertension, sweating and salivation. Toxicity has been observed in tobacco harvesters probably as a result of dermal absorption of nicotine (Gehlbach et al., 1975). The estimated minimal lethal dose of nicotine in man is 40 - 60 mg, an amount which will cause prostration, convulsions, respiratory paralysis and death within a few minutes to 1 hour after ingestion. A common means of exposure is by accidental or intentional ingestion of a solution which is commercially available for insecticidal purposes. Postmortem blood concentrations of 11 - 63 mg/L (average 29) were observed in 5 adult subjects who swallowed 20 - 25 g of nicotine in this manner and who died within 1 hour (Baselt and Cravey, 1977). In other fatal cases blood concentrations of 5 - 600 mg/L and urine concentrations of 17 - 58 mg/L have been reported (Clarke, 1969).

Biological Monitoring. Urine nicotine concentrations, although substantially higher than those of plasma, fluctuate greatly with changes in pH and are too variable to be reliably used as an index of exposure (Matsukura et al., 1979a). The plasma nicotine level correlates well with the absorbed dose and with pharmacological effect, and should provide a means of evaluating worker exposure to the chemical. Due to the short half-life of nicotine in plasma, specimens should be drawn during or just after the exposure period; tobacco use must be documented and pre-exposure specimens should be obtained in order to establish baseline nicotine concentrations for each individual.

Urine cotinine concentrations have been used as an index to nicotine exposure in tobacco harvesters. The concentrations of this metabolite were found to increase only slightly during the working day and to reach a maximum by 12 hours after the end of the exposure period. Cotinine averaged 35 μg/g creatinine (range 10 - 66) in control urine and 890 μg/g creatinine (range 26 - 2930) in the urine of 16 heavily exposed workers, 3 of whom manifested symptoms of nausea and dizziness after work (Gehlbach et al., 1975).

Analysis. Nicotine may be determined in plasma by gas chromatography using nitrogen-selective detection (Feyerabend et al., 1975; Hengen and Hengen, 1978). A flame-ionization gas chromatographic method is also presented for the measurement of nicotine and cotinine in urine (Beckett and Triggs, 1966).

References

A. K. Armitage, C. T. Dollery, C. F. George et al. Absorption and metabolism of nicotine from cigarettes. Brit. Med. J. 4: 313 - 316, 1975.

R. C. Baselt and R. H. Cravey. A compendium of therapeutic and toxic concentrations of toxicologically significant drugs in human biofluids. J. Anal. Tox. 1: 81 - 103, 1977.

A. H. Beckett and E. J. Triggs. Determination of nicotine and its metabolite, cotinine, in urine by gas chromatography. Nature 211: 1415 - 1417, 1966.

A. H. Beckett, J. W. Gorrod and P. Jenner. The analysis of nicotine-1′-N-oxide in urine, in the presence of nicotine and cotinine, and its application to the study of *in vivo* nicotine metabolism in man. J. Pharm. Pharmac. 23: 55S - 61S, 1971.

E. R. Bowman, L. B. Turnbull and H. McKennis, Jr. Metabolism of nicotine in the human and excretion of pyridine compounds by smokers. J. Pharm. Exp. Ther. 127: 92 - 95, 1959.

E. R. Bowman and H. McKennis, Jr. Studies on the metabolism of (-)- cotinine in the human. J. Pharm. Exp. Ther. 135: 306 - 311, 1962.

E. G. C. Clarke (ed.). *Isolation and Identification of Drugs,* Pharmaceutical Press, London, 1969, pp. 440 - 441.

C. Feyerabend, T. Levitt and M. A. H. Russell. A rapid gas-liquid chromatographic estimation of nicotine in biological fluids. J. Pharm. Pharmac. 27: 434 - 436, 1975.

S. H. Gehlbach, W. A. Williams, L. D. Perry and J. I. Freeman. Nicotine absorption by workers harvesting green tobacco. Lancet 1: 478 - 480, 1975.

N. Hengen and M. Hengen. Gas-liquid chromatographic determination of nicotine and cotinine in plasma. Clin. Chem. 24: 50 - 53, 1978.

W. C. Hinds and M. W. First. Concentrations of nicotine and tobacco smoke in public places. New Eng. J. Med. 292: 844 - 845, 1975.

P. F. Isaac and M. J. Rand. Cigarette smoking and plasma levels of nicotine. Nature 236: 308 - 310, 1972.

S. Matsukura, N. Sakamoto, K. Takahashi et al. Effect of pH and urine flow on urinary nicotine excretion after smoking cigarettes. Clin. Pharm. Ther. 25: 549 - 554, 1979a.

S. Matsukura, N. Sakamoto, Y. Seino et al. Cotinine excretion and daily cigarette smoking in habituated smokers. Clin. Pharm. Ther. 25: 555 - 561, 1979b.

M. A. H. Russell and C. Feyerabend. Blood and urinary nicotine in nonsmokers. Lancet 1: 179 - 181, 1975.

M. A. H. Russell, C. Feyerabend and P. V. Cole. Plasma nicotine levels after cigarette smoking and chewing nicotine gum. Brit. Med. J. 1: 1043 - 1046, 1976.

Plasma Nicotine by Nitrogen-Specific Gas Chromatography

Principle:

Nicotine is extracted from alkalinized plasma with ether, back extracted into aqueous acid and finally returned to an organic solvent. The extract is analyzed by nitrogen-specific gas chromatography, using quinoline as internal standard.

Reagents:

Stock solution — 1 mg/mL nicotine in methanol
Plasma standards — 0.005, 0.010, 0.020 and 0.040 mg/L
5 mol/L Sodium hydroxide
Ether
2 mol/L Hydrochloric acid
Internal standard — 0.5 mg/L quinoline in water
Heptane

Instrumental Conditions:

Gas chromatograph with nitrogen-phosphorus detector
2 m x 2 mm i.d. glass column containing 10% Apiezon L and 10% KOH on 80/100 mesh Chromosorb W (or 3% SP-2250 DB on 100/120 mesh Supelcoport)

Procedure:

1. Transfer 3 mL plasma to a 15 mL screw-cap tube. Add 2 mL 5 mol/L NaOH and 8 mL ether and shake to extract.
2. Centrifuge and transfer ether to a 12 mL centrifuge tube. Evaporate to low volume (0.2 - 0.5 mL) under a stream of nitrogen at room temperature.
3. Add 100 μL 2 mol/L HCl to the ether and vortex. Centrifuge and discard ether layer.
4. Wash aqueous phase with 0.5 mL ether, centrifuge and discard ether. Evaporate remaining traces of ether under a stream of nitrogen.
5. Add 100 μL internal standard and vortex. Transfer the solution to a 3 mL conical centrifuge tube with a narrow tapered end.
6. Add 400 μL 5 mol/L NaOH and 50 μL heptane and vortex for 1 min. Centrifuge and inject 5 μL of the heptane into the gas chromatograph.

	Retention time (min)
internal standard	2.8
nicotine	3.6

Calculation:

Calculation is based on a response factor derived from a standard curve. A quality control specimen containing 0.020 mg/L nicotine is analyzed daily.

Evaluation:

Sensitivity: 0.0001 mg/L
Linearity: 0.001 - 0.100 mg/L
C.V.: 6.5%
Relative recovery: 99 - 107%

Interferences:

Apparent nicotine concentrations of 0.0005 - 0.0040 mg/L were found in plasma from non-smokers who deliberately avoided exposure to cigarette smoking; it is believed that contamination may occur during the extraction process if smoking occurs in or near the laboratory. Fifteen other drugs were found not to interfere with the analysis.

Urine Nicotine and Cotinine by Gas Chromatography

Principle:

Nicotine and an internal standard are extracted from alkalinized urine. The extract is concentrated by evaporation and analyzed by flame-ionization gas chromatography. A parallel procedure is presented for cotinine, using less alkaline extraction conditions, a different internal standard and a higher column oven temperature.

Reagents:

Stock solutions — 1 mg/mL methanol solutions of nicotine and cotinine
Aqueous standards — 0.2, 0.5, 1.0, 2.0 and 5.0 mg/L for both compounds
5 mol/L Hydrochloric acid
Internal standard —
  5 mg/L chlorphentermine HCl in water (nicotine)
  5 mg/L lidocaine HCl in water (cotinine)
Ether
5 mol/L Sodium hydroxide
1 mol/L Ammonium hydroxide
Dichloromethane

Instrumental Conditions:

Gas chromatograph with flame-ionization detector
1 m x 2 mm i.d. glass column containing 5% KOH and 2% Carbowax 20 M on 80/100 mesh Diatoport S
Injector, 250° C.; column, 135° C. (nicotine) or 210° C. (cotinine); detector, 250° C.
Nitrogen flow rate, 33 mL/min

Procedure:

Nicotine

1. Transfer 5 mL urine to a 15 mL screw-cap tube and add 0.1 mL 5 mol/L HCl and 1 mL internal standard (chlorphentermine). Extract three times with 2.5 mL ether, centrifuging each time and discarding the upper ether layer.
2. Add 0.5 mL 5 mol/L NaOH to the aqueous layer. Extract three times with 2.5 mL ether, centrifuging each time and combining the ether layers in a 12 mL conical centrifuge tube.
3. Evaporate the ether extract to 50 μL at 40° C. under a stream of nitrogen. Inject 3-5 μL into the gas chromatograph at a column temperature of 135° C.

	Retention time (min)
nicotine	3.8
internal standard	4.5

Cotinine

1. Transfer 5 mL urine to a 15 mL screw-cap tube and add 1 mL internal standard (lidocaine) and 0.5 mL 1 mol/L NH_4OH. Extract with 7.5 mL dichloromethane and centrifuge to separate layers.
2. Discard the upper aqueous layer and transfer the lower organic layer to a 12 mL conical centrifuge tube. Evaporate to 50 μL at 40° C. under a stream of nitrogen and inject 3-5 μL into the gas chromatograph at a column temperature of 210° C.

	Retention time (min)
internal standard	4
cotinine	7

Calculation:

Calculation is based on a response factor derived from a standard curve. A quality control specimen containing 0.5 mg/L of each compound is analyzed daily.

Evaluation:

Sensitivity: 0.1 mg/L
Linearity: 0.2 - 10 mg/L
C.V.: 4 - 5%
Relative recovery: 95 - 100%

Interferences:

None are known. Nicotine and continine are stable in urine specimens for up to 2 weeks when stored at 4° C.

NITROBENZENE

Occurrence and Usage. Nitrobenzene is a chemical intermediate frequently employed in commercial organic syntheses. The substance is a liquid at room temperature, and is well absorbed after inhalation of the vapor or ingestion of or dermal contact with the liquid. The current threshold limit value for nitrobenzene in the industrial atmosphere is 1 ppm (5 mg/m^3).

Blood Concentrations. Nitrobenzene or its metabolites have not been measured in the blood of exposed persons at normally encountered levels. Methemoglobinemia, which is produced by exposure to nitrobenzene, does not exceed 2% in healthy non-smokers. Workers exposed daily for 8 hours to nitrobenzene at an average air concentration of 19 mg/m^3 were found to develop blood methemoglobin levels averaging 4.3% (Pacseri et al., 1958).

Metabolism and Excretion. Nitrobenzene is metabolized in man by oxidation to p-nitrophenol and by reduction to aniline, which is further oxidized to p-aminophenol. Nitrosobenzene and phenylhydroxylamine, highly toxic compounds, are believed to be produced as intermediates in the reduction of nitrobenzene to aniline. Only about 13 - 16% of a dose is excreted in the urine as p-nitrophenol, with probably less than 10% as p-aminophenol. Both of these substances are eliminated in the form of sulfate or glucuronide conjugates (Piotrowski, 1977).

In a subject exposed to 6 ppm of nitrobenzene for 6 hours, urine p-nitrophenol concentrations reached a maximum of about 5.2 mg/L at 2 hours after the end of the exposure and declined with a half-life of about 60 hours (Salmowa et al., 1963). With daily exposure to 1 - 6 ppm of nitrobenzene, urine p-nitrophenol concentrations reached a plateau after 3 days which was equivalent to 2.5 times the peak concentration achieved on the first day. p-Aminophenol was not found in urine in these studies, utilizing a colorimetric procedure with a sensitivity of 10 mg/L (Piotrowski, 1967).

Toxicity. Exposure to 3 - 6 ppm of nitrobenzene may cause headache and elevation of blood methemoglobin concentration. Chronic exposure has produced severe headache, cyanosis, anemia, dizziness, loss of appetite, nausea, loss of feeling in the extremities and severe weakness in a worker; methemoglobinemia at a level of 33% was observed initially, with peak urinary p-nitrophenol and p-aminophenol concentrations of 147 and 45 mg/L, respectively (Ikeda and Kita, 1964). One person has survived the acute ingestion of 50 mL of nitrobenzene; a methemoglobin level of 82% was attained on the first day, accompanied by severe cyanosis and unconsciousness, and peak urinary p-nitrophenol and p-aminophenol excretion rates of 512 mg/24 hr and 198 mg/24 hr were observed on the third and second days, respectively. The half-life for metabolite excretion was estimated at 84 hours and measurable excretion continued for 22 days (Myslak et al., 1977).

Biological Monitoring. An increase of blood methemoglobin concentration of 2% over an individual's baseline level is indicative of significant exposure to nitrobenzene.

The excretion rate of p-nitrophenol in urine collected over the last 2 - 3 hours of a work period on the fourth and fifth days of the week may be used to estimate the daily absorbed dose for a worker exposed to nitrobenzene. Using average values for pulmonary ventilation and vapor retention, the permissible daily dose has been calculated to be 35 mg of nitrobenzene at the TLV of 1 ppm (5 mg/m^3). The actual dose may be estimated by dividing the p-nitrophenol excretion rate in μg/hr by 7.9 and 10.8, factors which represent the extremes of experimental variation, to obtain a range (in mg) for the absorbed dose.

Another way to evaluate exposure is to use the calculated permissible urinary excretion rate of p-nitrophenol, 280 - 390 μg/hr, as a reference limit (Piotrowski, 1977).

Analysis. Procedures for blood methemoglobin and urine p-aminophenol are presented in the section on aniline (p. 20). A gas chromatographic procedure for the determination of p-nitrophenol in urine is presented in the section on parathion (p. 219) and is preferred for its accuracy and specificity. However, a more convenient colorimetric procedure is also applicable and is presented in this section (Piotrowski, 1967).

References

M. Ikeda and A. Kita. Excretion of p-nitrophenol and p-aminophenol in the urine of a patient exposed to nitrobenzene. Brit. J. Ind. Med. 21: 210 - 213, 1964.

Z. Myslak, J. K. Piotrowski and E. Musialowicz. Acute nitrobenzene poisoning. Arch. Tox. 28: 208 - 213, 1971.

I. Pacseri, L. Magos and L. A. Batskor. Threshold and toxic limits of some amino and nitro compounds. Arch. Ind. Health 18: 1 - 8, 1958.

J. Piotrowski. Further investigations on the evaluation of exposure to nitrobenzene. Brit. J. Ind. Med. 24: 60 - 65, 1967.

J. K. Piotrowski. *Exposure Tests for Organic Compounds in Industrial Toxicology,* U.S. Government Printing Office, Washington, D.C., 1977, pp. 76 - 80.

J. Salmowa, J. Piotrowski and U. Neuhorn. Evaluation of exposure to nitrobenzene. Brit. J. Ind. Med. 20: 41 - 46, 1963.

Urine p-Nitrophenol by Colorimetry

Principle:

p-Nitrophenol conjugates are hydrolyzed by heating in the presence of acid. After extraction into an organic solvent and re-extraction into dilute ammonium hydroxide, p-nitrophenol is reduced to p-aminophenol by treatment with zinc and hydrochloric acid. Aminophenol is then converted by reaction with phenol to indophenol, the absorbance of which is determined spectrophotometrically.

Reagents:

Stock solution — 1 mg/mL p-nitrophenol in methanol
Urine standards — 1, 2, 5 and 10 mg/L
Concentrated hydrochloric acid
40% Sodium hydroxide
30% Hydrogen peroxide
Extraction solvent — light petroleum ether/ether/isoamyl alcohol, 4/1/0.05 by volume
Oxalate buffer — 2.5% oxalic acid and 2.5% potassium oxalate
2 mol/L Ammonium hydroxide
Zinc powder
5% Phenol
Concentrated ammonium hydroxide

Instrumental Conditions:

Visible spectrophotometer set to 630 nm

Procedure:

1. Transfer 10 mL urine to a test tube and add 2 mL conc. HCl. Heat at 100° C. for 1 hour.
2. Cool, centrifuge and decant the supernatant into a 50 mL screw-cap tube. Adjust the pH to 10 with 40% NaOH, add 0.5 mL H_2O_2 and heat at 60° C. for 20 min.
3. Cool and adjust the pH to 4 with conc. HCl. Extract the solution twice with 25 mL portions of extraction solvent, centrifuging each time and transfering the organic layers to a 125 separatory funnel.
4. Rinse the combined solvent layers with 4 mL oxalate buffer and discard the lower aqueous layer. Extract the solvent with 4 mL of 2 mol/L NH_4OH and transfer the lower aqueous layer to a 50 mL beaker.
5. Add 2 mL conc. HCl and 1 g zinc powder to the beaker and rotate gently for 3 min (perform in fume hood). Filter the mixture into a 25 mL graduated cylinder, rinsing the filter paper with about 10 mL of water, and collect a total of 14 mL of filtrate.
6. Add 1 mL 5% phenol and 8 mL conc. NH_4OH to the cylinder and mix. Wait 30 min and measure the absorbance of the solution at 630 nm against a similarly prepared urine blank.

Calculation:

Calculation is based on a response factor derived from a standard curve. A quality control specimen containing 2 mg/L p-nitrophenol is analyzed daily.

Evaluation:

Sensitivity: 0.5 mg/L
Linearity: 0.5 - 10 mg/L
C.V.: 6%
Relative recovery: not established

Interferences:

p-Nitrophenol is not found as an endogenous urine component. Of 13 nitrobenzene congeners tested by administration to animals and analysis of urine, only o-chloronitrobenzene and 2,5-dichloronitrobenzene were found to interfere in the procedure, producing absorbances of 34% and 10%, respectively, of that produced by an equimolar dose of nitrobenzene.

OXALATE

Occurrence and Usage. Oxalic acid and oxalate salts may be encountered in industry and at home as cleaning and bleaching agents. Oxalate is also present in relatively high concentrations in certain dietary plants, including spinach, rhubarb and tea. Ingestion of the compounds produces local corrosive and irritant effects as well as hypocalcemia, due to the precipitation of calcium. Use is made of this latter property when oxalate is added to blood specimens as an anticoagulant. Oxalate is produced *in vivo* following the ingestion of ethylene glycol. The current threshold limit value for oxalic acid in the industrial atmosphere is 1 mg/m^3.

Blood Concentrations. Serum oxalate concentrations in 20 normal subjects were found to average 1.4 mg/L using a specific gas chromatographic procedure; a value of 2.4 mg/L was considered the upper limit for normal serum oxalate (Nuret and Offner, 1978). There is little or no binding of oxalic acid by plasma proteins at physiologic pH, and whole blood oxalate concentrations are only slightly higher (average, 1.7 mg/L) than plasma concentrations. Oxalate concentrations have not been measured in the blood of exposed workers.

Metabolism and Excretion. There is no evidence that oxalate is utilized or further metabolized by human tissues; up to 99% of an intravenously injected radiolabeled dose is excreted in the urine after 36 hours. Only 2 - 5% of ingested oxalic acid is absorbed in normal adults. Urinary oxalic acid, which usually ranges from 8 - 40 mg/day, is derived largely from dietary ascorbic acid (35 - 44%), from the metabolism of glycine (40%), and the remainder from minor metabolic sources and from dietary oxalic acid. Calcium oxalate is a major constituent of urinary calculi and also often occurs as crystals in freshly voided urine (Hodgkinson and Zarembski, 1968).

Toxicity. External contact with oxalic acid may cause eye and skin irritation. Systemic oxalate poisoning is characterized by local corrosive effects, renal damage and a marked fall in plasma calcium levels, with resulting shock, collapse and convulsions. By ingestion, the mean adult lethal dose is probably 15 - 30 g, although the intravenous injection of only 1.2 g of sodium oxalate caused the death of a 16 year old girl (Dvorackova, 1966). Following the ingestion of potassium hydrogen oxalate by 4 women, the plasma oxalate concentration at 6 hours in the one survivor was 3.7 mg/L, while those of the 3 who died ranged from 18 - 110 mg/L (average 68) (Zarembski and Hodgkinson, 1967). One case of poisoning due to chronic occupational exposure to oxalic acid fumes was reported in which the predominant symptoms were severe headache, vomiting, lower back pain, loss of weight, anemia and extreme exhaustion (Howard, 1932).

Biological Monitoring. Urinary oxalate excretion which is significantly increased over the normal upper limit of 40 - 50 mg/24 hr is indicative of excessive exposure to oxalic acid or oxalate salts. Exposure to ethylene glycol and certain dietary plants may also account for enhanced urine oxalate excretion.

Analysis. Oxalic acid may be determined in urine by colorimetry (Hodgkinson and Williams, 1972; Husdan et al., 1976).

References

I. Dvorackova. Todliche Vergiftung nach intravenoser Verabreichung von Natriumoxalat. Arch. Tox. 22: 63 - 67, 1966.

A. Hodgkinson and P. M. Zarembski. Oxalic acid metabolism in man: a review. Calc. Tiss. Res. 2: 115 - 132, 1968.

A. Hodgkinson and A. Williams. An improved colorimetric procedure for urine oxalate. Clin. Chim. Acta 36: 127 - 132, 1972.

C. D. Howard. Chronic poisoning by oxalic acid: with report of a case and results of a study concerning the volatilization of oxalic acid from aqueous solution. J. Ind. Hyg. 14: 283 - 290, 1932.

H. Husdan, M. Leung, D. Oreopoulos and A. Rapoport. Modified method for urinary oxalate. Clin. Chem. 22: 1538, 1976.

P. Nuret and M. Offner. A new method for determination of oxalate in blood serum by gas chromatography. Clin. Chim. Acta 82: 9 - 12, 1978.

P. M. Zarembski and A. Hodgkinson. Plasma oxalic acid and calcium levels in oxalate poisoning. J. Clin. Path. 20: 283 - 285, 1967.

Urine Oxalic Acid by Colorimetry

Principle:

Oxalic acid is precipitated from urine with calcium sulfate and ethanol. Oxalate is converted to glycollic acid by reduction with zinc, and chromotropic acid is added. The resulting chromophore is measured at 570 nm in a spectrophotometer.

Reagents:

Stock solution — 5 mg/mL oxalate ion (1.023 g $K_2C_2O_4 . H_2O$/100 mL water; stable for 1 month at 4° C.)
Aqueous standards — 25, 50 and 100 mg/L (prepare fresh)
Concentrated hydrochloric acid
1 mol/L Sodium hydroxide
Saturated calcium sulfate
Ethanol
1 mol/L Sulfuric acid
Zinc wire, 25 cm x 3 mm o.d., freshly cleaned by brief immersion in 10 mol/L HNO_3
1% Chromotropic acid solution (stable for 1 week at 4° C.)

Concentrated sulfuric acid
5 mol/L Sulfuric acid

Instrumental Conditions:

Visible spectrophotometer set to 570 nm

Procedure:

1. Acidify the urine specimen by adding 1 mL conc. HCl for each 100 mL of urine. Stir and transfer 1.0 mL urine to a 5 mL beaker.
2. Add 1 mL water and adjust the pH to 7.0 by adding 1 mol/L NaOH dropwise. Transfer the solution to a 30 mL conical centrifuge tube quantitatively by rinsing with a small amount of water.
3. Add 2 mL saturated $CaSO_4$ and 14 mL ethanol. Vortex briefly and allow to stand for at least 3 hours.
4. Centrifuge at 2000 rpm for 10 min. Carefully decant and discard the supernatant and allow the tube to drain onto a filter paper for several minutes.
5. Add 2 mL 1 mol/L H_2SO_4 to dissolve the precipitate. Add a piece of zinc wire and heat in a boiling water bath for 30 minutes or until the residual volume of the solution is less than 0.1 mL.
6. Remove the zinc wire, rinsing any adhering residue into the tube with 0.5 mL 1% chromotropic acid solution. Add 5 mL conc. H_2SO_4 slowly and heat in a boiling water bath for 30 min.
7. Cool and dilute to 20 mL with 5 mol/L H_2SO_4. Measure absorbance at 570 nm against a reagent blank (color is stable for several hours).

Calculation:

Calculation is based on a standard curve prepared each time an analysis is performed. This procedure cannot be controlled by the usual methods due to the instability of dilute oxalate solutions.

Evaluation:

Sensitivity: 20 mg/L
Linearity: 20 - 200 mg/L
C.V.: 5.2%
Relative recovery: not established

Interferences:

A glucose concentration of 30 g/L (such as might be present in diabetic urine) produced a 35% increase in the response of the method to a given amount of oxalic acid; oxaloacetic acid at a concentration of 10 mg/L (such as exists during hyperoxaluria) caused a 9% increase in response. Other normal urinary constituents were not found to cause significant interference.

PARAQUAT

Occurrence and Usage. Paraquat is a bis-quaternary ammonium compound which has seen widespread use since 1962 as a domestic and commercial herbicide. The compound was first synthesized in 1932, and under the name methyl viologen was used for many years as an oxidation-reduction indicator dye. The dichloride salt is supplied as a 5% powder for domestic use or a 10 - 30% aqueous concentrate for agricultural purposes; combinations of paraquat and diquat, an ortho-bipyridyl analogue, are also commercially available. The current threshold limit value for occupational exposure is 0.1 mg/m^3. The compound is known to be absorbed after dermal contact, inhalation and ingestion.

Blood Concentrations. Paraquat has not been measured in the blood of asymptomatic exposed persons. It is estimated that less than 5% of an oral dose is absorbed (Conning et al., 1969).

Metabolism and Excretion. Paraquat is not believed to be significantly biotransformed in man. An oral dose given to rats is eliminated in 3 days largely in feces (93 - 96%) and to a slight extent in urine (6%), whereas a subcutaneous dose appears to a much larger extent in urine (73 - 96%), indicating poor absorption from the gut. Unabsorbed paraquat appears to undergo substantial microbial degradation in the intestine (Daniel and Gage, 1966). The lung was the organ of highest paraquat concentration in the rats given an intravenous LD50 dose, from 4 hours until about 9 days after injection; plasma levels declined with a half-life of 56 hours (Sharp et al., 1972). An unidentified paraquat metabolite has been detected in rat lungs (Molnar and Hayes, 1971).

Concentrations of paraquat in the urine of 6 asymptomatic spray operators ranged from undetectable to 0.32 mg/L and averaged 0.04 mg/L during the daily agricultural application of large volumes of 0.25% paraquat solution over a 12 week period (Swan, 1969).

Toxicity. Occupational exposure to paraquat generally produces only skin rash, fingernail damage and epistaxis, although severe eye damage has occurred upon direct contact. There has been no report of long-term effects with routine exposures of up to several years' duration (Swan, 1969; Howard, 1979).

Several hundred deaths have occurred after the ingestion of paraquat, and it is believed that an oral dose of only 1 - 2 g is fatal to most adults. Victims of poisoning experience epigastric pain, vomiting, dyspnea, dysuria and jaundice; death usually follows, often after a period of many days, as a result of severe and extensive fibrotic lung changes and renal failure. Some subjects become comatose and die within a few hours, prior to the development of significant organ pathology.

Plasma paraquat concentrations exceeding 0.2 mg/L on the first day of poisoning are usually associated with an unfavorable prognosis (Davies et al.,

1977). Poisoning has been treated successfully with both forced diuresis (Kerr et al., 1968) and hemodialysis (van Dijk et al., 1975). In several episodes of nonfatal poisoning, maximal serum concentrations of 0.6 - 1.6 mg/L and urine concentrations of 0.9 - 64 mg/L have been noted (Tompsett, 1970; van Dijk et al., 1975). Paraquat has been detected in urine in concentrations exceeding 0.07 mg/L for up to 26 days after acute ingestion, even during forced diuresis (Beebeejaun et al., 1971).

In cases which eventually proved fatal, antemortem paraquat concentrations were initially as high as 19 mg/L in blood and 1766 mg/L in urine (van Dijk et al., 1975); often these are much lower, however, and when death is postponed for a period exceeding 18 days, autopsy specimens may yield negative results for paraquat by some analytical procedures (Tompsett, 1970; Carson and Carson, 1976).

Biological Monitoring. Urine concentrations of paraquat have been found to be useful in evaluating worker exposure to and absorption of the chemical. It has been calculated that complete absorption of the paraquat inhaled during exposure at the TLV of 0.1 mg/m^3 would lead to a urine paraquat concentration of 0.7 mg/L. In two studies of exposed workers, urine paraquat levels averaged less than 0.1 mg/L with individual excursions up to 0.15 and 0.32 mg/L. Absorption of paraquat is most likely to occur in workers with minor skin abrasions (Swan, 1969).

Analysis. Paraquat may be measured in urine using a visible spectrophotometric method based on sodium dithionite reduction of the ion under alkaline conditions; the analysis is performed after preliminary isolation by cation-exchange chromatography (Lott et al., 1978).

References

A. R. Beebeejaun, G. Beevers, and W. N. Rogers. Paraquat poisoning — prolonged excretion. Clin. Tox. 4: 397 - 407, 1971.

D. J. L. Carson and E. D. Carson. The increasing use of paraquat as a suicidal agent. For. Sci. 7: 151 - 160, 1976.

D. M. Conning, K. Fletcher and A. A. B. Swan. Paraquat and related bipyridyls. Brit. Med. Bull. 25: 245 - 249, 1969.

J. W. Daniel and J. C. Gage. Absorption and excretion of diquat and paraquat in rats. Brit. J. Ind. Med. 23: 133 - 136, 1966.

D. S. Davies, G. M. Hawksworth and P. N. Bennett. Paraquat poisoning. Proc. Eur. Soc. Tox. 18: 21 - 26, 1977.

J. K. Howard. A clinical survey of paraquat formulation workers. Brit. J. Ind. Med. 36: 220 - 223, 1979.

F. Kerr, A. R. Patel, P. D. R. Scott and S. L. Tompsett. Paraquat poisoning treated by forced diuresis. Brit. Med. J. 3: 290 - 291, 1968.

P. F. Lott, J. W. Lott and D. J. Doms. The determination of paraquat. J. Chrom. Sci. 16: 390 - 395, 1978.

I. G. Molnar and W. J. Hayes, Jr. Distribution and metabolism of paraquat in the rat. Tox. Appl. Pharm. 19: 405, 1971.

C. W. Sharp, A. Ottolenghi and H. S. Posner. Correlation of paraquat toxicity with tissue concentrations and weight loss of the rat. Tox. Appl. Pharm. 22: 241 - 251, 1972.

A. A. B. Swan. Exposure of spray operators to paraquat. Brit. J. Ind. Med. 26: 322 - 329, 1969.
S. L. Tompsett. Paraquat poisoning. Acta Pharm. Tox. 28: 346 - 358, 1970.
A. van Dijk, R. A. A. Maes, R. H. Drost et al. Paraquat poisoning in man. Arch. Tox. 34: 129 - 136, 1975.

Urine Paraquat by Colorimetry

Principle:

Urine is adjusted to an acid pH and passed through a cation exchange column. Paraquat is eluted from the column with saturated ammonium chloride. The eluate is treated with sodium dithionite with production of a blue color and the solution is analyzed in a visible spectrophotometer.

Reagents:

Stock solution — 1 mg/mL paraquat in water (store in the dark at 4° C.)
Aqueous standards — 0.01, 0.05, 0.10, 0.20 and 0.50 mg/L (prepare fresh)
Cation exchange column — 6 mL 50/100 mesh Dowex 50W-X8 in a 25 mL buret, rinsed with 50 mL water (prepare fresh for each sample)
2 mol/L Hydrochloric acid
10% Saturated ammonium chloride
Ammonium chloride
Saturated ammonium chloride
Dithionite solution — 0.2% sodium dithionite in 0.5 mol/L NaOH (prepare and use within 1.5 hours)

Instrumental Conditions:

Visible spectrophotometer
Determine absorbance at 390, 394 and 398 nm

Procedure:

1. Adjust the pH of a 100 mL urine specimen to 1 with conc. HCl. Transfer the solution to a separatory funnel connected to the cation exchange column with plastic tubing and pass the solution through the column at a flow rate of 5 - 10 mL/min.
2. Rinse the column in succession with 25 mL water, 25 mL 2 mol/L HCl, and 25 mL 10% saturated NH_4Cl. Add a small amount of solid NH_4Cl to the top of the column and elute the paraquat with saturated NH_4Cl at a rate of about 0.6 mL/min.
3. Collect 25 mL eluate, mix and transfer 15 mL to a test tube. Add 3 mL dithionite solution and mix.

4. Read immediately against a reagent blank in a spectrophotometer at the absorbance maximum (about 394 nm). Also determine the absorbance of the solution at 4 nm on either side of the maximum (390 and 398 nm).

Calculation:

Determine the correction factor (k) by preparing a standard solution of 0.5 mg/L paraquat in saturated NH_4Cl, adding 3 mL of dithionite solution and measuring the absorbance of this mixture at 390, 394 and 398 nm (or the appropriate absorption maximum ± 4 nm). Calculate k by the formula:

$$k = \frac{A_{394}}{2A_{394} - A_{390} - A_{398}}$$

Then use this factor to correct the absorbance of each specimen and aqueous standard with the formula:

$$A_{corr} = k(2A_{394} - A_{390} - A_{398})$$

Determine the concentration of each specimen from a standard curve of corrected absorbance of each standard versus concentration, prepared each time an analysis is performed. This procedure cannot be controlled by the usual methods due to the instability of dilute paraquat solutions.

Evaluation:

Sensitivity: 0.01 mg/L
Linearity: 0.01 - 1.0 mg/L
C.V.: not established
Relative recovery: not established

Interferences:

None are known. The transient nature of the chromogen formed by the reduction of paraquat requires that spectrophotometry be performed rapidly after the last reagent addition.

PARATHION

Occurrence and Usage. Parathion (nitrostigmine) is a highly toxic organophosphate insecticide which has been used frequently and in large quantities since 1949. Parathion and its dimethyl analogue, methylparathion, are yellow oily liquids in pure form which are supplied as dusts, wettable powders and aerosols in concentrations of up to 50% for agricultural purposes. The current threshold limit value for parathion is 0.1 mg/m^3. The compound is well absorbed after inhalation, dermal contact or ingestion.

Blood Concentrations. Dosages of 0.05 mg/kg (3.5 mg/70 kg) of parathion have been orally administered to humans daily for at least 3 weeks with no apparent effect on blood cholinesterase levels (Williams et al., 1958). An oral dose of 7.2 mg, when given daily to volunteers for 6 weeks, caused reduction of cholinesterase activity to levels of 84% of normal in erythrocytes and 63% in plasma; 28 days after the end of the experiment these values were only partially restored to pre-experiment control values (Edson, 1964). Parathion serum concentrations in 23 occupationally exposed asymptomatic workers ranged from 0.004 - 0.200 mg/L, with no correlation to erythrocyte or plasma cholinesterase activity. Paraoxon has occasionally been detected in the serum of persons exposed to parathion (Roan et al., 1969).

Metabolism and Excretion. Parathion must be activated by conversion via liver microsomal enzymes to paraoxon, a potent cholinesterase inhibitor; both compounds are rapidly hydrolyzed by plasma and tissue esterases, with production of diethylthiophosphoric acid (DETP), diethylphosphoric acid (DEP) and p-nitrophenol. These products are largely excreted in urine and represent the majority of a dose of parathion. Urinary DETP and DEP are known to be unstable in stored specimens (Comer et al., 1976) and thus p-nitrophenol, which is rapidly excreted in the urine as a conjugate within 48 hours of an exposure, has been used as a sensitive index of exposure to parathion. Urine p-nitrophenol concentrations ranged from 0.4 - 13.2 mg/L in 23 asymptomatic occupationally exposed workers and correlated well with serum parathion levels, but not with cholinesterase activity in blood (Roan et al., 1969). Due to slow absorption of parathion via the dermal route, p-nitrophenol excretion may be very prolonged after this type of exposure (Durham et al., 1972). Urine p-nitrophenol concentrations were found to average 0.11 mg/L (range 0.06 - 0.31) in residents living near orchards where parathion was used, 0.28 mg/L (range 0.10 - 0.72) in orchard workers, 2.0 mg/L (range 0.14 - 11.3) in parathion mixing-plant personnel and 4.7 mg/L (range 3.2 - 6.3) in parathion applicators (Arterberry et al., 1961).

Toxicity. Symptoms of exposure to parathion are similar to those produced by other cholinesterase inhibitors and include respiratory difficulty, excessive salivation, miosis, nausea, vomiting, muscle weakness and paralysis.

Food contamination by parathion has caused several epidemics of poisoning in which numerous deaths have occurred (Askew, 1968; Diggory et al., 1977). Several hundred deaths in Denmark over a 5 year period were attributed to the suicidal use of parathion (Frost and Poulsen, 1964). The estimated fatal dose of parathion for an adult by ingestion or inhalation is 10 - 300 mg. In a nonfatal poisoning of a worker following dermal exposure to parathion, diethylphosphate (DEP) concentrations in blood were as high as 0.28 mg/L; concentrations of monoethylphosphate reached 0.55 mg/L in blood and 7.0 mg/L in urine (Reichert et al., 1978). Urinary DETP and DEP concentrations in another nonfatal poisoning were initially 3.9 and 0.5 mg/L, respectively (Comer et al., 1976). Urinary p-nitrophenol concentrations in severe poisoning cases have ranged from 1.6 - 11.6 mg/L (Arterberry et al., 1961), lying within the range of concentrations observed in asymptomatic workers (Roan et al., 1969).

Biological Monitoring. The depression of cholinesterase activity in blood during daily worker exposure to parathion is considered to reflect the cumulative effects of numerous exposures, since cholinesterase activity reaches a steady state only after several weeks of repeated exposure to low levels, and it remains low for a period of weeks or months. Depression of an individual's erthyrocyte cholinesterase levels to 70% of his normal baseline activity is an indication of significant exposure to parathion, and depression to 60% of baseline requires removal from exposure and medical observation (NIOSH, 1976).

The measurement of urinary p-nitrophenol is a more sensitive index of exposure to parathion than cholinesterase inhibition. Since p-nitrophenol excretion reaches a maximum within several hours of the end of exposure, it reflects primarily recent exposure and does not necessarily correlate with cholinesterase activity. Concentrations of p-nitrophenol in urine do correlate with the absorbed dose of parathion, and should theoretically reach 0.5 mg/L during daily exposure to parathion at the TLV of 0.1 mg/m^3. Concentrations less than 0.2 mg/L in the daily urine have been found to be consistent with exposure to amounts of parathion which are without effect on blood cholinesterase activity (Piotrowski, 1977).

Preliminary studies have shown that measurement of intact parathion in serum may provide a more useful index of exposure to parathion than either cholinesterase inhibition or p-nitrophenol excretion (Roan et al., 1969).

While the phosphate metabolites of parathion have been measured in the blood and urine of poisoning victims, these determinations have not been performed routinely in the evaluation of exposed workers.

Analysis. Blood cholinesterase may be determined using the procedure presented in the section on carbaryl (p. 60). A method for measurement of the phosphate metabolites of parathion in urine was presented in the section on diazinon (p. 106). Urinary p-nitrophenol may be measured by colorimetry (see nitrobenzene, p. 206) or a more specific electron-capture gas chromatographic method presented here (Cranmer, 1970).

References

J. D. Arterberry, W. F. Durham, J. W. Elliott and H. R. Wolfe. Exposure to parathion. Arch. Env. Health. 3: 476-485, 1961.

A. B. Askew. History of assistance to Tijuana: acute parathion food poisoning. Clin. Tox. 1: 251 - 253, 1968.

S. W. Comer, H. E. Ruark and A. L. Robbins. Stability of parathion metabolites in urine samples collected from poisoned individuals. Bull. Env. Cont. Tox. 16: 618 - 625, 1976.

M. Cranmer. Determination of p-nitrophenol in human urine. Bull. Env. Cont. Tox. 5: 329 - 332, 1970.

H. J. P. Diggory, P. J. Landrigan, K. P. Latimer et al. Fatal parathion poisoning caused by contamination of flour in international commerce. Am. J. Epidemiol. 106: 145 - 153, 1977.

W. F. Durham, H. R. Wolfe and J. W. Elliott. Absorption and excretion of parathion by spraymen. Arch. Env. Health 24: 381 - 387, 1972.

E. F. Edson. No-effect levels of three organosphosphates in the rat, pig and man. Food Cosm. Tox. 2: 311 - 316, 1964.

J. Frost and E. Poulsen. Poisoning due to parathion and other organophosphorus insecticides in Denmark. Dan. Med. Bull. 11: 169 - 177, 1964.

NIOSH. *Occupational Exposure to Parathion,* National Institute for Occupational Safety and Health, Cincinnati, Ohio, 1976.

J. K. Piotrowski. *Exposure Tests for Organic Compounds in Industrial Toxicology,* U. S. Government Printing Office, Washington, D.C., 1977, pp. 107 - 111.

E. R. Reichert, H. W. Klemmer and T. J. Haley. A note on dermal poisoning from mevinphos and parathion. Clin. Tox. 12: 33 - 35, 1978.

C. C. Roan, D. P. Morgan, N. Cook and E. H. Paschal. Blood cholinesterases, serum parathion concentrations and urine p-nitrophenol concentrations in exposed individuals. Bull. Env. Cont. Tox. 4: 362 - 369, 1969.

M. W. Williams, J. W. Cook, J. R. Blake et al. The effect of parathion on human red blood cell and plasma cholinesterase. Arch. Ind. Health 18: 441 - 445, 1958.

Urine p-Nitrophenol by Electron-Capture Gas Chromatography

Principle:

Conjugated p-nitrophenol in urine is hydrolyzed by heating in the presence of acid. The released compound is extracted into an organic solvent. On-column derivatization to a less polar trimethylsilyl ether is performed, and analysis is by electron-capture gas chromatography.

Reagents:

Stock solution — 1 mg/mL p-nitrophenol in methanol
Urine standards — 1, 2, 5 and 10 mg/L
Hydrochloric acid — conc. HCl
20% Sodium hydroxide
Extraction solvent — benzene/ether, 80:20 by volume
Sodium sulfate — anhydrous Na_2SO_4
Derivatization reagent — hexamethyldisilazane/hexane, 20:80 by volume

Instrumental Conditions:

Gas chromatograph with electron-capture detector
2 m x 2 mm i.d. glass column containing 5% DC-200 on 80/100 mesh Gas Chrom Q
Injector, 200° C.; column, 140° C.; detector, 250° C.
Nitrogen flow rate, 30 mL/min

Procedure:

1. Transfer 3 mL urine to a 15 mL screw-cap tube. Add 0.3 mL conc. HCl, cap the tube and heat in a boiling water bath for 1 hour.
2. Cool and adjust the pH to 11 or higher with approximately 0.4 mL 20% NaOH. Extract twice with 5 mL extraction solvent and discard the solvent.
3. Adjust the pH of the aqueous layer to 2 or lower with conc. HCl. Extract with 5 mL extraction solvent.
4. Centrifuge and transfer the organic layer to a 15 mL centrifuge tube. Add a small amount of anhydrous Na_2SO_4 and vortex.
5. Transfer 1 mL of the organic layer to a 5 mL glass-stoppered centrifuge tube. Add 1 mL of the derivatization reagent and vortex.
6. Inject 5 μL of the mixture into the gas chromatograph.

Calculation:

Calculation is based on a response factor derived from a standard curve. A quality control specimen containing 1 mg/L p-nitrophenol is analyzed daily.

Evaluation:

Sensitivity: 0.05 mg/L
Linearity: 0.1 - 10 mg/L
C.V.: 2 - 5% within-run
Relative recovery: 92 - 100%

Interferences:

The method is relatively specific for p-nitrophenol in urine. Some loss of p-nitrophenol may occur during the hydrolysis step if the tube is not tightly capped. p-Nitrophenol is also a metabolite of methylparathion and EPN, and has been found at concentrations of 0.01 - 0.03 mg/L in the urine of members of the general population.

PENTACHLOROPHENOL

Occurrence and Usage. Pentachlorophenol and its sodium salt are frequently employed industrially and in the home as wood preservatives, contact herbicides, disinfectants and mildew retardants. The compound is often dissolved in hydrocarbon solvents for application by spraying, brushing or pressure treatment, and is known to be well-absorbed after oral, pulmonary or dermal exposure. Vaporization from treated wood is a source of chronic inhalation exposure in areas where pentachlorophenol is used extensively for termite control. The current threshold limit value for industrial exposure is 0.5 mg/m^3.

Blood Concentrations. Plasma concentrations of pentachlorophenol in members of the general population of Hawaii, where use of the chemical is high, ranged from 0.05 - 1.0 mg/L; plasma concentrations in healthy occupationally-exposed workers in a wood treatment plant were largely in the range of 1.0 - 10.0 mg/L, with several subjects attaining concentrations as high as 20 mg/L. Plasma contains 99% of the whole blood content of pentachlorophenol (Bevenue et al., 1968; Casarett et al., 1969). The plasma half-life of the compound in monkeys averaged 72 hours for males and 84 hours for females (Braun and Sauerhoff, 1976).

Metabolism and Excretion. The metabolism of pentachlorophenol has only been briefly studied in man. The chemical is known to be oxidized to tetrachlorohydroquinone, and this metabolite and its parent are excreted largely in urine in both free and conjugated form. Tetrachlorohydroquinone was found to be a potent inhibitor of β-glucuronidase, and urinary conjugates must therefore be hydrolyzed by boiling with strong acid prior to solvent extraction (Ahlborg et al., 1974). In monkeys from 69 - 78% of a single oral dose is eliminated as unchanged pentachlorophenol in the urine over a 15 day period, with 12 - 24% excreted in feces as pentachlorophenol or metabolites (Braun and Sauerhoff, 1976).

Free pentachlorophenol concentrations in members of the general population averaged 0.025 mg/kg (range 0.005 - 0.052) in fat (Shafik, 1973) and 0.044 mg/L (range 0.003 - 0.570) in urine. Persons with occupational exposure exhibited urine levels of 0.003 - 38.6 mg/L, averaging 0.465 mg/L (Bevenue et al., 1967). Morning urine specimens from workers with substantial dermal and respiratory exposure to pentachlorophenol averaged as high as 5.6 mg/L over one 10-day period; a direct correlation was observed between blood and urine concentrations of pentachlorophenol (Casarett et al., 1969).

Toxicity. Pentachlorophenol is a highly toxic substance which produces delirium, weakness, flushing, hyperpyrexia, tachycardia, tachypnea, coma and death within several hours of the absorption of approximately 2 g by an adult. Profound rigor mortis is often observed immediately after death, in both man and animals. Four men who developed excess sweating, facial flushing, fever and weight loss during occupational exposure to pentachlorophenol had urine concentrations of the chemical which ranged from 3.8 - 17.5 mg/L (Bergner et al., 1965). A young child exhibited symptoms of pentachlorophenol poisoning and a urine concentration of 60 mg/L following dermal exposure to contaminated bath water (Chapman and Robson, 1965). Contamination of nursery linens by pentachlorophenol was responsible for an epidemic of poisoning in a hospital; an initial serum pentachlorophenol concentration of 118 mg/L was noted in one infant, successfully treated by exchange transfusion, while concentrations of 28 mg/kg in kidney and 34 mg/kg in fat were determined in another child who died. Serum concentrations of 11.3 - 25.6 mg/L (average 18.7) and urine concentrations of 0.02 - 0.70 mg/L (average 0.34) were found in 6 healthy infants in the same nursery (Armstrong et al., 1969). The intentional ingestion of pentachlorophenol by an adult was successfully treated by forced diuresis; blood concentrations as high as 115 mg/L were observed and were noted to decline with half-lives of 116 and 42 hours before and after diuresis was instituted, respectively (Young and Haley, 1978). A blood concentration of 39 mg/L was measured in the case of an adult who ingested 11 g of the chemical and died within 4 hours (Burger, 1966). Blood concentrations of 46 - 173 mg/L (average 99) and urine concentrations of 28 - 520 mg/L (average 178) were observed in 7 fatalities resulting from pulmonary, oral or dermal exposure to pentachlorophenol (Gordon, 1956; Blair, 1961; Mason et al., 1965; Clarke, 1969; Cretney, 1976).

Biological Monitoring. Plasma and urine are equally acceptable specimens for monitoring exposure to pentachlorophenol. Concentrations of pentachlorophenol in plasma or urine which exceed 1 mg/L are indicative of excessive exposure to the chemical. With a half-life of 3 - 5 days, pentachlorophenol tends to accumulate in the body with repeated exposure. Possible domestic usage of the chemical should be considered when evaluating biological monitoring results.

Analysis. Pentachlorophenol may be determined in plasma or urine by electron-capture gas chromatography of a methyl derivative (Rivers, 1972). Flame-ionization detection is probably suitable for many routine applications of this method. Prior hydrolysis of urine specimens is not necessary for most routine industrial purposes, but has been found to yield pentachlorophenol levels up to 17 times as high as methods not incorporating this step (Edgerton and Moseman, 1979).

References

U. G. Ahlborg, J. E. Lindgren and M. Mercier. Metabolism of pentachlorophenol. Arch. Tox. 32: 271 - 281, 1974.

R. W. Armstrong, E. R. Eichner, D. E. Klein et al. Pentachlorophenol poisoning in a nursery for newborn infants. J. Pediat. 75: 317 - 325, 1969.

H. Bergner, P. Constantinidis and J. H. Martin. Industrial pentachlorophenol poisoning in Winnipeg. Can. Med. Asso. J. 92: 448 - 451, 1965.

A. Bevenue, J. Wilson, L. J. Casarett and H. W. Klemmer. A survey of pentachlorophenol content in human urine. Bull. Env. Cont. Tox. 2: 319 - 332, 1967.

A. Bevenue, M. L. Emerson, L. J. Casarett and W. L. Yauger, Jr. A sensitive gas chromatographic method for the determination of pentachlorophenol in human blood. J. Chrom. 38: 467 - 472, 1968.

D. M. Blair. Dangers in using and handling sodium pentachlorophenate as a molluscicide. Bull. WHO 25: 597 - 601, 1961.

W. H. Braun and M. W. Sauerhoff. The pharmacokinetic profile of pentachlorophenol in monkeys. Tox. Appl. Pharm. 38: 525 - 533, 1976.

E. Burger. Akute tödliche Vergiftung mit Pentachlorphenolnatrium. Deut. Z. Gericht. Med. 58: 240 - 247, 1966.

L. J. Casarett, A. Bevenue, W. L. Yauger, Jr. and S. A. Whalen. Observations on pentachlorophenol in human blood and urine. Am. Ind. Hyg. Asso. J. 30: 360 - 366, 1969.

J. B. Chapman and P. Robson. Pentachlorophenol poisoning from bathwater. Lancet 1: 1266 - 1267, 1965.

E. G. C. Clarke (ed.). *Isolation and Identification of Drugs,* Pharmaceutical Press, London, 1969, pp. 471 - 472.

M. J. Cretney. Personal communication, 1976.

T. R. Edgerton and R. F. Moseman. Determination of pentachlorophenol in urine: the importance of hydrolysis. J. Agr. Food Chem. 27: 197 - 199, 1979.

D. Gordon. How dangerous is pentachlorophenol. Med. J. Aust. 2: 485 - 488, 1956.

M. F. Mason, S. M. Wallace, E. Foerster and W. Drummond. Pentachlorophenol poisoning: report of two cases. J. For. Sci. 10: 136 - 147, 1965.

J. B. Rivers. Gas chromatographic determination of pentachlorophenol in human blood and urine. Bull. Env. Cont. Tox. 8: 294 - 296, 1972.

T. M. Shafik. The determination of pentachlorophenol and hexachlorophene in human adipose tissue. Bull. Env. Cont. Tox. 10: 57 - 63, 1973.

J. F. Young and T. J. Haley. A pharmacokinetic study of pentachlorophenol poisoning and the effect of forced diuresis. Clin. Tox. 12: 41 - 48, 1978.

Plasma and Urine Pentachlorophenol by Electron-Capture Gas Chromatography

Principle:

Pentachlorophenol is extracted from the acidified specimen with benzene. Diazomethane is used to form the methyl ether of pentachlorophenol and the derivative is analyzed by electron-capture gas chromatography.

Reagents:

Stock solution — 1 mg/mL pentachlorophenol in methanol
Plasma standards — 0.1, 1, 10 and 50 mg/L
Urine standards — 0.1, 1, 10 and 50 mg/L
Benzene
Sulfuric acid — conc. H_2SO_4
Diazomethane reagent — add 0.5 g N-methyl-N′-nitro-N-nitrosoguanidine slowly in small increments to a mixture of 25 mL hexane and 2 mL 20% NaOH in a flask; decant the hexane layer and store frozen for up to one week (prepare in well-ventilated hood)
Isooctane

Instrumental Conditions:

Gas chromatograph with electron-capture detector
1.8 m x 2 mm i.d. glass column containing 4% OV-1 and 6% QF-1 on 80/100 mesh Chromosorb W
Injector, 220° C.; column, 190° C.; detector, 280° C.
Nitrogen flow rate, 85 mL/min

Procedure:

1. Transfer 2 mL plasma or urine to a 15 mL screw-cap tube. Add 6 mL benzene and 2 drops conc. H_2SO_4 and place on a tilted rotator for 2 hours at 50 rpm.
2. Centrifuge and transfer 3 mL of the benzene layer to a 10 mL volumetric flask. Add 200 μL diazomethane reagent and allow to stand for 15 min.
3. Remove excess diazomethane by bubbling nitrogen through the solution until the yellow color disappears.
4. Dilute to 10 mL with isooctane and inject 2 - 8 μL into the gas chromatograph.

	Retention time (min)
pentachlorophenol derivative	2.2

Calculation:

Calculation is based on a response factor derived from a standard curve. A quality control specimen containing 10 mg/L pentachlorophenol is analyzed daily.

Evaluation:

Sensitivity: 0.01 mg/L
Linearity: 0.1 - 50 mg/L
C.V.: 1 - 7%
Relative recovery: 89 - 99%

Interferences:

Normal plasma and urine components do not interfere with the assay. The use of excess diazomethane solution can lead to interferences due to reagent impurities.

PHENOL

Occurrence and Usage. Phenol is used commercially as a disinfectant and as an intermediate in chemical syntheses. Exposure may occur by inhalation of the vapor, by cutaneous absorption or by oral ingestion. The current threshold limit value is 5 ppm (19 mg/m^3).

Blood Concentrations. Phenol is present as acid-labile conjugates in the serum of normal persons at an average level of 0.1 mg/L (Wengle and Hellstrom, 1972). The chemical has not been measured in the blood of occupationally exposed individuals.

Metabolism and Excretion. An oral dose of phenol is efficiently eliminated in the 24 hour urine as the sulfate and glucuronide conjugates, representing 77% and 16% of the dose, respectively (Capel et al., 1972). The excretory half-life of phenol has been variously reported to be 1 - 2 hours and 4.5 hours (Sherwood, 1972; Docter and Zielhuis, 1967).

A subject exposed to phenol vapor at a concentration of 24 mg/m^3 for 6 hours developed a total urine phenol level of 100 mg/L within 2 hours of the end of exposure (Piotrowski, 1971). Urine phenol concentrations of 100 - 400 mg/L have been observed in workers exposed to phenol at air concentrations of 4.2 - 12.5 mg/m^3 (Ohtsuji and Ikeda, 1972). By comparison, phenol levels in urine are generally less than 75 mg/L during worker exposure to 10 ppm of benzene, which yields phenol as a metabolite, and endogenous phenol in the urine of normal persons averages 5 - 10 mg/L (Docter and Zielhuis, 1967; Piotrowski, 1971).

Toxicity. Phenol causes severe irritation and corrosion on contact with skin or other tissue. Absorption of the chemical may produce cyanosis, shock, weakness, collapse, convulsions, liver and kidney damage, coma and death. Phenol is rapidly absorbed upon dermal contact; one subject developed a urine phenol concentration of 100 mg/L with 30 minutes of accidental dermal exposure to the substance (Sherwood, 1972).

Biological Monitoring. Piotrowski (1971) has found that the excretion rate of phenol in urine sampled during the last 2 hours of an exposure is proportional to the absorbed dose in an exposed worker. The absorbed dose (D) may be accurately calculated using the equation:

$$R = 0.44 + 0.108D$$

where R is the excretion rate of phenol in mg/hr. This equation corrects for the presence of endogenous phenol in urine, which is excreted at an average daytime rate of 0.44 mg/hr. Exposure to phenol at the current TLV of 19 mg/m^3 for 8 hours results in the absorption of 135 mg of the chemical and the excretion of phenol in urine (during the last 2 hours of exposure) at a rate of 15.3 mg/hr. Phenol does not appear to accumulate in the body with repeated exposure, since morning pre-exposure urine specimens are not elevated in phenol content over normal values even after a week of exposure (Ohtsuji and Ikeda, 1972).

Analysis. Procedures involving both colorimetry and gas chromatography for the analysis of total phenol in urine specimens were presented in the section on benzene (p. 37).

References

I. D. Capel, M. R. French, P. Millburn et al. The fate of (^{14}C) phenol in various species. Xenobiotica 2: 25 - 34, 1972.

H. J. Docter and R. L. Zielhuis. Phenol excretion as a measure of benzene exposure. Ann. Occ. Hyg. 10: 317 - 326, 1967.

H. Ohtsuji and M. Ikeda. Quantitative relationship between atmospheric phenol vapour and phenol in the urine of workers of Bakelite factories. Brit. J. Ind. Med. 29: 70-73, 1972.

J. K. Piotrowski. Evaluation of exposure to phenol: absorption of phenol vapour in the lungs and through the skin and excretion of phenol in urine. Brit. J. Ind. Med. 28: 172 - 178, 1971.

R. J. Sherwood. Benzene: the interpretation of monitoring results. Ann. Occ. Hyg. 15: 409 - 421, 1972.

B. Wengle and K. Hellstrom. Volatile phenols in serum of uraemic patients. Clin. Sci. 43: 493 - 498, 1972.

POLYBROMINATED BIPHENYLS

Occurrence and Usage. Polybrominated biphenyls (PBB), usually with 4-8 bromine atoms per molecule, are used commercially as fire retardants. One such mixture, consisting primarily of 2,2′,4,4′,5,5′-hexabromobiphenyl, was inadvertently added to cattle feed in Michigan, leading to widespread contamination. The compounds are believed to be well absorbed after ingestion or dermal contact. There is no assigned threshold limit value for the polybrominated biphenyls.

Blood Concentrations. In a study conducted in 1976 - 1977, a group of unexposed farmers had nearly uniformly undetectable serum PBB concentrations, while Michigan farmers and consumers showed concentrations ranging from undetectable to greater than 100 μg/L, with most in the 1 - 5 μg/L range (Anderson et al., 1979). Serum PBB levels ranged from 1 - 1530 μg/L in 14 workers at a PBB production plant (Wolff et al., 1979).

Metabolism and Excretion. PBB metabolites have not been identified in man. The compounds are very lipid soluble and tend to accumulate in fat with continued exposure. In rats, hexabromobiphenyl is apparently not metabolized; it primarily localizes in adipose tissue and is excreted very slowly over a 42 day period in urine (0.1%) and feces (6.6%). It was estimated that less than 10% of a single dose would be excreted by a rat in its lifetime (Matthews et al., 1977).

PBB concentrations in adipose tissue of most members of the general population are below detectable levels, but in 1975 averaged 226 μg/kg in urban residents of Michigan, 516 μg/kg in non-quarantined farmers and 1965 μg/kg in quarantined farmers. After 1974, fat PBB levels were found to decline by an average of 39% (range 11 - 72) in 16 persons over a six-month period. No consistent relationship was found between PBB concentrations in fat and serum. The ratio of PBB in fat to that in breast milk averaged about 2 (Meester and McCoy, 1977; Meester, 1979).

Toxicity. Symptoms observed in persons exposed to PBB in their diets have included fatigue, joint pain and stiffness, headache, muscle pain, dizziness, sleepiness and skin rash. Abnormal serum enzyme levels suggestive of liver damage were especially noted in farmers whose serum PBB concentrations exceeded 1 μg/L, and a positive correlation was noted between serum PBB concentrations and urinary porphyrin excretion (Anderson et al., 1979; Meester, 1979). Animals severely poisoned by PBB developed anorexia, alopecia, abnormal growth of the hooves, fatty metamorphosis of the liver, and kidney damage (Meester and McCoy, 1977).

Biological Monitoring. Exposure to PBB may be evaluated by determination of PBB concentrations in serum or biopsy fat. Serum concentrations greater than 0.2 μg/L or fat concentrations greater than 100 μg/kg are indicative of significant absorption of PBB. Serum PBB levels in excess of 1 μg/L are associated with a 14% incidence of abnormal serum SPGT values.

Analysis. A procedure is presented for the analysis of hexabromobiphenyl, the major component of a commercial PBB mixture, in serum utilizing electron-capture gas chromatography (Burse et al., 1979).

References

H. A. Anderson, M. S. Wolff, R. Lilis et al. Symptoms and clinical abnormalities following ingestion of polybrominated-biphenyl-contaminated food products. Ann. N.Y. Acad. Sci. 320: 684 - 702, 1979.

V. W. Burse, L. L. Needham, J. A. Liddle et al. Interlaboratory comparison for results of analyses for polybrominated biphenyls in human serum. J. Anal. Tox. 4: 22 - 26, 1980.

H. B. Matthews, S. Kato, N. M. Morales and D. B. Tuey. Distribution and excretion of 2,4,5,2′,4′,5′-hexabromobiphenyl, the major component of firemaster BP-6. J. Tox. Env. Health 3: 599 - 605, 1977.

W. D. Meester and D. J. McCoy, Sr. Human toxicology of polybrominated biphenyls. In *Management of the Poisoned Patient* (B. H. Rumack and A. R. Temple, eds.), Science Press, Princeton, 1977, pp. 32 - 61.

W. D. Meester. The effect of polybrominated biphenyls on man: the Michigan PBB disaster. Vet. Hum. Tox. 21: 131 - 135, 1979.

M. S. Wolff, H. A. Anderson, K. D. Rosenman and I. J. Selikoff. Equilibrium of polybrominated biphenyl (PBB) residues in serum and fat of Michigan residents. Bull. Env. Cont. Tox. 21: 775 - 781, 1979.

Serum Hexabromobiphenyl by Electron-Capture Gas Chromatography

Principle:

Hexabromobiphenyl and its isomers are extracted from serum with an organic solvent mixture. The extract is purified by passage through a Florisil column. After concentration of the eluate, an aliquot is analyzed by electron-capture gas chromatography. Calculation is based on the peak height of the predominant polybrominated biphenyl isomer.

Reagents:

Stock solution — 1 mg/mL Firemaster FF-1 PBB mixture (U.S. Food and Drug Administration) in methanol

Serum standards — 1, 5, 10, 20 and 50 μg/L (prepare fresh)

Methanol (nanograde)

Extraction solvent — hexane/ethyl ether, 1:1

Hexane (nanograde)

Florisil column — 1.6 g Florisil (activated by heating at 130° C. for 16 hours) in a 6 mm i.d. glass column topped with 0.5 g anhydrous Na_2SO_4 and washed with 12 mL hexane

Instrumental Conditions:

Gas chromatograph with electron-capture detector
1.8 m x 2 mm i.d. glass column containing 1% OV-101 on 100/120 mesh Gas Chrom Q
Injector, 250° C.; column, 235° C.; detector, 300° C.
Nitrogen flow rate, 20 mL/min

Procedure:

1. Transfer 2 mL serum to a 15 mL screw-cap tube. Add 1 mL methanol and vortex briefly.
2. Extract three times with 5 mL extraction solvent by placing on a rotary mixer for 10 min at 50 rpm. Centrifuge each time and transfer the upper organic layer to a clean tube.
3. Evaporate the combined extracts to approximately 0.5 mL under a stream of nitrogen at 50° C. Apply this concentrate to the Florisil column, using additional extraction solvent to rinse the tube.
4. Elute the PBB by adding three 5 mL portions of hexane to the column. Collect the eluate and evaporate to 1.0 mL under a stream of nitrogen at 50° C.
5. Inject 5 μL of the concentrated extract into the gas chromatograph.

	Retention time (min)
hexabromobiphenyl	6.8

Calculation:

Calculation is based on a standard curve prepared each time an analysis is performed. This procedure cannot be controlled by the usual methods due to the instability of dilute PBB solutions.

Evaluation:

Sensitivity: <1 μg/L
Linearity: 1 - 100 μg/L
C.V.: 2.2 - 10.0%
Relative recovery: 95 - 99%

Interferences:

None have been reported.

POLYCHLORINATED BIPHENYLS

Occurrence and Usage. The polychlorinated biphenyls (PCB) were produced in the United States from 1929 until 1977 for use as coolant and insulator fluids for transformers and capacitors, as heat transfer fluids and as flame retardants for wood products. Their manufacture continues in a number of European countries. The substances are extremely persistent and heavy industrial usage has led to widespread contamination of the environment. The current FDA limit for PCB in edible freshwater fish is 5 mg/kg, although examples of certain species have been found to contain as much as 900 mg/kg. Exposure can be dietary or by inhalation, dermal contact or ingestion in occupational situations. The current threshold limit value is 1 mg/m^3 for PCB containing 42% chlorine and 0.5 mg/m^3 for mixtures containing 54% chlorine.

Blood Concentrations. PCB residues were found in 43% of 616 plasma specimens from residents of the southeastern United States, in concentrations up to 29 $\mu g/L$ (Finklea et al., 1972). These levels ranged from 1.8 - 3.8 $\mu g/L$ in the blood of 10 members of the Japanese population in 1975 (Fukano and Doguchi, 1977). Blood PCB levels were observed to increase by 50% in two volunteers within several hours after the ingestion of a fish meal containing 128 - 181 μg of PCB (Kuwabara et al., 1979).

Metabolism and Excretion. The metabolism of the PCB isomers has not been studied in humans. In animals, the compounds are biotransformed by oxidation and dechlorination, and the hydroxylated metabolites and their conjugates are excreted in urine, feces and milk. The rate of metabolism of each isomer is a function of the number and position of chlorine atoms; the fully chlorinated compound, decachlorobiphenyl, is apparently not metabolized. All of the PCB isomers are highly lipid soluble and tend to accumulate in adipose tissue with repeated exposure (NIOSH, 1977). The extent of elimination of an isomer is a function of its rate of metabolism such that the more highly chlorinated compounds are extremely long-lived in mammals (Matthews and Anderson, 1975).

Of 637 specimens of adipose tissue obtained from members of the U.S. population, 69% contained less than 1 mg/kg of PCB, 26% contained from 1 - 2 mg/kg and 5%, more than 2 mg/kg (Yobs, 1972). In 30 Japanese citizens, these levels averaged 1.0 mg/kg and ranged from 0.4 - 2.5 mg/kg (Fukano and Doguchi, 1977).

Toxicity. Workers exposed to PCB air concentrations of only 0.1 mg/m^3 have developed skin irritation characterized by an acneform eruption (chloracne). In 34 workers, air concentrations of up to 2.2 mg/m^3 have produced skin irritation, nausea and an average blood PCB level of 400 $\mu g/L$ (Ouw et al., 1976). In a study of 326 capacitor manufacturing workers, the most prevalent symptoms of PCB exposure were the dermatologic effects together with such neurologic effects as headache, nervousness, fatigue and dizziness; these workers had total PCB concentrations in plasma which averaged 172 μg/L and ranged up to 2530 μg/L. A positive correlation was found between plasma PCB level and plasma SGOT concentration (Fischbein et al., 1979).

A mass poisoning in Japan which affected nearly 2000 persons has been attributed to the dietary use of PCB-contaminated rice oil. The symptoms of the disease, known as Yusho, includes those mentioned above as well as brown pigmentation of the skin and nails, increased eye secretions, weakness, swelling of the joints and numbness in the extremities. The average blood PCB concentration in 72 of these patients was 5.9 μg/L (Urabe et al., 1979), and in 6 other patients the PCB fat concentration ranged from 0.7 - 4.3 mg/kg (Masuda et al., 1974). These concentrations are relatively low and it has been suggested that polychlorinated dibenzofurans also present in the Japanese oil contributed significantly to the toxic effects observed in these patients (Fischbein et al., 1979).

Biological Monitoring. The extent of exposure to PCB may be estimated by measuring the PCB concentration of blood, plasma or adipose tissue. Most of the industrial experience in the United States has been with plasma PCB concentrations, which appear to relate well to the degree and duration of worker exposure. Plasma PCB levels which exceed 2 - 4 μg/L are indicative of significant exposure to PCB, although the possible contribution of non-occupational exposure should be assessed when elevated plasma levels are present. Ouw et al. (1976) suggested 200 μg/L PCB in blood as an upper acceptable limit for occupationally exposed individuals.

Analysis. Plasma PCB levels may be estimated by electron-capture gas chromatography, using a commercial PCB mixture as a standard (Doguchi and Fukano, 1975).

References

M. Doguchi and S. Fukano. Residue levels of polychlorinated terphenyls, polychlorinated biphenyls and DDT in human blood. Bull. Env. Cont. Tox. 13: 57 - 63, 1975.

J. Finklea, L. E. Priester, J. P. Creason et al. Polychlorinated biphenyl residues in human plasma expose a major urban pollution problem. Am. J. Pub. Health 62: 645 - 651, 1972.

A. Fischbein, M. S. Wolff, R. Lilis et al. Clinical findings among PCB-exposed capacitor manufacturing workers. Ann. N.Y. Acad. Sci. 320: 703 - 714, 1979.

S. Fukano and M. Doguchi. PCT, PCB and pesticide residues in human fat and blood. Bull. Env. Cont. Tox. 17: 613 - 617, 1977.

K. Kuwabara, T. Kakushiji, I. Watanabe et al. Increase in the human blood PCB levels promptly following ingestion of fish containing PCBs. Bull. Env. Cont. Tox. 21: 273 - 278, 1979.

Y. Masuda, R. Kagawa, and M. Kuratsune. Comparison of polychlorinated biphenyls in Yusho patients and ordinary persons. Bull. Env. Cont. Tox. 11: 213 - 216, 1974.

H. B. Matthews and M. W. Anderson. Effect of chlorination on the distribution and excretion of polychlorinated biphenyls. Drug Met. Disp. 3: 371 - 380, 1975.

NIOSH. *Occupational Exposure to Polychlorinated Biphenyls (PCBs),* National Institute for Occupational Safety and Health, Cincinnati, Ohio, 1977.

H. K. Ouw, G. R. Simpson and D. W. Siyali. Use and health effects of Aroclor 1242, a polychlorinated biphenyl, in an electrical industry. Arch. Env. Health 31: 189 - 194, 1976.

H. Urabe, H. Koda and M. Asahi. Present state of Yusho patients. Ann. N.Y. Acad. Sci. 320: 273 - 276, 1979.

A. R. Yobs. Levels of polychlorinated biphenyls in adipose tissue of the general population of the nation. Env. Health Persp. 1: 79 - 81, 1972.

Plasma PCB by Electron-Capture Gas Chromatography

Principle:

PCB isomers are extracted from plasma with hexane following alkaline hydrolysis of the specimen. The extract is purified by passage through a silicic acid/ Florisil column, and the eluate is analyzed by electron-capture gas chromatography.

Reagents:

Stock solution — 1 mg/mL Arochlor 1260 (Environmental Protection Agency, Research Triangle Park, NC or Applied Science Labs) in methanol
Plasma standards — 10, 20, 50, 100 and 200 μg/L (prepare fresh)
Ethanol
Potassium hydroxide
Hexane (nanograde)
Concentrated sulfuric acid
Glass column packed to contain 1 g each of silicic acid, Florisil and anhydrous Na_2SO_4 in that order

Instrumental Conditions:

Gas chromatograph with electron-capture detector
2 m x 3 mm i.d. glass column containing 2% OV-1 on 80/100 mesh Gas Chrom Q
Injector, 225° C.; column, 200° C.; detector, 250° C.
Nitrogen flow rate, 30 mL/min

Procedure:

1. Transfer 5 mL plasma to a 50 mL glass-stoppered centrifuge tube, add 20 mL ethanol and vortex. Add 5 g KOH and heat at 90° C. for one hour.
2. Cool and extract the solution twice with 20 mL portions of hexane. Centrifuge each time and transfer the hexane extracts to a 100 mL separatory funnel.
3. Carefully add 20 mL conc. H_2SO_4 to the funnel and gently shake. Discard the lower aqueous layer.
4. Pass the hexane layer through the clean-up column and add an additional 60 mL hexane, collecting the eluate.

5. Evaporate the total eluate to 1.0 mL at 60° C. under a stream of nitrogen and inject 5 μL into the chromatograph. Record the 10 - 14 major PCB isomers which elute over a period of about 20 minutes.

Calculation:

Quantitation is performed by comparing the peak heights of one or more representative peaks in the chromatogram of the sample with those of corresponding peaks in the standards. This procedure cannot be controlled by the usual methods due to the instability of PCB in dilute solutions.

Evaluation:

Sensitivity: 1 μg/L
Linearity: 5 - 200 μg/L
C.V.: not established
Relative recovery: not established

Interferences:

Many of the organochlorine pesticides have retention times similar to those of PCB isomers; it is therefore preferable to base quantitation on several of the major PCB peaks in order to reduce the inaccuracy caused by interfering compounds. The equipment used for blood collection and storage should be checked for the presence of interfering substances. If a sample of the actual PCB mixture to which workers are exposed is available, this should be used as the analytical standard for the method. Quantitation is most accurate when recent exposure is involved, since the passage of time results in metabolism of some of the PCB isomers and a shift in the chromatographic pattern of the plasma extract away from that of the standard.

SELENIUM

Occurrence and Usage. Selenium is produced largely as a by-product of copper refining. It has numerous applications in industry, including its use in electronic semiconductors, as a decolorizer for ceramics and glass, a vulcanizing agent for rubber and an antidandruff agent in shampoos. It is considered an essential trace element and is supplied in the diet at an average rate of 60 - 150 μg/day. The current threshold limit value for occupational exposure to selenium, as the metal or its compounds, is 0.2 mg/m^3.

Blood Concentrations. Selenium concentrations in the blood and plasma of 250 normal subjects have been found to average 0.182 mg/L and 0.144 mg/L, respectively, by neutron activation analysis (Dickson and Tomlinson, 1967). In a study of 210 residents of various areas of the United States, blood selenium concentrations averaged 0.206 mg/L and ranged from 0.100 - 0.340 mg/L (Allaway et al., 1968). Blood selenium concentrations did not correlate with domestic water selenium content in a community where selenium levels in water (range 26 - 1800 μg/L) were substantially elevated over the U.S. standard of 10 μg/L (Valentine et al., 1978).

Metabolism and Excretion. The body burden of selenium in normal humans has been estimated to range from 13 - 20 mg, with the highest concentrations found in kidney, liver and spleen. Nearly all of the daily dietary intake of selenium can be accounted for in the daily urine (20 - 50 μg), feces (8 - 30 μg) and miscellaneous excreta (32 - 80 μg). The selenium body burden does not appear to increase with age (Schroeder et al., 1970).

In animals given relatively large doses of selenium, urinary and pulmonary excretion became increasingly important; from 50 - 80% of a dose may be excreted in urine, largely as trimethylselenonium ion, and up to 30% in the exhaled air, largely as dimethylselenium. These organic metabolites of selenium are formed regardless of the original nature of the selenium administered and are much less toxic than either selenite or selenate (Gunn et al, 1976).

Urine selenium concentrations have been found to range from undetectable to 150 μg/L (average 34) in normal persons, from 22 - 203 μg/L (average 79) in persons living in an area with high water selenium content, and from 120 - 350 μg/L in asymptomatic selenium workers. Urine concentrations of the metal correlate well with dietary intake and with air concentrations of selenium; the urine concentrations decline rapidly when exposure to selenium is curtailed (Glover, 1967; Glover, 1970; Valentine et al., 1978).

Toxicity. Selenium and its compounds cause irritation of the skin and mucous membranes on contact. Workers in a selenium plant exposed to air concentrations of 0.2 - 3.6 mg/m^3 and excreting urine containing up to 430 μg/L selenium had symptoms limited to garlic odor of the breath (probably due to *in vivo* formation of dimethylselenium), metallic taste, dermatitis and indigestion (Glover, 1967; Glover, 1970). Acute exposure to selenium fumes in a group of workers at a smelting plant produced irritation of the mucous membranes, headache, sore throat and, in one worker, severe dyspnea (Clinton, 1947).

Selenium which accumulates in certain plants growing in alkaline soil has been held responsible for a chronic disease in cattle known as "blind staggers," causing impaired vision, stumbling and respiratory distress. Alkaline disease in domestic animals is believed due to excessive amounts of selenium in feed, and is manifested by lameness, loss of hair and hoof malformation (Gunn et al., 1976).

Biological Monitoring. Both urine and hair have been found to contain selenium in amounts which are proportional to the extent of selenium intake as a result of dietary or occupational exposure (Valentine, 1978; Glover, 1967). Since hair is often subject to contamination in an industrial situation, urine is a preferred specimen for routine monitoring purposes. Glover (1970) has proposed a biological threshold limit value of 100 $\mu g/L$ selenium in the urine of exposed workers. This value is achieved when air selenium concentrations are restricted to 0.1 mg/m^3.

Analysis. Selenium in urine may be analyzed by atomic absorption spectrometry using the hydride generation technique described for antimony (p. 27), with the spectrometer wavelength set to 196.0 nm. The sensitivity of this procedure is about 2 $\mu g/L$.

Alternatively, a method is presented for determination of urinary selenium by fluorimetry (Olson et al., 1973), which offers a sensitivity of 20 $\mu g/L$.

References

W. H. Allaway, J. Kubota, F. Losee and M. Roth. Selenium, molybdenum, and vanadium in human blood. Arch. Env. Health 16: 342 - 348, 1968.

M. Clinton, Jr. Selenium fume exposure. J. Ind. Hyg. Tox. 29: 225-226, 1947.

R. C. Dickson and R. H. Tomlinson. Selenium in blood and human tissues. Clin. Chim. Acta 16: 311 - 321, 1967.

J. R. Glover. Selenium in human urine: a tentative maximum allowable concentration for industrial and rural populations. Ann. Occ. Hyg. 10: 3 - 14, 1967.

J. R. Glover. Selenium and its industrial toxicology. Ind. Med. 39: 50 - 54, 1970.

O. E. Olson, I. S. Palmer and E. I. Whitehead. Determination of selenium in biological materials. Meth. Biochem. Anal. 21: 39 - 78, 1973.

H. A. Schroeder, D. V. Frost and J. J. Balassa. Essential trace metals in man: selenium. J. Chron. Dis. 23: 227 - 243, 1970.

J. L. Valentine, H. K. Kang and G. H. Spivey. Selenium levels in human blood, urine, and hair in response to exposure via drinking water. Env. Res. 17: 347 - 335, 1978.

Urine Selenium by Fluorescence Spectrophotometry

Principle:

Urine is digested to destroy the organic constituents and the digest is heated with hydrochloric acid to convert selenium to the tetravalent state. A fluorescent complex is formed with diaminonaphthalene and extracted into cyclohexane. The fluorescence of the extract is measured in a spectrophotofluorometer.

Reagents:

Stock solution — 1 mg/mL selenium ion (Fisher reference standard)
Aqueous standards — 20, 50 and 100 μg/L (prepare fresh)
Concentrated nitric acid
70% Perchloric acid
20% Hydrochloric acid
5 mol/L Ammonium hydroxide
EDTA solution — slowly add 5 mol/L NH_4OH to a suspension of 4 g ethylenediaminetetracetic acid in 20 mL water until the solid dissolves; further add 100 mL water and 12 g NH_2OH . HCl, stir to dissolve and adjust the final volume to 500 mL with water
Cresol red indicator — add 1 drop 5% NaOH to 20 mg cresol red and mix; dissolve in 100 mL water
0.1 mol/L Hydrochloric acid
DAN solution — in a darkened room, dissolve 100 mg 2,3-diaminonaphthalene in 100 mL 0.1 mol/L HCl; incubate at 50° C. for 15 min, cool to room temperature and extract twice with 10 mL cyclohexane, discarding extracts; filter through wet filter paper and use immediately (prepare fresh at step 5 of procedure)

Instrumental Conditions:

Fluorescence spectrophotometer set to excite at 370 nm
Measure fluorescence at 525 nm

Procedure:

1. Transfer 3 mL urine to a 30 mL Kjeldahl flask and add 10 mL conc. HNO_3 and a glass bead. Boil gently for 10 - 15 minutes.
2. Carefully add 2 mL 70% $HClO_4$ and continue heating until white fumes appear. If the solution darkens upon cooling, add additional HNO_3 and heat again until all HNO_3 is eliminated.
3. Cool the solution and add 1 mL water and 1 mL 20% HCl. Heat for 30 minutes in a boiling water bath and allow to cool.
4. Add 5 mL EDTA solution and 2 drops of cresol red indicator. Add 5 mol/L NH_4OH with mixing to a yellow color and 20% HCl to an orange-pink color.

5. In a semidarkened room, or in yellow light, prepare the DAN solution and add 5 mL to the flask. Place in a 50° C. water bath for 25 min and cool to room temperature.
6. Transfer the solution to a 125 mL separatory funnel, rinsing with 5 - 10 mL water. Extract by shaking for 30 seconds with 10 mL cyclohexane.
7. Allow layers to separate and discard the lower aqueous layer. Wash the cyclohexane by shaking twice with 25 mL portions of 0.1 mol/L HCl, discarding the washings.
8. Transfer the cyclohexane to a 12 mL centrifuge tube and centrifuge to clarify. Decant the cyclohexane into a cuvette and read against a reagent blank in the fluorometer.

Calculation:

Calculation is based on a standard curve prepared each time an analysis is performed. This procedure cannot be controlled by the usual methods due to the instability of selenium in dilute solutions.

Evaluation:

Sensitivity: 20 μg/L
Linearity: 20 - 150 μg/L
C.V.: <4%
Relative recovery: 101%

Interferences:

No major interferences were observed from other inorganic ions normally present in biological materials. The loss of selenium during the digestion process is very low and is reproducible.

STYRENE

Occurrence and Usage. Styrene (phenylethylene, vinylbenzene) is used as an intermediate for chemical synthesis, a solvent for synthetic resins and in the manufacture of polymeric plastics. The compound is volatile (b.p. 146° C.) and is readily absorbed following inhalation or dermal contact. The current threshold limit value for styrene in the industrial atmosphere is 100 ppm (420 mg/m^3), although this level is pending revision to 50 ppm.

Blood Concentrations. Three volunteers exposed to styrene at an air concentration of approximately 50 ppm for 1 hour developed blood styrene concentrations of 0.2 - 0.7 mg/L; exposure to approximately 100 ppm for 8 hours produced maximal blood concentrations of 0.9 - 1.4 mg/L (Stewart et al., 1968).

Metabolism and Excretion. Styrene is extensively metabolized in man by oxidation of the vinyl sidechain. Mandelic acid and phenylglyoxylic acid are produced as major metabolites and represent 85% and 10%, respectively, of an inhaled dose of styrene as urinary excretion products. About 1 - 2% of a dose is exhaled unchanged. The half-life of styrene as determined by mandelic acid excretion is 4 - 7 hours, whereas by excretion in breath it varies from 1 - 7 hours (Bardodej and Bardodejova, 1970; Stewart et al., 1968). Other authors have found that mandelic acid elimination follows biphasic kinetics, with an initial half-life of 4 hours and a terminal half-life of 25 hours (Guillemin and Bauer, 1979); this model is consistent with the known prolonged storage of styrene in body fat (Engstrom et al., 1978). Hippuric acid may be a minor metabolite of styrene in man (Ikeda et al., 1974).

Mandelic acid concentrations in the urine of exposed workers have ranged from physiological levels (<5 mg/L) to as high as 3000 mg/L. The concentrations tend to increase during the exposure period and usually reach a peak within an hour after the end of exposure. Phenylglyoxylic acid concentrations are often one-sixth to one-half of the mandelic acid concentrations (Piotrowski, 1977). Breath styrene concentrations average about 25% of the corresponding air styrene concentration during constant exposure, but decline very rapidly after cessation of exposure (Stewart et al., 1968).

Toxicity. At lower atmospheric levels, styrene produced irritation of the mucous membranes. The substance is absorbed upon dermal contact and may cause dermatitis (Dutkiewicz and Tyras, 1968). Higher concentrations cause central nervous system depression, nausea, headache and fatigue. Organ toxicity due to chronic exposure is rare, although the compound is potentially hepatotoxic on the basis of its metabolism to an epoxide intermediate (Leibman, 1975).

Biological Monitoring. The urinary concentrations of the two primary styrene metabolites have been used more or less successfully as indices to the extent of styrene exposure. Most investigators agree that the metabolite concentrations in urine taken immediately after an 8 hour exposure correlate well with the average styrene air concentration, as long as the latter does not exceed 150 ppm.

In workers exposed to the current TLV of 100 ppm, mandelic acid concentrations average 2300 mg/g creatinine (Engstrom et al., 1976) or 3000 mg/L (Harkonen et al., 1974). At a level of 50 ppm, this concentration is about 1000 mg/L (Gotell et al., 1972). Phenylglyoxylic acid concentrations during exposure to 100 ppm styrene should not exceed 350 mg/g creatinine (Lauwerys, 1975). Mandelic acid derivatives are used as antispasmodic and vasodilator drugs and can produce urinary mandelic acid and phenylglyoxylic acid concentrations similar to those seen after styrene exposure (Schaller et al., 1977).

The measurement of blood styrene concentrations has also been proposed as a routine monitoring technique (Astrand et al., 1974).

Analysis. A gas chromatographic procedure for measurement of mandelic acid and phenylglyoxylic acid in urine was presented in the section on ethylbenzene (p. 138). Urine specimens should be analyzed or frozen immediately after collection to avoid a steady loss of phenylglyoxylic acid by spontaneous decarboxylation.

References

I. Astrand, A. Kilbom, P. Ovrum et al. Exposure to styrene. Work Env. Health. 11: 69 - 85, 1974.

Z. Bardodej and E. Bardodejova. Biotransformation of ethyl benzene, styrene, and alpha-methylstyrene in man. Am. Ind. Hyg. Asso. J. 31: 206 - 209, 1970.

T. Dutkiewicz and H. Tyras. Skin absorption of toluene, styrene, and xylene by man. Brit. J. Ind. Med. 25: 243, 1968.

K. Engstrom, H. Harkonen, P. Kalliokoski and J. Rantanen. Urinary mandelic acid concentration after occupational exposure to styrene and its use as a biological exposure test. Scand. J. Work Env. Health 2: 21 - 26, 1976.

J. Engstrom, R. Bjurstrom, J. Astrand and P. Ovrum. Uptake, distribution and elimination of styrene in man. Scand J. Work Env. Health 4: 315 - 323, 1978.

P. Gotell, O. Axelson and B. Lindelof. Field studies on human styrene exposure. Work Env. Health 9: 76-83, 1972.

M. P. Guillemin and D. Bauer. Human exposure to styrene. III. Elimination kinetics of urinary mandelic and phenylglyoxylic acids after single experimental exposure. Int. Arch. Occ. Env. Health 44: 249 - 263, 1979.

H. Harkonen, P. Kalliokoski, S. Hietala and S. Hernberg. Concentrations of mandelic and phenylglyoxylic acid in urine as indicators of styrene exposure. Work Env. Health 11: 162 - 169, 1974.

M. Ikeda, T. Imamura, M. Hayashi et al. Evaluation of hippuric, phenylglyoxylic and mandelic acids in urine as indices of styrene exposure. Int. Arch. Arbeitsmed. 32: 93 - 101, 1974.

R. Lauwerys. Biological criteria for selected industrial toxic chemicals: a review. Scand. J. Work Env. Health 1: 139 - 172, 1975.

K. C. Liebman. Metabolism and toxicity of styrene. Env. Health Persp. 11: 115 - 119, 1975.

J. K. Piotrowski. *Exposure Tests for Organic Compounds in Industrial Toxicology*, U.S. Government Printing Office, Washington, D.C., 1977, pp. 60 - 65.

K. H. Schaller, H. W. Schutz, G. V. Mallinckrodt et al. The qualitative and quantitative determination of mandelic acid in urine in clinical and occupational medical toxicology. Acta. Pharm. Tox. 41 (Suppl. 2): 230 - 238, 1977.

R. D. Stewart, H. C. Dodd, E. D. Baretta and A. W. Schaffer. Human exposure to styrene vapor. Arch. Env. Health 16: 656 - 662, 1968.

H. K. Wilson, J. Cocker, C. J. Purnell et al. The time course of mandelic and phenylglyoxylic acid excretion in workers exposed to styrene under model conditions. Brit. J. Ind. Med. 36: 235 - 237, 1979.

TETRACHLOROETHYLENE

Occurrence and Usage. Tetrachloroethylene (perchloroethylene) is widely used as a solvent, dry-cleaning agent and degreasing fluid. Pulmonary absorption constitutes the primary route of entry into the body under industrial conditions, although the liquid is also known to penetrate the intact skin. The current threshold limit value for tetrachloroethylene in the industrial atmosphere is 100 ppm (670 mg/m^3).

Blood Concentrations. Blood tetrachloroethylene concentrations in six subjects reached an average peak level of 2.6 mg/L at the end of a 3 hour exposure to 194 ppm of the vapor; the compound was rapidly cleared from the blood when the exposure ended and was not detectable (at a sensitivity limit of 1 mg/L) after 30 minutes (Stewart et al., 1961a). Blood concentrations were found to correlate with the atmospheric tetrachloroethylene concentration as well as the degree of physical activity of an individual (Monster et al., 1979).

Metabolism and Excretion. The disposition of tetrachloroethylene in man is poorly understood. Of an inhaled dose, about 25% is eliminated unchanged in the breath during the 40 hours after exposure and only a very minor amount through the skin (Bolanowska and Golacka, 1972). The biological half-life of the compound has been estimated from pulmonary excretion data as 72 hours (Guberan and Fernandez, 1974), and it is therefore likely that the major portion of a dose (at least 80%) is eventually exhaled unchanged. Urinary metabolites, consisting of trichloroacetic acid and an unknown compound, have been found to account for less than 3% of a dose over a 67 hour period (Ogata et al., 1971). Trichloroethanol as determined by colorimetry was thought to be a minor urinary metabolite (Ikeda and Ohtsuji, 1972), but other investigators using a gas chromatographic technique have not found this compound in human urine (Fernandez et al., 1976).

Alveolar breath concentrations of tetrachloroethylene approach 50% of the atmospheric concentration of the chemical during constant exposure (Guberan and Fernandez, 1974). In subjects exposed to 100 ppm of the vapor, breath concentrations average 15 ppm during the first hour after exposure, 8 ppm after 15 hours and 4.5 ppm after 71 hours (Stewart et al., 1961a; Stewart et al., 1970).

Chlorinated metabolites of tetrachloroethylene generally do not exceed concentrations of 100 mg/L in the urine of workers exposed to the vapor at air concentrations of up to 400 ppm (Ikeda et al., 1972).

Toxicity. Acute exposure to tetrachloroethylene may cause blistering of the skin on contact and symptoms of central nervous system depression, including confusion, irritability, nausea, numbness and coma, upon absorption of the compound into the body. Chronic exposure has been associated with peripheral neuropathy, chemical hepatitis and damage to liver, kidneys and spleen.

Tetrachloroethylene is known to cause hepatocellular carcinoma in mice and is suspected of being a human carcinogen (NIOSH, 1978).

Breath tetrachloroethylene concentrations of 85 - 110 ppm were measured shortly after accidental inhalation exposure to the chemical in two subjects who developed unconsciousness as a result; in one of these situations it was estimated that exposure to 1100 ppm of the vapor for 30 minutes had been sufficient to produce coma (Stewart, 1969; Stewart et al., 1961b). In experimental human exposures, it has been found that vapor concentrations of 1000 ppm may be tolerated for up to 1.5 hours, but that levels of 1500 ppm and above quickly produce faintness and dizziness (Carpenter, 1937).

Biological Monitoring. Urine concentrations of tetrachloroethylene metabolites appear to be of only limited usefulness in monitoring exposure to the chemical, inasmuch as the metabolic pathways are saturated at very low levels. The data of Ikeda et al. (1972) indicate that saturation takes place at a vapor concentration of about 50 ppm, and that above this level no correlation exists between urinary metabolites and vapor concentrations.

Breath concentrations of tetrachloroethylene measured after the end of exposure relate quite well to the amount of chemical absorbed, and possibly to the blood level as well. During chronic exposure, breath concentrations measured at the same time each day eventually increase on the order of only 20% over the initial level. Immediately after a 7 hour exposure to 100 ppm of the vapor, breath tetrachloroethylene concentrations average about 20 ppm (Piotrowski, 1977). Guberan and Fernandez (1974) have published a nomograph for determination of the average ambient tetrachloroethylene vapor level from the expired breath concentration, duration of exposure and time of sampling.

Blood concentrations have not been used in monitoring worker exposure, but may prove useful when a method of sufficient sensitivity is applied to their determination.

Analysis. Blood and breath concentrations of tetrachloroethylene may be measured using the gas chromatographic procedure described for benzene (p. 39). Methods for determination of trichloroacetic acid in urine are presented in the section on trichloroethylene (p. 261).

References

W. Bolanowska and J. Golacka. Absorption and excretion of tetrachloroethylene in humans under experimental conditions. Med. Prac. 23: 109 - 119, 1972.

C. P. Carpenter. The chronic toxicity of tetrachloroethylene. J. Ind. Hyg. Tox. 19: 323 - 336, 1937.

F. Fernandez, E. Guberan and J. Caperos. Experimental human exposures to tetrachloroethylene vapor and elimination in breath after inhalation. Am. Ind. Hyg. Asso. J. 37: 143 - 150, 1976.

E. Guberan and J. Fernandez. Control of industrial exposure to tetrachloroethylene by measuring alveolar concentrations: theoretical approach using a mathematical model. Brit. J. Ind. Med. 31: 159 - 167, 1974.

M. Ikeda and H. Ohtsuji. A comparative study of the excretion of Fujiwara reaction-positive substances in urine of humans and rodents given trichloro- or tetrachloro-derivatives of ethane and ethylene. Brit. J. Ind. Med. 29: 99 - 104, 1972.

M. Ikeda, H. Ohtsuji, T. Imamura and Y. Komoike. Urinary excretion of total trichloro-compounds, trichloroethanol, and trichloroacetic acid as a measure of exposure to trichloroethylene and tetrachloroethylene. Brit. J. Ind. Med. 29: 328 - 333, 1972.

A. C. Monster, G. Boersma and H. Steenweg. Kinetics of tetrachloroethylene in volunteers; influence of exposure concentration and work load. Int. Arch. Occ. Env. Health 42: 303 - 309, 1979.

NIOSH. *Current Intelligence Bulletin 20, Tetrachloroethylene,* National Institute for Occupational Safety and Health, Cincinnati, Ohio, January 20, 1978.

M. Ogata, Y. Takatsuka and K. Tomokuni. Excretion of organic chlorine compounds in the urine of persons exposed to vapours of trichloroethylene and tetrachloroethylene. Brit. J. Ind. Med. 28: 386 - 391, 1971.

J. K. Piotrowski. *Exposure Tests for Organic Compounds in Industrial Toxicology,* U. S. Government Printing Office, Washington, D.C., 1977, pp. 98 - 101.

R. D. Stewart, H. H. Gay, D. S. Erley et al. Human exposure to tetrachloroethylene vapor. Arch. Env. Health 2: 40 - 46, 1961a.

R. D. Stewart, D. S. Erley, A. W. Schaffer and H. H. Gay. Accidental vapor exposure to anesthetic concentrations of a solvent containing tetrachloroethylene. Ind. Med. Surg. 30: 327 - 330, 1961b.

R. D. Stewart. Acute tetrachloroethylene intoxication. J. Am. Med. Asso. 208: 1490 - 1492, 1969.

R. D. Stewart, E. D. Baretta, H. C. Dodd and T. R. Torkelson. Experimental human exposure to tetrachloroethylene. Arch. Env. Health 20: 224 - 229, 1970.

TETRAETHYLLEAD

Occurrence and Usage. Tetraethyllead is a volatile (b.p. 199° C.) and flammable liquid which is used to improve the octane rating of automotive and aviation gasoline. It is found in most premium grade fuels at a concentration not exceeding 0.1%. The compound slowly decomposes in the atmosphere to inorganic lead, although most atmospheric lead is derived from tetraethyllead which is oxidized in automotive engines and is discharged as inorganic lead salts. The average urban adult inhales 20 - 40 μg of lead daily, retaining 30 - 45%, and ingests about 300 μg in the diet, absorbing only 5 - 10%. The current threshold limit value for tetraethyllead is 0.100 mg/m^3. It is well absorbed after inhalation, ingestion or dermal contact.

Blood Concentrations. In healthy suburban adults, a range of 0.07 - 0.22 mg/L was observed for blood lead, 7 - 14% of which was derived from atmospheric sources (Manton, 1977). Blood lead concentrations in 104 healthy tetraethyllead workers averaged 0.43 mg/L (range 0.10 - 1.19) over an 8 - 10 year period (Robinson, 1976). Generally, 0.40 mg/L is considered the upper limit for blood lead levels in normal subjects.

Metabolism and Excretion. The disposition of tetraethyllead in man has been only briefly studied. The compound is quite lipid-soluble and is well distributed throughout the body, tending to localize in liver, kidney, brain and adipose tissue. Tetraethyllead is known to be slowly metabolized to triethyllead, to which is attributed the toxic effects of the parent compound. However, little is known about the extent of metabolism, further metabolic products or the kinetics of elimination (Kehoe, 1976). It is believed that eventually the alkyl compounds are converted to inorganic lead and largely excreted in urine.

Urinary lead concentrations averaged 0.04 mg/L (range 0.01 - 0.19) in 60 urban adult males (Barry, 1975) and 0.09 mg/L (range 0.03 - 0.17) in 153 healthy tetraethyllead workers (Robinson, 1976). Urine lead concentrations did not exceed 0.15 mg/L in workers exposed to an average atmospheric tetraethyllead level of 0.121 mg/m^3 (ACGIH, 1971).

Toxicity. Acute exposure to tetraethyllead causes symptoms of central nervous system toxicity which include insomnia, anxiety, lassitude, tremor, hallucinations, psychotic behavior and convulsions. Absorption of only 1 g of the chemical may be sufficient to cause death within 3 - 30 days due to the slow degradation of the compound to triethyllead. In intoxicated workers, blood lead concentrations are rarely elevated to significant levels yet urine lead concentrations generally exceed 0.2 mg/L (Fleming, 1964).

Numerous cases of acute and chronic poisoning due to the inhalation of tetraethyllead have occurred, usually as a result of accidental or intentional exposure to gasoline (Beattie et al., 1972; Boeckx et al., 1977; Hansen and Sharp, 1978; Robinson, 1978; Stasik et al., 1969). Subjects with chronic exposure may demonstrate symptoms of inorganic lead poisoning as well as the central nervous system effects of organic lead intoxication.

Biological Monitoring. The blood lead concentration is a relatively insensitive indicator of acute exposure to tetraethyllead. However, during gross overexposure or following chronic exposure to the compound, the level of inorganic lead in blood is markedly elevated.

The measurement of inorganic lead in urine is the most useful biologic parameter in monitoring tetraethyllead exposure. It has been proposed that a urine lead concentration exceeding 0.11 mg/L (corrected to a specific gravity of 1.024) be considered an indication of overexposure in workers, and that persons with urine concentrations exceeding 0.15 mg/L be removed from exposure (Hygienic Guide Series, 1963).

Analysis. Two methods for determination of lead in blood by atomic absorption spectrometry were presented in the section on lead (p. 159). These methods are also applicable to urine specimens.

References

ACGIH. *Documentation of the Threshold Limit Values,* American Conference of Governmental Industrial Hygienists, Cincinnati, Ohio, 1971, pp 251 - 252.

A. D. Beattie, M. R. Moore and A. Goldberg. Tetraethyl-lead poisoning. Lancet 2: 12 - 15, 1972.

R. L. Boeckx, B. Posti and F. J. Coodin. Gasoline sniffing and tetraethyl lead poisoning in children. Pediat. 60: 140 - 145, 1977.

A. J. Fleming. Industrial hygiene and medical control procedures. Arch. Env. Health 8: 266 - 270, 1964.

K. S. Hansen and F. R. Sharp. Gasoline sniffing, lead poisoning, and myoclonus. J. Am. Med. Asso. 240: 1375 - 1376, 1978.

Hygienic Guide Series. Tetraethyllead. Am. Ind. Hyg. Asso. J. 24: 423 - 426, 1963.

R. A. Kehoe. Pharmacology and toxicology of heavy metals: lead. Pharm. Ther. A. 1: 161 - 188, 1976.

W. I. Manton. Sources of lead in blood. Arch. Env. Health 32: 149 - 159, 1977.

T. R. Robinson. The health of long service tetraethyl lead workers. J. Occ. Med. 18: 31 - 40, 1976.

R. O. Robinson. Tetraethyl lead poisoning from gasoline sniffing. J. Am. Med. Asso. 240: 1373 - 1374, 1978.

M. Stasik, Z. Byczkowska, S. Szendzikowski and Z. Fiedorczuk. Acute tetraethyllead poisoning. Arch. Tox. 24: 283 - 291, 1969.

THALLIUM

Occurrence and Usage. Thallium salts are currently used as insecticides and rodenticides; the amount of the monovalent metal, usually as the sulfate, in these commercially available products is limited to 1% in the United States. Thallium also has a number of minor industrial uses, and has been employed externally as a dipilatory. It was once administered orally to children in doses of 8 mg/kg as the acetate salt to produce alopecia during treatment of ringworm of the scalp. The current threshold limit value for soluble thallium salts in the industrial atmosphere is 0.1 mg/m^3.

Blood Concentrations. In 320 young urban children, normal blood thallium concentrations averaged 0.003 mg/L, with a range of 0 - 0.080 mg/L; over 79% of the blood specimens contained less than 0.005 mg/L of thallium (Singh et al., 1975). The half-life of thallium in blood is approximately two days (Hologgitas et al., 1980).

Metabolism and Excretion. Thallium salts are well absorbed after inhalation, ingestion or dermal contact. When thallium was administered orally in small doses to an adult, it was found to localize primarily in the soft tissues with the highest concentrations in scalp hair, kidney and heart. Excretion was primarily via the kidney and proceeded at the rate of about 3% daily of the amount remaining in the body (Barclay et al., 1953). The slow elimination of thallium from the body has been attributed to a persistent cycle of intestinal secretion and reabsorption (Rauws, 1974). Following thallium overdosage, elimination is largely via the feces (Stevens et al., 1974). Thallium, if present in normal urine, is in concentrations of less than 0.002 mg/L (Kubasik and Volosin, 1973).

Toxicity. Many fatal and non-fatal poisonings have resulted from the medicinal, cosmetic and pesticidal application of thallium salts. Symptoms of intoxication include colic, nausea, vomiting, tremors and paralysis, with alopecia occurring only after a period of approximately 1 - 3 weeks. The average lethal dose in an adult is about 1 g of a soluble thallium salt. No single chelating agent has been shown to be especially effective in treating thallium poisoning although dithiocarb and Prussian blue have been shown to hasten excretion of the metal; trihexyphenidyl is frequently used to control tremors in victims. Blood thallium concentrations of 1.0 - 8.0 mg/L and urine concentrations of 1.8 - 20 mg/L have been measured 1 to 21 days after hospital admission in several young children who survived the poisoning episode (Grossman, 1955; Chamberlain et al., 1958; Stein and Perlstein, 1959; Taber, 1964; Arena et al., 1965). In 5 adults who survived the accidental or intentional ingestion of thallium sulfate, blood concentrations of 0.08 - 1.0 mg/L and urine concentrations of 1.4 - 4.1 mg/L were observed within 1 - 30 days after admission (Gettler and Weiss, 1943; Grunfeld and Hinostroza, 1964). Postmortem blood concentrations of 1.9 and 2.6 mg/L were determined in 2 adults who died 5 and 15 days after the intentional ingestion of 3.3 and 1.3 g, respectively, of thallium sulfate (Grunfeld and Hinostroza, 1964; van Peteghem, 1974).

Industrial exposure to excessive amounts of thallium has caused albuminuria, sensory changes, polyneuritis, speech impairment, weakness and visual disturbances to the point of permanent blindness. Workers who manifested symptoms of chronic thallium intoxication had urine thallium concentrations of 0.2 - 1.0 mg/L (Richeson, 1958).

Biological Monitoring. Investigations have not been conducted on urine thallium concentrations which are produced in persons exposed to thallium at the current TLV of 0.1 mg/m^3. However, the monitoring of urine thallium in exposed workers is recommended as a preventive measure, since any amount exceeding the normal limit of 0.005 mg/L is indicative of significant absorption of the metal.

Determination of thallium concentrations in both blood and urine has been found to be of value in the diagnosis and management of acute and chronic thallium poisoning.

Analysis. A procedure is presented for the analysis of thallium in blood and urine which utilizes atomic absorption spectrometry following chelation and extraction (Berman, 1967; Amore, 1974).

References

F. Amore. Determination of cadmium, lead, thallium, and nickel in blood by atomic absorption spectrometry. Anal. Chem. 46: 1597 - 1599, 1974.

J. M. Arena, G. A. Watson and S. S. Sakhadeo. Fatal thallium poisoning. Clin. Pediat. 4: 267 - 270, 1965.

R. K. Barclay, W. C. Peacock and D. A. Karnofsky. Distribution and excretion of radioactive thallium in the chick embryo, rat, and man. J. Pharm. Exp. Ther. 107: 178 - 187, 1953.

E. Berman. Determination of cadmium, thallium and mercury in biological materials by atomic absorption. At. Abs. Newsl. 6: 57 - 60, 1967.

P. H. Chamberlain, W. B. Stavinoha, H. Davis et al. Thallium poisoning. Pediat. 22: 1170 - 1182, 1958.

A. O. Gettler and L. Weiss. Thallium poisoning. III. Clinical toxicology of thallium. Am. J. Clin. Path. 13: 422 - 429, 1943.

H. Grossman. Thallotoxicosis. Report of a case and a review. Pediat. 16: 868 - 872, 1955.

O. Grunfeld and G. Hinostroza. Thallium poisoning. Arch. Int. Med. 114: 132 - 138, 1964.

J. Hologgitas, P. Ullucci, J. Driscoll et al. Thallium elimination kinetics in acute thallotoxicosis. J. Anal. Tox. 4: in press, 1980.

N. P. Kubasik and M. T. Volosin. A simplified determination of urinary cadmium, lead, and thallium, with use of carbon rod atomization and atomic absorption spectrophotometry. Clin. Chem. 19: 954 - 958, 1973.

A. G. Rauws. Thallium pharmacokinetics and its modification by Prussian blue. Naunyn-Schmiedeberg's Arch. Pharm. 284: 295 - 306, 1974.

E. M. Richeson. Industrial thallium intoxication. Ind. Med. Surg. 27: 607 - 619, 1958.

N. P. Singh, J. D. Bodgen and M. M. Joselow. Distribution of thallium and lead in children's blood. Arch. Env. Health 30: 557 - 558, 1975.

M. D. Stein and M. A. Perlstein. Thallium poisoning. Am. J. Dis. Child. 98: 80 - 85, 1959.

W. Stevens, C. van Peteghem, A. Heyndrickx and F. Barbier. Eleven cases of thallium intoxication treated with Prussian blue. Int. J. Clin. Pharm. 10: 1 - 22, 1974.
P. Taber. Chronic thallium poisoning: rapid diagnosis and treatment. J. Pediat. 65: 461 - 463, 1964.
C. van Peteghem. Personal communication, 1974.

Blood and Urine Thallium by Atomic Absorption Spectrometry

Principle:

Blood and urine are treated with diethyldithiocarbamate to chelate ionic thallium. The chelate is extracted into methylisobutylketone and the extract is analyzed by flame atomic absorption spectrometry.

Reagents:

Stock solution — 1 mg/mL thallium ion
Aqueous standards — 0.2, 0.5, 1.0, 2.0 and 4.0 mg/L (prepare fresh)
2.5 mol/L Sodium hydroxide
DDC solution — 1% sodium diethyldithiocarbamate in water
5% Triton X-100
MIBK — methylisobutylketone

Instrumental Conditions:

Atomic absorption spectrometer with air-acetylene oxidizing flame
Thallium hollow cathode lamp
Measure absorption at 276.7 nm

Procedure:

Blood:

1. Transfer 5 mL citrated or heparinized whole blood to a 15 mL screw-cap tube. Add 1 mL DDC solution and 1 mL 5% Triton X-100 and vortex.
2. Let stand for 10 min. Add 3 mL MIBK and shake to extract.
3. Centrifuge and aspirate the MIBK layer into the flame of the spectrometer. Compare to aqueous standards processed in the same manner.

Urine:

4. Transfer 5 mL urine to a 15 mL screw-cap tube. Adjust to pH 6.0 - 7.5 by adding 2.5 mol/L NaOH.
5. Add 1 mL DDC solution and vortex. Add 3 mL MIBK and shake to extract.
6. Centrifuge and aspirate the MIBK layer into the flame of the spectrometer. Compare to aqueous standards processed in the same manner.

Calculation:

Calculation is based on a standard curve prepared with each set of specimens. This procedure cannot be controlled by the usual methods due to the instability of thallium in dilute solutions.

Evaluation:

Sensitivity: 0.1 mg/L
Linearity: 0.2 - 4.0 mg/L
C.V.: 3 - 5% within-run
Relative recovery: not established

Interferences:

Normal biological fluids contain only trace amounts of thallium. Other metals do not interfere, but to prevent thallium contamination all glassware should be soaked overnight in 25% nitric acid and reagent blanks should be analyzed frequently. The use of EDTA as a blood anticoagulant causes a slight reduction in the recovery of thallium.

TIN

Occurrence and Usage. In man, tin is a trace element for which there is apparently no biological requirement. The metal and its inorganic salts have numerous applications in metallurgy and other industries, including their use as tanning agents, polishing compounds and metal coatings ("tin" cans). The organic compounds of tin, usually ethyl, butyl or phenyl derivatives, are widely used as fungicides, pesticides, antihelmintics and stabilizers for plastics. The current threshold limit values (expressed as Sn) for industrial usage are 10 mg/m^3 for tin oxide, 2 mg/m^3 for other inorganic compounds and 0.1 mg/m^3 for organic compounds of tin. The soluble compounds are well-absorbed after ingestion or inhalation, and the organic forms are known to be absorbed through the skin as well.

Blood Concentrations. The average concentration of tin in the blood of normal subjects is 0.14 mg/L, although not all specimens contain detectable amounts of the metal. Most or all of this amount, which resides primarily in the erythrocytes, is believed to originate in the daily diet. A typical daily diet contains 3.6 mg of tin, the major portion of which is derived from canned foods (Schroeder et al., 1964).

Metabolism and Excretion. Of an approximate 4 mg of tin which is ingested daily in the diet by urban adults, over 99% is excreted unabsorbed in the feces and less than 1% is eliminated in the urine. Tin accumulates to only a small extent in the body with age and when present in tissues, is rather randomly distributed. Lung, liver and kidney specimens from Americans usually contain from 0.2 - 1.2 mg/kg of the metal. Specimens from primitive peoples may contain little or none. Tin concentrations in the urine of Americans have been estimated to average 23 μg/L, with a range of 0 - 40 μg/L (Schroeder et al., 1964).

The organic forms of tin behave as liposoluble compounds and, unlike inorganic tin, are rapidly distributed to the central nervous system. The compounds are believed to undergo slow degradation via oxidative dealkylation (Barnes and Stoner, 1959).

Toxicity. Tin and its inorganic compounds are relatively nontoxic and are not considered important industrial hazards. Some of the compounds cause skin and mucous membrane irritation due to their acidity or alkalinity in aqueous solution. Exposure to tin oxide dust has caused benign pneumoconiosis in workers (Oyanguren et al., 1958; Schuler et al., 1958).

The organotin compounds, especially the tri- and tetraalkyl derivatives, present a more serious hazard. Exposure to these substances can cause local irritation, cerebral edema, hepatic necrosis and death. Severe skin lesions have been observed in workers exposed to butyl tin derivatives (Lyle, 1958). A clinical trial of a diethyltin preparation for the treatment of furunculosis ended in disaster when 217 subjects developed tin poisoning and 100 of these persons died. The medication, found to contain the more toxic triethyltin as an impurity, was administered orally in doses of 90 mg/day for 8 days. The symptoms of poisoning appeared after a period of 4 days and included persistent headache, vertigo, visual disturbances, abdominal pain, vomiting and psychic disturbances. The more severely poisoned subjects developed partial paralysis and convulsions and died of respiratory or cardiac failure. Interstitial edema of the white matter of the brain was a characteristic finding at autopsy (Barnes and Stoner, 1959). Similar effects were produced by trimethyltin in two subjects who survived the poisoning episode (Fortemps et al., 1978).

Biological Monitoring. It has been proposed that urinary tin concentrations be used as an index of exposure to and absorption of soluble forms of inorganic tin, although no studies have been performed to confirm the usefulness of this procedure (Lauwerys, 1975). Likewise, the excretion of organotin compounds in urine has not been investigated.

Analysis. A colorimetric method is presented for the determination of inorganic and organic compounds of tin in urine (Corbin, 1973).

References

J. M. Barnes and H. B. Stoner. The toxicology of tin compounds. Pharm. Rev. 11: 211 - 231, 1959.

H. B. Corbin. Rapid and selective pyrocatechol violet method for tin. Anal. Chem. 45: 534 - 537, 1973.

E. Fortemps, G. Amand, A. Bomboir et al. Trimethyltin poisoning: report of two cases. Int. Arch. Occ. Env. Health 41: 1 - 6, 1978.

R. Lauwerys. Biological criteria for selected industrial toxic chemicals: a review. Scand. J. Work Env. Health 1: 139 - 172, 1975.

W. H. Lyle. Lesions of the skin in process workers caused by contact with butyl tin compounds. Brit. J. Ind. Med. 15: 193 - 196, 1958.

H. Oyanguren, R. Haddad and H. Maass. Stannosis. I. Environmental and experimental studies. Ind. Med. Surg. 27: 427 - 431, 1958.

H. A. Schroeder, J. J. Balassa and I. H. Tipton. Abnormal trace metals in man: tin. J. Chron. Dis. 17: 483 - 502, 1964.

P. Schuler, E. Cruz, C. Guijon et al. Stannosis. II. Clinical study. Ind. Med. Surg. 27: 432 - 435, 1958.

Urine Tin by Colorimetry

Principle:

Urine samples are acid-digested to destroy organic matter and to oxidize organic and inorganic tin to the tetravalent form. Tin is converted to its tetraiodide, extracted into hexane and then returned to aqueous acid solution. Sensitized pyrocatechol violet is added and the resulting chromogenic complex is analyzed by colorimetry.

Reagents:

Stock solution — 1 mg/mL tin (Fisher reference standard)
Aqueous standards — 0.05, 0.10, 0.20, 0.50 and 1.00 mg/L (prepare fresh)
Concentrated sulfuric acid
Concentrated nitric acid
20% Potassium iodide
Hexane
Acid solution — 5% sulfuric acid and 2.5% citric acid
Standard tin solution — transfer 50 mL of the stock solution of tin to a 250 mL beaker; add 50 mL conc. H_2SO_4 and 5 mL conc. HNO_3 and heat until fumes of SO_3 are evolved; adjust the volume to about 50 mL with conc. H_2SO_4 and transfer to a 500 mL volumetric flask; rinse the beaker several times with water and add to the flask until the volume is about 250 mL; cool and add 100 mL of a 50% citric acid solution; finally dilute to 500 mL with water (prepare fresh)
5% Ascorbic acid (prepare fresh)
CTAB solution — 1.1 g cetyltrimethylammonium bromide in 100 mL water
Pyrocatechol violet solution — dissolve 45 mg pyrocatechol violet in about 10 mL of water in a 250 mL volumetric flask; add 5 mL CTAB solution and dilute to volume with water (prepare fresh)

All glassware used in this procedure should be soaked overnight in 30% nitric acid and rinsed in distilled-deionized water

Instrumental Conditions:

Visible spectrophotometer set to 660 nm
10 cm pathlength sample cell

Procedure:

1. Transfer 10 mL urine to a 250 mL flask and add 10 mL conc. H_2SO_4 and 15 mL conc. HNO_3. Heat gently, adding additional amounts of conc. HNO_3 as needed to destroy organic matter.
2. Heat solution until fumes of SO_3 are evolved and then cool. Add 20 mL water and 10 mL of 20% KI.
3. Transfer the solution to a 125 mL separatory funnel and extract with 30 mL of hexane. Allow the phases to separate and discard the lower aqueous layer.
4. Add 15 mL acid solution and 5 mL standard tin solution. Shake the funnel for 1 min, allow layers to separate and transfer the lower aqueous layer to a 50 mL volumetric flask.
5. Wash the hexane layer twice with 10 mL portions of water, adding each to the volumetric flask. Allow the solution in the flask to stand for at least 2 hours.
6. Add 2 mL 5% ascorbic acid, 5 mL pyrocatechol violet solution and adjust to volume with water. Mix, wait 30 min and determine the absorbance of the solution against a reagent blank.

Calculation:

Calculation is based on a standard curve of concentration (excluding the 5 μg of tin added to all samples) versus absorbance. This procedure cannot be controlled by the usual methods due to the instability of dilute tin solutions.

Evaluation:

Sensitivity: 0.05 mg/L
Linearity: 0.05 - 1.0 mg/L
C.V.: 8 - 10%
Relative recovery: 98 - 106%

Interferences:

The two step extraction procedure makes this method relatively specific for tin. However, very high concentrations of many other metals will produce positive interference and high concentrations of anions such as fluoride, chloride or phosphate will cause negative interference.

TOLUENE

Occurrence and Usage. Toluene (toluol) is an aromatic petroleum hydrocarbon which has many important commercial and industrial applications as a solvent and starting material for organic syntheses. It is present in numerous paints, paint thinners, glues, and other products likely to be found in the household. The acute narcotic effects of toluene are similar to those of benzene, although chronic toxicity is much less a problem. The current threshold limit value for atmospheric toluene is 100 ppm (375 mg/m^3). Industrial exposure generally occurs by inhalation of the vapor or dermal contact with the liquid.

Blood Concentrations. Blood toluene concentrations in workers exposed to air concentrations of 100 ppm for 2 hours can exceed 0.9 mg/L (Sato et al., 1975). Subjects exposed for 30 minutes to a level of 100 ppm toluene had blood concentrations which averaged 0.4 mg/L when resting and 1.2 mg/L during light exercise (Astrand et al., 1972).

Metabolism and Excretion. Approximately 80% of an absorbed dose of toluene is oxidized to benzoic acid, which is then conjugated with glucuronic acid or glycine and excreted in the urine. The glycine conjugate (hippuric acid) accounts for about 68% of a dose in the 24 hour urine, and has an excretion half-life of 2 - 3 hours. Glucuronic acid conjugation of the metabolically produced benzoic acid is relatively unimportant until large amounts of toluene are absorbed. Up to 20% of a dose is eliminated unchanged in the expired air and less than 0.1% in the urine (Piotrowski, 1977).

Urinary hippuric acid concentrations were found to average 0.8 g/L (range 0.4 - 1.4) in nonexposed persons (Pagnotto and Lieberman, 1967) and were found to parallel the intensity of the toluene exposure in industrial workers. For instance, workers exposed to an average daily level of 50 ppm developed urinary concentrations of 1.26 - 2.93 g/L (average 1.92) by late afternoon, and those exposed to 200 ppm had hippuric acid concentrations of 4.12 - 8.65 g/L (average 5.97). These urine values are uncorrected for specific gravity (Ikeda and Ohtsuji, 1969).

Alveolar air concentrations of toluene reach a plateau within 15 - 30 minutes after the start of an exposure and decline rapidly after cessation of exposure; in persons exposed to 100 ppm of toluene, these levels were found to average 18 ppm at rest, 31 ppm during light exercise and 38 ppm during moderate exercise (Astrand et al., 1972).

Toxicity. Concern over excessive exposure to toluene is based primarily on the acute depressant effects of the chemical rather than on any chronic or residual effects on organ systems (von Oettingen et al., 1942). Employee exposure to toluene vapor at concentrations of 200 - 500 ppm for several weeks produced symptoms of headache, nausea, lassitude, impairment of coordination and loss of memory; concentrations of 500 - 1500 ppm caused similar but more severe effects (Wilson, 1943). Exposure to air concentrations of 10,000 - 30,000 ppm of toluene may cause mental confusion, drunkenness and unconsciousness within a few minutes (Longley et al., 1967).

Toluene has been frequently abused for its intoxicating effects by teenagers or adults who inhale the vapors of paint and glue solvents. A report of 7 such persons who were either hospitalized or arrested while intoxicated showed blood toluene concentrations of 0.3 - 7.0 mg/L and urine concentrations of 0 - 5.0 mg/L (Bonnichsen et al., 1966). Two cases of long-term habituation to toluene were shown to result in electroencephalographic abnormalities, encephalopathy and one confirmed diagnosis of permanent cerebral atrophy (Satran and Dodson, 1963; Knox and Nelson, 1966). Another 6 persons who died as a result of accidental or intentional acute exposure to toluene fumes exhibited postmortem blood concentrations of 10 - 20 mg/L, averaging 13 mg/L (Bonnichsen et al., 1966; Collom and Winek, 1970; Bidanset, 1973; Luskus et al, 1977).

Biological Monitoring. Blood and breath concentrations of toluene measured during exposure correlate quite well to atmospheric toluene levels in subjects at rest, but this relationship varies according to the degree of physical activity. The determination of these concentrations has not yet found routine application in industrial chemical monitoring (Astrand et al., 1972; Piotrowski, 1977).

The measurement of hippuric acid in urine as an index to toluene exposure is widely practiced, although its usefulness is limited to evaluating moderate to heavy exposure, due to the relatively high and variable levels of endogenous urinary hippuric acid (up to 1.4 g/L). Using the spectrophotometric method of Pagnotto and Lieberman (1967), an exposure to 100 ppm of toluene would produce a urinary hippuric acid concentration of about 4 g/L in specimens collected at the end of a shift. The same exposure conditions using the more specific gas chromatographic method would produce a hippuric acid value of 2.8 - 3.5 g/L. Alternatively, the hippuric acid excretion rate, obtained from a timed specimen collected during the period from 4 hours after exposure has started to not more than 1 hour after exposure ends, has been shown to be a more accurate index of toluene exposure. The excretion rate should lie between 2.0 and 2.5 mg/min during exposure to 100 ppm of the vapor (Veulemans and Masschelein, 1979; Veulemans et al., 1979). NIOSH (1973) recommended that a level of 5 g/L of hippuric acid in an end-of-shift urine specimen be considered as an indication of exposure to toluene at an average concentration of 200 ppm and of unacceptable absorption of toluene.

Analysis. Toluene determination in blood or breath may be accomplished with the flame-ionization gas chromatographic method described for benzene (p. 39). A method for analysis of hippuric acid in urine by ultraviolet spectrophotometry (Pagnotto and Lieberman, 1967) is presented and may be used to assess exposure to toluene in the absence of xylene. A more specific gas chromatographic method for both hippuric acid and the methylhippuric acids is described in the section on ethylbenzene (p. 138) and is recommended for use when both toluene and xylene vapors are encountered.

References

I. Astrand, H. Ehrner-Samuel, A. Kilbom and P. Ovrum. Toluene exposure I. Concentration in alveolar air and blood at rest and during exercise. Work-Env.-Health 9: 119 - 130, 1972.

J. Bidanset. Presented at the 25th Annual Meeting of the American Academy of Forensic Sciences, Las Vegas, February 22, 1973.

R. Bonnichsen, A. C. Maehly and M. Moeller. Poisoning by volatile compounds. I. Aromatic hydrocarbons. J. For. Sci. 11: 186 - 204, 1966.

W. D. Collom and C. L. Winek. Detection of glue constituents in fatalities due to "glue sniffing." Clin. Tox. 3: 125 - 130, 1970.

M. Ikeda and H. Ohtsuji. Significance of urinary hippuric acid determination as an index of toluene exposure. Brit. J. Ind. Med. 26: 244 - 246, 1969.

J. W. Knox and J. R. Nelson. Permanent encephalopathy from toluene inhalation. New Eng. J. Med. 275: 1494 - 1496, 1966.

E. O. Longley, A. T. Jones, R. Welch and O. Lomaev. Two acute toluene episodes in merchant ships. Arch. Env. Health 14: 481 - 487, 1967.

L. J. Luskus, H. J. Kilian, W. W. Lackey and J. D. Biggs. Gases released from tissue and analyzed by infrared and gas chromatography/mass spectroscopy techniques. J. For. Sci. 22: 500 - 507, 1977.

L. D. Pagnotto and L. M. Lieberman. Urinary hippuric acid excretion as an index of toluene exposure. Am. Ind. Hyg. Asso. J. 28: 129 - 134, 1967.

J. K. Piotrowski. *Exposure Tests for Organic Compounds in Industrial Toxicology,* U.S. Government Printing Office, Washington, D.C., 1977, pp. 48 - 54.

A. Sato, T. Nakajima and F. Fujiwara. Determination of benzene and toluene in blood by means of syringe-equilibration method using a small amount of blood. Brit. J. Ind. Med. 32: 210 - 214, 1975.

R. Satran and U. N. Dodson. Toluene habituation — report of a case. New Eng. J. Med. 268: 719 - 721, 1963.

H. Veulemans and R. Masschelein. Experimental human exposure to toluene, III. Int. Arch. Occ. Env. Health 43: 53 - 62, 1979.

H. Veulemans, E. Van Vlem, H. Janssens and R. Masschelein. Exposure to toluene and urinary hippuric acid excretion in a group of heliorotagravure printing workers. Int. Arch. Occ. Env. Health 44: 99 - 107, 1979.

W. F. von Oettingen, P. A. Neal and D. D. Donahue. The toxicity and potential dangers of toluene. J. Am. Med. Asso. 118: 579 - 584, 1942.

R. H. Wilson. Toluene poisoning. J. Am. Med. Asso. 123: 1106 - 1108, 1943.

Urine Hippuric Acid by Ultraviolet Spectrophotometry

Principle:

Hippuric acid is extracted from acidified urine into an organic solvent mixture. The ultraviolet absorbance of the compound is measured directly in the solvent extract at 230 nm.

Reagents:

Stock solution — 4 g/L hippuric acid in water
Aqueous standards — 1, 2 and 4 g/L
3 mol/L Sulfuric acid
Extraction solvent — diethyl ether/isopropanol, 80:20 by volume

Instrumental Conditions:

Ultraviolet spectrophotometer capable of scanning from 320 - 220 nm
Measure absorbance at 230 nm

Procedure:

1. Transfer from 0.1 - 0.5 mL of urine, depending on hippuric acid concentration, to a 100 mL volumetric flask and dilute to volume with water. Transfer 20 mL of this solution to a 50 mL screw-cap centrifuge tube.
2. Add 1 mL of 3 mol/L H_2SO_4 and extract with 20 mL of extraction solvent by shaking for 1 min. Centrifuge and transfer the upper organic layer to a 50 mL glass-stoppered graduated cylinder.
3. Repeat the extraction with another 20 mL of solvent, centrifuging and combining the organic layers in the cylinder. Mix the contents of the cylinder and record the volume (approximately 32 mL).
4. Determine the ultraviolet spectrum of the organic extract against a reagent blank, recording the absorbance at 230 nm.

Calculation:

Calculation is based on a response factor derived from a standard curve. A quality control specimen containing 2 g/L hippuric acid is analyzed daily. Correction should be made for the volume of organic extract recovered if it differs substantially from 32 mL. Results may be corrected for specific gravity or creatinine content of the urine specimen.

Evaluation:

Sensitivity: 0.5 g/L
Linearity: 0.5 - 8.0 g/L (with proper volume adjustment of urine specimen)
C.V.: not established
Relative recovery: not established

Interferences:

The methylhippuric acid metabolites of xylene will contribute to the absorbance of hippuric acid in this procedure. Other possible interfering compounds include phenol, p-cresol and urea.

TRICHLOROETHANE

Occurrence and Usage. 1,1,1-Trichloroethane (methyl chloroform) was introduced commercially in 1954 as a substitute for the more toxic carbon tetrachloride. It is encountered frequently in both industrial and domestic use as a degreaser, dry cleaning agent, and solvent in paints, glues and aerosol products. The compound has received clinical trials as an inhalation anesthetic, but is not currently used for this purpose. Air concentrations of trichloroethane in the workplace are not to exceed an average 8-hour level of 350 ppm (1900 mg/m^3), which is approximately 3 times the odor threshold for this chemical.

Blood Concentrations. Trichloroethane blood concentrations in 12 resting subjects averaged 1.4 mg/L during a 30 minute exposure to 250 ppm of the vapor (Astrand et al., 1973). Blood concentrations of trichloroethane ranged from 1.5 - 6.5 mg/L (average 3 - 4) during a 78 minute exposure to 500 ppm, but fell to 1 mg/L or less within 25 minutes after cessation of exposure. Maximum blood concentrations of 7 - 10 mg/L were achieved 65 minutes after the start of a 73 minute exposure to 955 ppm by asymptomatic subjects (Stewart et al., 1961).

Metabolism and Excretion. Trichloroethane is slowly metabolized in man by oxidation to trichloroethanol, which is excreted as a glucuronide conjugate (urochloralic acid) in urine over a period of 5 - 12 days and which accounts for only about 2% of an absorbed dose. Trichloroacetic acid is formed from trichloroethanol as a further oxidation product and is also found in urine to the extent of about 0.5% of a dose. Both of these metabolites are also biotransformation products of chloral hydrate, tetrachloroethylene and trichloroethylene. Trichloroethane is largely exhaled unchanged, 60 - 80% of a dose appearing within one week, and traces may be found in the post-exposure expired breath for as long as one month (Stewart et al., 1969; Monster et al., 1979). In the rat, 98.7% of a single dose is exhaled unchanged in 25 hours, with 0.5% as CO_2, and much of the balance is found as urinary trichloroethanol glucuronide (Hake et al., 1960).

Alveolar air concentrations in subjects exposed to 350 ppm of trichloroethane were found to average 179 ppm at rest and 239 ppm during light exercise; these concentrations were obtained within 20 - 30 minutes after the start of exposure and declined rapidly upon cessation of exposure (Astrand et al., 1973).

Urinary concentrations of trichloroethanol in workers exposed daily to 53 ppm of trichloroethane were found to average 9.9 mg/L (range 6.8 - 14.5) in specimens collected toward the end of the week; the corresponding values for trichloroacetic acid were 3.6 mg/L and a range of 2.4 - 5.5 mg/L. The half-life of trichloroethane as calculated from urinary metabolite excretion data was 8.7 hours (Seki et al., 1975).

Toxicity. The anesthetic effects of trichloroethane, such as lightheadedness and loss of coordination, are displayed by persons exposed to vapor concentrations exceeding 1000 ppm. The compound has only slight capacity to cause liver or kidney damage with repeated exposure to high concentrations (Torkelson et al., 1958), although there is some indication that liver abnormalities may be experienced by abusers of trichloroethane (Litt and Cohen, 1969). Only a small number of non-fatal and fatal acute episodes of poisoning have been reported (Stewart and Andrews, 1966; Stewart, 1971). A postmortem trichloroethane blood concentration of 60 mg/L was determined in a man who succumbed while exposed to a vapor concentration of 500 ppm (Hatfield and Maykoski, 1970). The blood concentrations found in 10 fatal cases show a wide variation ranging from 1.5 - 720 mg/L and averaging 140 mg/L; it is conceivable that in certain instances, cardiac arrest following ventricular fibrillation may occur prior to the absorption of significant quantities of the vapor (Hall and Hine, 1966; Stahl et al., 1969; Bidanset, 1973; Caplan et al., 1976).

Biological Monitoring. Venous blood concentrations of trichloroethane relate to both the intensity of exposure to the chemical and the level of physical activity of the individual, when specimens are taken during an exposure. However, blood has not been considered a realistic specimen for routine monitoring purposes (Astrand et al., 1973).

The use of alveolar air specimens has been suggested for monitoring exposure to trichloroethane. Astrand et al. (1973) proposed an upper limit of 150 ppm for alveolar trichloroethane in specimens taken during an exposure as a level which would avoid significant central nervous system impairment of workers. Stewart (1971) demonstrated the use of serial breath specimens obtained after an exposure to estimate the amount of trichloroethane absorbed by an individual.

While the concentrations of urinary metabolites of trichloroethane appear to correlate with both intensity and duration of exposure, the data yet available are not sufficient to propose a biological threshold limit value for these substances (Stewart et al., 1969; Seki et al., 1975; NIOSH, 1976).

Analysis. Blood and breath concentrations of trichloroethane may be measured using the gas chromatographic procedure described for benzene (p. 39). Methods for determination of trichloroethanol and trichloroacetic acid in urine are presented in the section of trichloroethylene (p. 261).

References

I. Astrand, A. Kilbom, I. Wahlberg and P. Ovrum. Methylchloroform exposure. Work-Env.-Health 10: 69 - 81, 1973.

J. Bidanset. Presented at the 25th Annual Meeting of the American Academy of Forensic Sciences, Las Vegas, February 22, 1973.

Y. H. Caplan, R. C. Backer and J. Q. Whitaker. 1,1,1-Trichloroethane: report of a fatal intoxication. Clin. Tox. 9: 69 - 74, 1976.

C. L. Hake, T. B. Waggoner, D. N. Robertson and V. K. Rowe. The metabolism of 1,1,1-trichloroethane by the rat. Arch. Env. Health 1: 101 - 105, 1960.

F. B. Hall and C. H. Hine. Trichloroethane intoxication: a report of two cases. J. For. Sci. 11: 404 - 413, 1966.

T. R. Hatfield and R. T. Maykoski. A fatal methyl chloroform (trichloroethane) poisoning. Arch. Env. Health 20: 279 - 281, 1970.

I. F. Litt and M. I. Cohen. "Danger . . . vapor harmful:" spot-remover sniffing. New Eng. J. Med. 281: 543 - 544, 1969.

A. C. Monster, G. Boersma and H. Steenweg. Kinetics of 1,1,1-trichloroethane in volunteers; influence of exposure concentration and work load. Int. Arch. Occ. Env. Health 42: 293 - 301, 1979.

NIOSH. *Occupational Exposure to 1,1,1-Trichloroethane (Methyl Chloroform)*, National Institute for Occupational Safety and Health, Cincinnati, Ohio, 1976.

Y. Seki, Y. Urashima, H. Aikawa et al. Trichloro-compounds in the urine of humans exposed to methyl chloroform at sub-threshold levels. Int. Arch. Arbeitsmed. 34: 39 - 49, 1975.

C. J. Stahl, A. V. Fatteh and A. M. Dominguez. Trichloroethane poisoning: observations on the pathology and toxicology in six fatal cases. J. For. Sci. 14: 393 - 397, 1969.

R. D. Stewart, H. H. Gay, D. S. Erley et al. Human exposure to 1,1,1-trichloroethane vapor: relationship of expired air and blood concentrations to exposure and toxicity. Am. Ind. Hyg. Asso. J. 22: 252 - 262, 1961.

R. D. Stewart and J. T. Andrews. Acute intoxication with methylchloroform. J. Am. Med. Asso. 195: 904 - 906, 1966.

R. D. Stewart, H. H. Gay, A. W. Schaffer et al. Experimental human exposure to methyl chloroform vapor. Arch. Env. Health 19: 467 - 472, 1969.

R. D. Stewart. Methyl chloroform intoxication. J. Am. Med. Asso. 215: 1789 - 1792, 1971.

T. R. Torkelson, F. Oyen, D. D. McCollister and V. K. Rowe. Toxicity of 1,1,1-trichloroethane as determined on laboratory animals and human subjects. Am. Ind. Hyg. Asso. J. 19: 353 - 362, 1958.

TRICHLOROETHYLENE

Occurrence and Usage. Trichloroethylene, first described in 1864, has been used industrially as a solvent, degreaser and dry cleaning agent for over 60 years; since 1934 it has also been employed as an induction agent and sole anesthetic in surgical procedures, but has largely been replaced by the less toxic fluorinated ethers. The current threshold limit value for trichloroethylene is 100 ppm (535 mg/m^3), which is approximately the odor threshold for the compound. The TLV is expected to be lowered to 50 ppm in the near future.

Blood Concentrations. Blood concentrations of trichloroethylene and trichloroethanol, a metabolite, reached average peak levels of 1 and 6 mg/L, respectively, in 5 subjects exposed to 100 ppm trichloroethylene for 6 hours; this was approximately the same trichloroethanol level seen 2 hours after the ingestion of a hypnotic dose (15 mg/kg) of chloral hydrate by 2 subjects (Müller et al., 1974). During a 3 hour exposure to a vapor concentration of 211 ppm, blood trichloroethylene concentrations in 7 subjects rose to an average maximum of 6 mg/L (range 4.5 - 7) within 2 hours (Stewart et al., 1962). Trichloroethylene blood concentrations in 22 surgical patients anesthesized with an induction level of 1% trichloroethylene for 30 minutes averaged 64 mg/L (range 33 - 90); blood concentrations upon waking ranged from 16 - 57 mg/L (Prior, 1972).

Metabolism and Excretion. Trichloroethylene is extensively metabolized in man, probably via an epoxide intermediate which rearranges with migration of a chlorine atom; chloral hydrate has been identified as a transient metabolite, achieving a blood concentration of 0.17 mg/L during trichloroethylene anesthesia (Cole et al., 1975). The major urinary metabolites are trichloroacetic acid and trichloroethanol, the latter appearing largely as a glucuronide conjugate (urochloralic acid). Both chloral hydrate and free trichloroethanol have hypnotic activity in man. Trichloroacetic acid is a hypnotically inactive metabolite, but its presence in plasma should be recognized due to its possible interference in colorimetric assays for trichloroethylene or trichloroethanol; plasma trichloroacetic acid concentrations of 9 - 40 mg/L (average 24) were observed on the third day after exposure of subjects to a trichloroethylene concentration of 194 ppm for 5 hours (Bartonicek, 1962).

From 51 - 64% of an inhaled dose of trichloroethylene is retained; of this, an average of 45% is slowly excreted as trichloroethanol glucuronide and 32% as trichloroacetic acid in the urine over a 3 week period. The excretion half-lives of these metabolites in persons exposed to trichloroethylene are 12 and 100 hours, respectively (Müller et al., 1974). An additional 8% as both metabolites is eliminated in feces (Bartonicek, 1962), and a small amount (4%) is reportedly found as monochloroacetic acid in urine (Soucek and Vlachova, 1960). Approximately 16% of a dose is excreted unchanged in the expired breath (Nomiyama and Nomiyama, 1971).

Urine concentrations of trichloroethanol and trichloroacetic acid in subjects chronically exposed to trichloroethylene air concentrations of 120 - 250 ppm averaged 133 and 72 mg/L, respectively, in specimens obtained on a Friday afternoon (Tanaka and Ikeda, 1968). Other investigators using similar conditions have found average values of 682 and 230 mg/L for trichloroethanol and trichloroacetic acid, respectively, in urine of workers exposed to an average air concentration of 120 ppm (Ikeda et al., 1972).

Toxicity. Trichloroethylene has been implicated in numerous chronic and acute poisonings. The compound is addicting in chronic usage (Ikeda et al., 1971), and is known to produce hepatic and renal abnormalities in abusers, probably as a result of its metabolites (Baerg and Kimberg, 1970). Acute toxic episodes may be due to the anesthetic effects of trichloroethylene, hypnotic effects of trichloroethanol or to cardiac arrhythmia produced by high concentrations of the vapor (Kleinfeld and Tabershaw, 1954; Ertle et al., 1972). Postmortem blood concentrations of trichloroethylene averaged 28 mg/L and ranged from 3 - 110 mg/L in 16 fatal cases due to the ingestion or inhalation of this agent (Alha, 1974; Bonnichsen and Maehly, 1966; Cravey and Baselt, 1968; Le Breton et al., 1963).

Workers chronically exposed to trichloroethylene vapor concentrations of 40 - 270 ppm often exhibit symptoms of fatigue, headache, irritability, vomiting, flushing of the skin, intolerance to alcohol and electrocardiographic changes. These symptoms are first noted when urinary trichloroacetic acid concentrations are on the order of 100 mg/L, and become pronounced at concentrations of 200 mg/L (ACGIH, 1971).

Biological Monitoring. Numerous procedures have been proposed for evaluating exposure to trichloroethylene by measuring the chemical or its metabolites in biological specimens. The determination of trichloroethylene itself in blood is generally not considered desirable as a routine practice, although this view may be based more on the difficulty encountered in obtaining specimens rather than on the usefulness of blood concentration data.

Alveolar air concentrations of the chemical, however, have been shown to correlate well with both the actual environmental trichloroethylene level as well as the time-weighted average exposure for an individual, depending on when the breath specimen is obtained. Most investigators agree that for routine monitoring purposes alveolar air samples should be taken at least 6 hours after the end of an exposure and, for convenience, may be obtained just prior to the start of the next working day. In this case, the concentration of trichloroethylene in such a specimen should not exceed 1 ppm in persons exposed to 100 ppm of the chemical for 8 hours daily (Droz and Fernandez, 1978; Lowry et al., 1974; Nomiyama, 1971; Pfaffli and Backman, 1972; Stewart et al., 1974).

Determination of urinary metabolites of trichloroethylene has not been fully successful as an index of exposure, due to the interindividual variation in metabolism, the tendency toward accumulation of metabolites during chronic exposure and delayed urinary excretion (especially for trichloroacetic acid), and the fact that other chemicals (chloral hydrate, tetrachloroethylene and trichloroethane) produce the same metabolic products in man. However, several standards have been proposed in relation to these metabolites in urine. These include the British Occupational Hygiene Society recommendation (1974) that a trichloroacetic acid concentration of 100 mg/L in urine (corrected to a specific gravity of 1.016) be considered consistent with exposure to 100 ppm of trichloroethylene. Total trichlorocompounds have been measured by several investigators and found to offer an approximate guide to exposure; trichlorocompounds in a urine specimen collected at the end of a work shift from a person who is chronically exposed to 100 ppm trichloroethylene should average 500 - 600 mg/g creatinine (Tanaka and Ikeda, 1968; Nomiyama, 1971). Finally, urine trichloroethanol concentrations have been claimed to be a fairly accurate index of exposure, and should be measured in a specimen collected just before the start of the next work period; trichloroethanol in such a specimen should not exceed 300 mg/L in persons exposed to 100 ppm of trichloroethylene on a daily basis (Droz and Fernandez, 1978; Ikeda et al., 1972).

Monster et al. (1979) found that blood trichloroacetic acid concentrations exhibited the least interindividual variability of any of the above parameters, and concluded that this measurement was the most promising for monitoring purposes. However, trichloroacetic acid tends to accumulate with repeated exposure and, after exposure ceases, leaves the blood slowly ($t\frac{1}{2}$ = 70 - 90 hrs).

Analysis. Trichloroethylene concentrations in blood or breath may be estimated using the gas chromatographic method described for benzene (p. 39). A colorimetric method is described in this section for urinary total trichlorocompounds, trichloroacetic acid and trichloroethanol (Tanaka and Ikeda, 1968). Additionally, more sensitive and specific electron-capture gas chromatographic methods are presented for conjugated trichloroethanol in urine (Ertle et al., 1972) and for trichloroacetic acid as its methyl derivative (Ehrner-Samuel et al., 1973).

References

ACGIH. *Documentation of the Threshold Limit Values,* American Conference of Governmental Industrial Hygienists, Cincinnati, Ohio, 1971, pp. 263 - 265.

A. Alha. Personal communication, 1974.

R. D. Baerg and D. V. Kimberg. Centrilobular hepatic necrosis and acute renal failure in "solvent sniffers." Ann. Int. Med. 73: 713 - 720, 1970.

V. Bartonicek. Metabolism and excretion of trichloroethylene after inhalation by human subjects. Brit. J. Ind. Med. 19: 134 - 141, 1962.

R. Bonnichsen and A. H. Maehly. Poisoning by volatile compounds. II. Chlorinated aliphatic hydrocarbons. J. For. Sci. 11: 414 - 427, 1966.

British Occupational Hygiene Society. Biochemical threshold for trichloroethylene. Ann. Occ. Hyg. 17: 169, 1974.

W. J. Cole, R. G. Mitchell and R. F. Salamonsen. Isolation, characterization and quantitation of chloral hydrate as a transient metabolite of trichloroethylene in man using electron capture gas chromatography and mass fragmentography. J. Pharm. Pharmac. 27: 167 - 171, 1975.

R. H. Cravey and R. C. Baselt. Unpublished results, 1968.

P. O. Droz and J. G. Fernandez. Trichloroethylene exposure. Biological monitoring by breath and urine analyses. Brit. J. Ind. Med. 35: 35 - 42, 1978.

H. Ehrner-Samuel, K. Balmer and W. Thorsell. Determination of trichloroacetic acid in urine by a gas chromatographic method. Am. Ind. Hyg. Asso. J. 34: 93-96, 1973.

T. Ertle, D. Henschler, G. Müller and M. Spassowski. Metabolism of trichloroethylene in man. Arch. Tox. 29: 171 - 188, 1972.

M. Ikeda, H. Ohtsuji, H. Kawai and M. Kuniyoshi. Excretion kinetics of urinary metabolites in a patient addicted to trichloroethylene. Brit. J. Ind. Med. 28: 203 - 206, 1971.

M. Ikeda, H. Ohtsuji, T. Imamura and Y. Komoike. Urinary excretion of total trichloro-compounds, trichloroethanol, and trichloroacetic acid as a measure of exposure to trichloroethylene and tetrachloroethylene. Brit. J. Ind. Med. 29: 328 - 333, 1972.

M. Kleinfeld and I. R. Tabershaw. Trichloroethylene toxicity. Arch. Ind. Hyg. Occ. Med. 10: 134 - 141, 1954.

R. Le Breton, J. Le Bourhis and J. Garat. Un cas d'empoisonnement criminel par le trichloroethylene. Ann. Med. Leg. 43: 281 - 283, 1963.

L. K. Lawry, R. Vandervort and P. L. Polakoff. Biological indicators of occupational exposure to trichloroethylene. J. Occ. Med. 16: 98 - 101, 1974.

A. C. Monster, G. Boersma and W. C. Duba. Kinetics of trichloroethylene in repeated exposure of volunteers. Int. Arch. Occ. Env. Health 42: 283 - 292, 1979.

G. Müller, M. Spassovski and D. Henschler. Metabolism of trichloroethylene in man. Arch. Tox. 32: 283 - 295, 1974.

K. Nomiyama. Estimation of trichloroethylene exposure by biological materials. Int. Arch. Arbeitsmed. 27: 281 - 292, 1971.

K. Nomiyama and H. Nomiyama. Metabolism of trichloroethylene in human. Int. Arch. Arbeitsmed. 28: 37 - 48, 1971.

P. Pfaffli and A. Backman. Trichloroethylene concentrations in blood and expired air as indicators of occupational exposure. A preliminary report. Work Env. Health 9: 140 - 144, 1972.

F. N. Prior. Blood levels of trichloroethylene during major surgery. Anaesthesia 27: 379 - 389, 1972.

B. Soucek and D. Vlachova. Excretion of trichloroethylene metabolites in human urine. Brit. J. Ind. Med. 17: 60 - 64, 1960.

R. D. Stewart, H. H. Gay, D. S. Erley et al. Observations on the concentrations of trichloroethylene in blood and expired air following exposure of humans. Am. Ind. Hyg. Asso. J. 23: 167 - 170, 1962.

R. D. Stewart, C. L. Hake and J. E. Peterson. Use of breath analysis to monitor trichloroethylene exposures. Arch. Env. Health 29: 6 - 13, 1974.

S. Tanaka and M. Ikeda. A method for determination of trichloroethanol and trichloroacetic acid in urine. Brit. J. Ind. Med. 25: 214 - 219, 1968.

Urine Trichloroacetic Acid and Trichloroethanol by Colorimetry

Principle:

Total trichlorocompounds in urine are determined by chromic acid oxidation of trichloroethanol to trichloroacetic acid, and colorimetric analysis of the latter compound using the Fujiwara reaction. Trichloroacetic acid itself is measured by omitting the oxidation step, and trichloroethanol is estimated from the difference between the two values.

Reagents:

Stock solutions —

1 mg/mL trichloroacetic acid in water

1 mg/mL trichloroethanol in water

Urine standards — 50, 100, 200 and 400 mg/L of each compound

Oxidizing agent — 8 g CrO_3 in 5 mL water and 15 mL conc. HNO_3

7.8 mol/L Potassium hydroxide

Pyridine

Toluene

Instrumental Conditions:

Visible spectrophotometer set to 530 nm

Procedure:

Total Trichlorocompounds:

1. Transfer 0.5 mL urine to a 15 mL screw-cap centrifuge tube and add 0.5 mL oxidizing agent. Cap tightly and heat at 65° C. for 4 hours.
2. Cool the tube in ice water and add 2.5 mL 7.8 mol/L KOH, 5 mL pyridine and 0.5 mL toluene. Vortex, cap tightly and heat at 65° C. for 50 minutes.
3. Cool and transfer 3 mL of the pyridine layer to a 12 mL conical centrifuge tube. Add 0.6 mL water and vortex.
4. Transfer the solution to a cuvette and read the absorbance at 530 nm against a urine blank.

Trichloroacetic Acid:

5. Transfer 0.5 mL urine to a 15 mL screw-cap centrifuge tube and add 2.5 mL 7.8 mol/L KOH. Cool in ice water and add 0.5 mL oxidizing agent, 5 mL pyridine and 0.5 mL toluene.
6. Vortex, cap tightly and heat at 65° C. for 50 minutes. Cool and transfer 3 mL of the pyridine layer to a 12 mL conical centrifuge tube.
7. Add 0.6 mL water and vortex. Transfer the solution to a cuvette and read the absorbance at 530 nm against a urine blank.

Calculation:

Calculation is based on a response factor derived from a standard curve. A quality control specimen containing 200 mg/L of both trichloroacetic acid and trichloroethanol is analyzed daily. Determine the trichloroethanol concentration by subtracting the trichloroacetic acid concentration from the concentration of total trichlorocompounds.

Evaluation:

Sensitivity: <1 mg/L
Linearity: 50 - 400 mg/L
C.V.: not established
Relative recovery: 97 - 99%

Interferences:

The method gives apparent trichloroacetic acid and trichloroethanol concentrations of 0.1 mg/L or less in the urine of normal subjects. Other halogenated hydrocarbons which are present in the specimen will give a positive response.

Urine Trichloroethanol by Electron-Capture Gas Chromatography

Principle:

The glucuronide conjugate of trichloroethanol is hydrolyzed by incubating the specimen overnight in the presence of β-glucuronidase. The solution is diluted with acetone and analyzed directly by electron-capture chromatography.

Reagents:

Stock solution — 1 mg/mL trichloroethanol in water
Urine standards — 50, 100, 200 and 400 mg/L
β-Glucuronidase — 3000 Fishman units/mL; dilute 1 mL of Type H-2 β-glucuronidase solution (Sigma Chemical Co.) to 30 mL with pH 4.5 acetate buffer
Acetone (nanograde)

Instrumental Conditions:

Gas chromatograph with electron-capture detector
4 ft. x 2 mm i.d. glass column containing 10% Carbowax 20 M on 60/80 mesh Chromosorb W
Injector, 150° C.; column, 150° C.; detector, 200° C.
5% Methane in argon flow rate, 75 mL/min

Procedure:

1. Transfer 1 mL urine into a 15 mL screw-cap tube and add 1 mL β-glucuronidase solution. Cap tightly and incubate at 37° C. for 18 hours.

2. Transfer the solution to a 50 mL volumetric flask, rinsing with acetone to achieve a quantitative transfer. Adjust to volume with acetone, mix and inject 1 μL into the gas chromatograph.

	Retention time (min)
trichloroethanol	1

Calculation:

Calculation is based on a response factor derived from a standard curve. A quality control specimen containing 100 mg/L trichloroethanol is analyzed daily.

Evaluation:

Sensitivity: 1 mg/L
Linearity: 10 - 400 mg/L
C.V.: not established
Relative recovery: not established

Interferences:

Trichloroethylene, trichloroacetic acid and normal urinary constituents were not found to interfere with the procedure.

Urine Trichloroacetic Acid by Electron-Capture Gas Chromatography

Principle:

Trichloroacetic acid is extracted into toluene from acidified urine. Boron trifluoride-methanol reagent is used to form the methyl derivative of the acid directly in the toluene extract, and the resulting solution is analyzed by electron-capture gas chromatography.

Reagents:

Stock solution — 1 mg/mL trichloroacetic acid in water
Urine standards — 50, 100, 200 and 400 mg/L
1 mol/L Sulfuric acid
Toluene
Derivatizing reagent — 14% boron trifluoride in methanol (Sigma Chemical Co.)

Instrumental Conditions:

Gas chromatograph with electron-capture detector
1.5 m x 2 mm i.d. glass column containing 5% QF-1 on 60/80 mesh Chromosorb W
Injector, 185° C.; column, 110° C.; detector, 160° C.
Nitrogen flow rate, 45 mL/min

Procedure:

1. Transfer 50 μL urine to a 15 mL screw-cap tube and add 0.5 mL 1 mol/L H_2SO_4. Extract with 8 mL of toluene using mechanical shaking for 4 minutes.
2. To separate phases, heat the closed tube at 80° C. for 10 minutes and cool to room temperature. Transfer 2 mL of the toluene phase to a clean tube.
3. Add 0.2 mL derivatizing reagent and vortex. Cap the tube and heat at 80° C. for exactly 1 hour.
4. Cool to room temperature and add 1 mL water. Vortex for 30 seconds, centrifuge if necessary to separate phases, and inject 2 μL of the upper toluene layer into the gas chromatograph.

	Retention time (min)
trichloroacetic acid derivative	1.8

Calculation:

Calculation is based on a response factor derived from a standard curve. A quality control specimen containing 100 mg/L trichloroacetic acid is analyzed daily.

Evaluation:

Sensitivity: 3 mg/L
Linearity: 5 - 400 mg/L
C.V.: 5.2%
Relative recovery: not established

Interferences:

Neither trichloroethylene nor its other metabolites interfere with this procedure. Endogenous urinary constituents have not been found to interfere.

2,4,5-TRICHLOROPHENOXYACETIC ACID

Occurrence and Usage. 2,4,5-Trichlorophenoxyacetic acid (2,4,5-T) and its salts have been extensively used as herbicides for the control of broadleaf plants, often in combination with 2,4-dichlorophenoxyacetic acid. 2,4,5-T in pure form is of relatively low toxicity, but some commercial preparations have been found to contain traces of the highly toxic dioxin. For this reason, the U.S. Environmental Protection Agency banned most major uses of 2,4,5-T in early 1979. The current threshold limit value for occupational exposure to 2,4,5-T is 10 mg/m^3.

Blood Concentrations. A single oral dose of 5 mg/kg (350 mg/70 kg) given to volunteers who remained asymptomatic produced maximal plasma concentrations of 40 - 88 mg/L, averaging about 60 mg/L, within 4 hours. The levels declined with an average half-life of 23 hours. Approximately 65% of whole blood 2,4,5-T resides in plasma, and of this amount 98.7% is protein bound. The apparent volume of distribution of the compound is 6.1 L/kg (Gehring et al., 1973).

Metabolism and Excretion. An average of 89% of a single 5 mg/kg dose of 2,4,5-T was excreted in the urine of asymptomatic volunteers over a 4 day period as unchanged compound. The urine collected during the first 12 hours after administration contained 27% of the dose, producing estimated urine concentrations of 100 - 300 mg/L. No metabolites are known, although it is possible that a small amount is eliminated as a glucuronide conjugate. Less than 1% of a dose is excreted in feces (Gehring et al., 1973).

Urine concentrations of 2,4,5-T in 8 asymptomatic herbicide spray operators were found to range from 0.05 - 3.6 mg/L (Shafik et al., 1971).

Toxicity. 2,4,5-T in pure form is considered to be of relatively low toxicity. In overdosage, the compound causes muscular weakness and stiffness, nausea, vomiting and diarrhea. One human fatality occurred due to combined ingestion of 2,4-D and 2,4,5-T; postmortem blood concentrations of these agents were 83 and 18 mg/L, respectively (Coutselinis et al., 1977).

2,4,5-T is not believed to be carcinogenic or teratogenic in animals or man; these effects, produced by technical grades of the chemical, are believed due to the dioxin which is present as an impurity. Early technical grades of 2,4,5-T contained up to 30 ppm of dioxin, although recent samples have contained as little as 0.04 ppm (Courtney and Moore, 1971; American Farm Bureau Federation, 1980).

Biological Monitoring. Both plasma and urine concentrations of 2,4,5-T appear to be directly related to the amount of the chemical absorbed by an individual. Limits have not been proposed for 2,4,5-T in specimens from exposed workers, but routine measurement of plasma or urine woud be a useful tool in an industrial monitoring program.

Analysis. 2,4,5-T may be analyzed in plasma or urine at concentrations greater than 1 mg/L using the gas chromatographic assay described in the section on 2,4-D (p. 116). 2,4-D, if not present in the specimen, may be used as internal standard.

References

American Farm Bureau Federation. Dispute resolution conference on 2,4,5-T. Vet. Hum. Tox. 22: 40-42, 1980.

K. D. Courtney and J. A. Moore. Teratology studies with 2,4,5-trichlorophenoxyacetic acid and 2,3,7,8-tetrachlorodibenzo-p-dioxin. Tox. App. Pharm. 20: 396 - 403, 1971.

A. Coutselinis, R. Kentarchou and D. Boukis. Concentration levels of 2,4-D and 2,4,5-T in forensic material. For. Sci. 10: 203 - 204, 1977.

P. J. Gehring, C. G. Kramer, B. A. Schwetz et al. The fate of 2,4,5-trichlorophenoxyacetic acid (2,4,5-T) following oral administration to man. Tox. App. Pharm. 26: 352 - 361, 1973.

M. T. Shafik, H. C. Sullivan and H. F. Enos. A method for determination of low levels of exposure to 2,4-D and 2,4,5-T. Int. J. Env. Anal. Chem. 1: 23 - 33, 1971.

URANIUM

Occurrence and Usage. Uranium and its compounds are encountered primarily during the processing of uranium ore for nuclear fuel uses. This process is potentially capable of producing uranium dusts during the crushing of the ore and machining of the metal, and fumes of metallic uranium or its more volatile compounds. Exposure is generally by inhalation of these substances, which are currently assigned a threshold limit value of 0.2 mg/m^2 (as U). Uranium is encountered in the daily diet in amounts which average 1 - 2 μg.

Blood Concentrations. Uranium concentrations have not been measured in the blood or plasma of exposed workers. The uranium content of whole blood from normal individuals averages 0.84 μg/L (Hamilton, 1970).

Metabolism and Excretion. Only about 1% of an oral dose of a soluble uranium salt is absorbed into the body, although both soluble and insoluble uranium compounds appear to be reasonably well-absorbed following their inhalation as dusts or fumes. The more insoluble compounds tend to accumulate in the lungs and to be absorbed into the bloodstream at a slow rate. Absorbed uranium is believed to localize in soft tissues and to a certain extent in bone, with up to 66% of a dose being excreted in urine within 24 hours. Uranium which appears in feces is mainly a result of insoluble dust which has been mobilized up the respiratory tract and swallowed (Fischoff, 1965; Lippmann et al., 1964).

Baseline urinary uranium levels in 26 non-exposed persons ranged from 0.03 - 0.30 μg/L (Welford et al., 1960). Industrial uranium oxide workers were found to excrete urine containing uranium at concentrations of 3 - 389 μg/L, with a level of about 50 μg/L expected at an air uranium concentration of 0.05 mg/m^3. Workers exposed chronically to uranium continue to excrete the metal in their urine for years after termination of exposure; storage in bone probably accounts for the long terminal half-life of uranium, which has been estimated at 450 days (Eisenbud and Quigley, 1956). Urine concentrations as high as 13,200 μg/L have been observed in asymptomatic workers exposed to soluble compounds of uranium (Lippmann, 1959).

Toxicity. Inhalation of uranium compounds may cause respiratory irritation and lung damage; following absorption of the compounds, renal toxicity characterized by albuminuria and hematuria occurs. With chronic exposure, radiation damage may lead to malignancies at sites where uranium accumulates, including the lungs, lymph nodes and bone marrow. Uranium mill workers have been found to have an increased incidence of death due to lymphatic and hematopoietic cancer (Archer et al., 1973).

A number of massive acute and chronic exposures of workers to various forms of uranium have occurred in which urine concentrations as high as 13,200 μg/L were observed. Often these cases involved only minimal transient renal damage, with apparent full recovery after several days or weeks (Eisenbud and Quigley, 1956; Lippmann, 1959; Lippmann et al., 1964).

Biological Monitoring. In controlled studies, it has been shown that urinary uranium concentrations are a function of environmental air levels of the element. Urine concentrations average about 50 μg/L at constant daily exposure to 0.05 mg/m^3 of uranium and about 100 μg/L at a level of 0.25 mg/m^3. However, due to the relatively rapid absorption and elimination of uranium, spot urine samples taken during a shift often show a wide variation in concentrations. Several alternatives to spot samples have been suggested, including collecting specimens just prior to beginning a shift, collecting just prior to the Monday shift, or collection of all urine voided from the end of one shift to the beginning of the next. Each of these methods has its advantages and disadvantages, but the most important features of any monitoring program for uranium exposure are that sampling times be consistent for each worker and that sampling be performed on a frequent basis. In this way, a pattern of uranium excretion can be established for each individual which may be used to assess the significance of an apparently high value (Eisenbud and Quigley, 1956; Fischoff, 1965; Lippmann et al., 1964).

Analysis. A method is presented for the determination of uranium in urine by spectrophotofluorometry (Price et al., 1953). Neutron activation techniques, not presented here, have also been recommended for their precision and freedom from interferences (Kramer et al., 1967; Picer and Strohal, 1968). An alternative procedure involves persulfate oxidation of the specimen followed by analysis in a nitrogen laser fluorometer. This instrument and the detailed procedure are available from the manufacturer (Scintrex, Inc., Salt Lake City, Utah 84116).

References

V. E. Archer, J. K. Wagoner and F. E. Lundin, Jr. Cancer mortality among uranium mill workers. J. Occ. Med. 15: 11 - 14, 1973.

M. Eisenbud and J. A. Quigley. Industrial hygiene of uranium processing. Arch. Ind. Health 14: 12 - 22, 1956.

R. L. Fischoff. The relationship between and the importance of the dimensions of uranium particles dispersed in air and the excretion of uranium in the urine. Am. Ind. Hyg. Asso. J. 26: 26 - 33, 1965.

E. I. Hamilton. Uranium content of normal blood. Nature 227: 501 - 502, 1970.

H. H. Kramer, V. J. Molinski and H. W. Nass. Urinalysis for uranium-235 and uranium-238 by neutron activation analysis. Health Physics 13: 27 - 30, 1967.

M. Lippmann. Environmental exposure to uranium compounds. Arch. Ind. Health 20: 211 - 226, 1959.

M. Lippmann, L. D. Y. Ong and W. B. Harris. The significance of urine uranium excretion data. Am. Ind. Hyg. Asso. J. 25: 43 - 54, 1964.

M. Picer and P. Strohal. Determination of thorium and uranium in biological materials. Anal. Chim. Acta. 40: 131 - 136, 1968.

G. R. Price, R. J. Ferretti and S. Schwartz. Fluorophotometric determination of uranium. Anal. Chem. 25: 322 - 331, 1953.

G. A. Welford, R. S. Morse and J. S. Alercio. Urinary uranium levels in non-exposed individuals. Am. Ind. Hyg. Asso. J. 21: 68 - 70, 1960.

Urine Uranium by Fluorescence Spectrometry

Principle:

An aliquot of urine is dried and fused with solid sodium fluoride. The fluorescence of the uranium compound which is formed is measured in a specially designed photoelectric fluorometer.

Reagents:

Stock solution — 1 mg/mL uranium ion in water
Urine standards — 50, 100, 200, 500 and 1000 μg/L (prepare fresh)
Sodium fluoride
Platinum dishes

Instrumental Conditions:

Fluorescence spectrophotometer for uranium analysis, designed and constructed by the Argonne National Laboratory, Argonne, Illinois (Price et al., 1953). Excite at 365 nm and measure the yellow-green fluorescence.

Procedure:

1. Transfer 100 μL of urine to a shallow platinum dish of 1.5 cm diameter. Evaporate the specimen to dryness under a heat lamp.
2. Add 90 mg NaF and fuse by holding the dish in the flame of a Meker burner, or by placing in a muffle furnace with an oxygen-free atmosphere.
3. Allow the disc of fused salt to cool and measure the fluorescence produced when the disc is irradiated at 365 nm in the fluorometer. Subtract the fluorescence of a urine blank from that of each standard and specimen.

Calculation:

Calculation is based on a standard curve prepared each time an analysis is performed. This procedure cannot be controlled by the usual methods due to the instability of dilute uranium solutions.

Evaluation:

Sensitivity: 5 μg/L
Linearity: 5 - 1000 μg/L
C.V.: <10%
Relative recovery: not established

Interferences:

With the possible exception of cerium, no element besides uranium has been shown to produce measurable fluorescence under the conditions employed. Urine blanks should be analyzed in each of the platinum dishes to be used in order to verify uniformly low background fluorescence. The method of standard additions may improve the accuracy of the procedure by correcting for the variations in fluorescent behavior of each specimen.

VANADIUM

Occurrence and Usage. Vanadium has many minor industrial uses, including its incorporation into dyes, paints and insecticides, but its primary use is as an alloying agent in the production of hard steel. In this process, it is encountered as vanadium pentoxide, which may be inhaled by workers as a dust or fume. The current threshold limit values for vanadium as a dust or fume are 0.5 and 0.05 mg/m^3, respectively. Vanadium is a trace element in biological systems, but is not considered essential for higher animals. The estimated average daily dietary intake of the metal is 20 μg.

Blood Concentrations. Using an indirect colorimetric method, blood vanadium concentrations in normal subjects were found to be generally less than 10 $\mu g/L$ (Allaway et al., 1968). Schroeder et al. (1963) reported serum vanadium concentrations averaging 420 $\mu g/L$ (range 350 - 480) in normal subjects; no vanadium was found in erythrocytes. Schroeder's very high values have been questioned by other authors (Myron et al., 1978), and are apparently the result of using a nonspecific analytical method.

Metabolism and Excretion. Of the 20 μg of vanadium which is ingested in the daily diet, most is believed to be excreted in feces, apparently unabsorbed. Normal urine averages less than 8 $\mu g/24$ hr of the metal, with an upper concentration limit of 22 $\mu g/L$. Vanadium is found in only trace amounts in most tissues in the body and data regarding body accumulation with age are inconclusive. Fat contains up to 90% of the total body burden of vanadium (Schroeder et al., 1963; Myron et al., 1978).

In subjects given 4.5 mg daily of a soluble form of vanadium, urinary excretion over 24 hours accounted for 5% of a dose; urine vanadium concentrations ranged from 53 - 296 $\mu g/L$ in the asymptomatic subjects (Schroeder et al., 1963).

Toxicity. Vanadium compounds are irritants of the skin and mucous membranes, and when encountered in toxic amounts cause primarily symptoms of pulmonary dysfunction. Workers exposed to vanadium pentoxide for only a few days may develop irritation of the conjunctivae, rhinitis, dryness of the throat, hoarseness, bronchitis with coughing and wheezing, dyspnea and pneumonitis (Sjoberg, 1956). Green coloration of the tongue is also associated with vanadium toxicity and is believed to be due to the deposition of vanadium salts (Lewis, 1959). Few systemic effects are seen in this disease and, once the worker has been removed from exposure, the prognosis is very favorable (Sjoberg, 1951).

Eighteen workers who were exposed to vanadium pentoxide dust at concentrations in excess of 0.5 mg/m^3 for a period of up to 2 weeks developed acute respiratory symptoms which persisted for nearly 2 weeks after removal from exposure; vanadium was demonstrable in urine at elevated levels, and it continued to be excreted for up to 14 days after exposure had ended (Zenz et al., 1962). Controlled human exposure to vanadium pentoxide at a concentration of 0.1 mg/m^3 for 8 hours produced mucous formation in the lungs and cough which subsided within 3 days, while a concentration of 0.25 mg/m^3 caused a loose cough which persisted for 7 - 10 days. The peak urinary vanadium concentration observed was 130 μg/L at 3 days after exposure; vanadium was undetectable in all urine specimens by 7 days following exposure (Zenz and Berg, 1967). Vanadium is a natural component of fuel oil, and workers have developed vanadium poisoning during cleaning operations on oil-fired furnaces. Several of the most severely affected men were found to have urine vanadium concentrations of 43 - 380 μg/L (Williams, 1952; Thomas and Stiebris, 1956).

Volunteers given oral doses of 50 - 125 mg of ammonium vanadyl tartrate for periods of up to six weeks developed green tongue, intestinal cramps, diarrhea and black stools; urinary vanadium concentrations ranged from 38 - 1300 μg/L and correlated roughly with the dosage administered (Dimond et al., 1963).

Biological Monitoring. Urine vanadium concentrations appear to correlate reasonably well with the degree of absorption of the metal. Normal urine concentrations were found to average 12 μg/L in control subjects and 47 μg/L in workers exposed to 0.1 - 0.9 mg/m^3 of vanadium as the pentoxide (Lewis, 1959).

Analysis. An indirect colorimetric procedure for determination of vanadium in urine is presented (Welch and Allaway, 1972).

References

W. H. Allaway, J. Kubota, F. Losee and M. Roth. Selenium, molybdenum, and vanadium in human blood. Arch. Env. Health 16: 342 - 348, 1968.

E. G. Dimond, J. Caravaca and A. Benchimol. Vanadium. Excretion, toxicity, lipid effect in man. Am. J. Clin. Nutr. 12: 49 - 53, 1963.

C. E. Lewis. The biological effects of vanadium. II. The signs and symptoms of occupational vanadium exposure. Arch. Ind. Health 19: 497 - 503, 1959.

D. R. Myron, T. J. Zimmerman, T. R. Shuler et al. Intake of nickel and vanadium by humans. A survey of selected diets. Am. J. Clin. Nutr. 31: 527 - 531, 1978.

H. A. Schroeder, J. J. Balassa and I. H. Tipton. Abnormal trace metals in man — vanadium. J. Chron. Dis. 16: 1047 - 1071, 1963.

S. G. Sjoberg. Health hazards in the production and handling of vanadium pentoxide. Arch. Ind. Health 3: 631 - 646, 1951.

S. G. Sjoberg. Vanadium dust, chronic bronchitis and possible risk of emphysema. Acta Med. Scand. 154: 381 - 386, 1956.

D. L. G. Thomas and K. Stiebris. Vanadium poisoning in industry. Med. J. Aust. 43: 607 - 609, 1956.

R. M. Welch and W. H. Allaway. Vanadium determination in biological materials at nanogram levels by a catalytic method. Anal. Chem. 44: 1644 - 1647, 1972.

N. Williams. Vanadium poisoning from cleaning oil-fired boilers. Brit. J. Ind. Med. 9: 50 - 55, 1952.

C. Zenz, J. P. Bartlett and W. H. Thiede. Acute vanadium pentoxide intoxication. Arch. Env. Health 5: 542 - 546, 1962.

C. Zenz and B. A. Berg. Human responses to controlled vanadium pentoxide exposure. Arch. Env. Health 14: 709 - 712, 1967.

Urine Vanadium by Catalytic Colorimetry

Principle:

An acid digest of urine is extracted with 8-quinolinol/chloroform solution to remove vanadium from interfering ions. The element is then back-extracted into aqueous alkaline buffer and mercuric ion is added to complex interfering halides. A reaction between gallic acid and persulfate ion is allowed to occur in which vanadium acts as a catalyst. The oxidation of gallic acid produces a red color which is measured spectrophotometrically.

Reagents:

Stock solution — 1 mg/mL vanadium ion (Fisher reference standard)
Aqueous standards — 10, 25, 50 and 100 μg/L (prepare fresh)
Concentrated nitric acid
70% Perchloric acid
Glacial acetic acid
Concentrated ammonium hydroxide
Quinolinol solution — 0.5% 8-quinolinol in chloroform
4 mol/L Ammonium hydroxide
pH 9.5 Buffer — add 100 mL 4 mol/L HNO_3 to 200 mL 4 mol/L NH_4OH and dilute to 2 L with water
0.035% Mercuric nitrate
Acid persulfate solution — dissolve 2.5 g $(NH_4)_2S_2O_8$ in 25 mL water, heat to a boil, and add 25 mL conc. H_3PO_4; let stand for 24 hours before use
2% Gallic acid — dissolve 1 g of gallic acid in 50 mL water at a near boil, cool and filter (prepare fresh)

Instrumental Conditions:

Visible spectrophotometer set to 415 nm

Procedure:

1. Transfer 10 mL urine to a 125 mL flask containing several glass beads. Add 10 mL conc. HNO_3 and heat at a boil for 15 min.
2. Add 2 mL 70% $HClO_4$ and continue heating for 20 minutes after white fumes of $HClO_4$ appear. If, after cooling, the solution turns dark, repeat the above steps until a clear digestate is obtained.
3. Transfer the solution to a 125 mL separatory funnel with water rinsing. Add 5 mL glacial acetic acid and adjust pH to 4.0 with conc. NH_4OH dropwise.
4. Extract the solution by shaking for 5 min with 10 mL of quinolinol solution. Drain the chloroform phase into a clean separatory funnel and repeat the extraction twice more, combining the chloroform layers.

5. Add 25 mL pH 9.5 buffer to the chloroform and shake for 30 min in a mechanical shaker. Readjust the pH of the aqueous phase to 9.5 with 4 mol/L NH_4OH, recording the volume added, and continue shaking for 90 minutes.
6. Transfer a 10 mL aliquot of the aqueous phase into a 15 mL screw-cap tube. Add 1 mL 0.035% mercuric nitrate to the tube, mix and incubate at 30° C. for 30 min.
7. Add 1 mL acid persulfate solution (prewarmed to 30° C.) to the tube and mix. Add 1 mL 2% gallic acid (prewarmed at 30° C.) to the tube and mix.
8. Continue incubation at 30° C. for an additional 60 min. Measure absorbance of the solution at 415 nm against a reagent blank.

Calculation:

Calculation is based on a standard curve prepared each time an analysis is performed. The standard curve is non-linear at the concentrations used in this application of the method, and so the standards must bracket the concentration of the unknown. This procedure cannot be controlled by the usual methods due to the instability of dilute vanadium solutions.

Evaluation:

Sensitivity: 2.5 μg/L
Linearity: not applicable
C.V.: 8.4%
Relative recovery: 94 - 98%

Interferences:

Molybdenum was the only element found to seriously interfere with this procedure. A 1000 μg/L molybdenum concentration will cause a 28% increase in the value obtained for a specimen containing 10 μg/L of vanadium.

VINYL CHLORIDE

Occurrence and Usage. Vinyl chloride is an intermediate in the synthesis of several major commercial chemicals, including polyvinyl chloride, and has been used as an aerosol propellant. The compound is a gas at room temperature and therefore industrial exposure is by inhalation. Prior to recognition of the carcinogenic effect of vinyl chloride, the threshold limit value was set as high as 500 ppm. Currently, this value is 1 ppm.

Blood Concentrations. Vinyl chloride has not been measured in the blood of exposed workers.

Metabolism and Excretion. The disposition kinetics of vinyl chloride have not been studied in humans. In rats, 69% of an absorbed dose of the compound is excreted in the 24 hour urine as products of metabolism, and an additional 1.7% is found in the 24 - 48 hour urine (Bolt et al., 1976). The half-life for urinary excretion in rats is about 4 hours. As much as 12% of a dose is excreted unchanged in the breath after exposure to 1000 ppm of the chemical in air, while only 2% is exhaled after exposure to 10 ppm. The urinary excretion products were found to consist of N-acetyl-S-(2-hydroxyethyl)cysteine, thiodiglycolic acid and an unidentified compound (Watanabe et al., 1976).

Urinary thiodiglycolic acid concentrations average 0.5 - 0.7 mg/L in unexposed persons and range up to 4 mg/L in workers exposed to 1 - 7 ppm of vinyl chloride (Müller et al., 1978).

Vinyl chloride concentrations in the breath of exposed workers, when measured from one to twenty hours post-exposure, tend to decline relatively slowly; the initial one-hour post-exposure concentrations in workers exposed to 25, 50 or 100 ppm of the chemical for 8 hours were less than 0.6, 1.5 and 3.0 ppm, respectively (Baretta et al., 1969).

Toxicity. Acute exposure to high concentrations ($>$10,000 ppm) of vinyl chloride causes central nervous system depression in man, with symptoms of dizziness, lightheadedness, nausea, dulling of the senses and headache (Lester et al., 1963). At least two fatalities have occurred in workers exposed for only a few minutes to vinyl chloride vapor while cleaning polymerization tanks; the chemical was not found in postmortem specimens of tissue during toxicological testing (Danziger, 1960).

Chronic exposure to lower levels of vinyl chloride has been found to cause degenerative bone changes in workers (Cook et al., 1971). Other significant chronic effects include circulatory disturbances, thrombocytopenia, splenomegaly, hepatomegaly and hepatic fibrosis; this condition is quite persistent following removal from exposure to vinyl chloride (Veltman et al., 1975; Berk et al., 1975). Angiosarcoma of the liver was first reported in vinyl chloride workers in

1974; the very high incidence of this rare disease prompted the reduction of the TLV for vinyl chloride to the current level of 1 ppm (Falk et al., 1974; Lloyd, 1975).

Biological Monitoring. Breath is one of two specimens which have been preliminarily investigated from the standpoint of monitoring worker exposure to vinyl chloride. The lowest atmospheric level studied in the single report on this application was 25 ppm; an 8 hour exposure to this concentration produced breath vinyl chloride concentrations which averaged less than 0.6 ppm when sampled at 1 hour after exposure ceased (Baretta et al., 1969). Whether such an approach is feasible at the current TLV of 1 ppm has not been determined.

Urine thiodiglycolic acid concentrations have been found to correlate roughly with atmospheric vinyl chloride at much lower levels, 1 - 7 ppm. However, this metabolite is found as a normal urinary component and is also a metabolite of other industrial chemicals and some drugs. Its measurement cannot yet be recommended for routine monitoring purposes (Müller et al., 1978; Müller et al., 1979).

Analysis. Flame- ionization gas chromatography, such as described for benzene and other volatile compounds (p. 39), has been found suitable for measuring breath vinyl chloride concentrations as low as 0.01 ppm (Baretta et al., 1969). It may be necessary to use more sensitive detection methods, such as electron-capture or mass spectrometric detectors, in order to apply this technique to exposures at the level of 1 ppm of vinyl chloride in the atmosphere.

References

E. D. Baretta, R. D. Stewart and J. E. Mutchler. Monitoring exposures to vinyl chloride vapor: breath analysis and continuous air sampling. Am. Ind. Hyg. Asso. J. 30: 537 - 544, 1969.

P. D. Berk, J. F. Martin and J. G. Waggoner. Persistence of vinyl chloride-induced liver injury after cessation of exposure. Ann. N.Y. Acad. Sci. 246: 70 - 77, 1975.

H. M. Bolt, H. Kappus, A. Buchter and W. Bolt. Disposition of (1,2-^{14}C) vinyl chloride in the rat. Arch. Tox. 35: 153 - 162, 1976.

W. A. Cook, P. M. Giever, B. D. Dinman and H. J. Magnuson. Occupational acroosteolysis. II. An industrial hygiene study. Arch. Env. Health 22: 74 - 82, 1971.

H. Danziger. Accidental poisoning by vinyl chloride: report of two cases. Can. Med. Asso. J. 82: 828 - 830, 1960.

H. Falk, J. L. Creech, Jr., C. W. Heath, Jr. et al. Hepatic disease among workers at a vinyl chloride polymerization plant. J. Am. Med. Asso. 230: 59 - 63, 1974.

D. Lester, L. A. Greenberg and W. R. Adams. Effects of single and repeated exposures of humans and rats to vinyl chloride. Am. Ind. Hyg. Asso. J. 24: 265 - 275, 1963.

J. W. Lloyd. Angiosarcoma of the liver in vinyl chloride/polyvinyl chloride workers. J. Occ. Med. 17: 333 - 334, 1975.

G. Müller, K. Norpoth, E. Kusters et al. Determination of thiodiglycolic acid in urine specimens of vinyl chloride exposed workers. Int. Arch. Occ. Env. Health 41: 199 - 205, 1978.

G. Müller, K. Norpoth and R. H. Wickramasinghe. An analytical method, using GC - MS, for the quantitative determination of urinary thiodiglycolic acid. Int. Arch. Occ. Env. Health 44: 185 - 191, 1979.

P. G. Watanabe, G. R. McGowan, E. O. Madrid and P. J. Gehring. Fate of (^{14}C) vinyl chloride following inhalation exposure in rats. Tox. App. Pharm. 37: 49 - 59, 1976,

G. Veltman, C. E. Lange, S. Jühe et al. Clinical manifestations and course of vinyl chloride disease. Ann. N.Y. Acad. Sci. 246: 6 - 17, 1975.

WARFARIN

Occurrence and Usage. Warfarin is a synthetic vitamin K antagonist which was first developed at the Wisconsin Alumni Research Foundation in 1947. It is available as the sodium salt of the racemic mixture for use as an anticoagulant in oral doses of 2 - 25 mg daily; loading doses of 40 - 75 mg are sometimes administered when initiating therapy. The compound is also found in commercial animal baits in a concentration of 0.025%. Industrial exposure is generally by inhalation or absorption through the skin. The current threshold limit value is 0.1 mg/m^3.

Blood Concentrations. A single oral dose of 20 mg of warfarin produced a plasma concentration of 2.7 mg/L at 1 hour, declining to 2.1 mg/L by 5 hours and 1.2 mg/L by 24 hours (Midha et al., 1974). Following a single oral loading dose of 1.5 mg/kg (105 mg/70 kg) administered to 30 subjects, plasma warfarin concentrations averaged 8.8 mg/L (range 6.4 - 11.8) after 24 hours and 4.3 mg/L (range 2.4 - 6.0) after 72 hours, with a mean half-life of 47 hours. Fifteen subjects who received chronic oral doses of 10 or 15 mg of the drug daily developed steady-state plasma concentrations of 2.0 mg/L (range 1.4 - 3.5) and 3.1 mg/L (range 1.7 - 6.8), respectively, by the fourth day (O' Reilly and Aggeler, 1968). Steady-state plasma concentrations in 23 controlled patients on long-term therapy with warfarin (0.04 - 0.22 mg/kg/day) ranged from 0.6 - 3.1 mg/L (Breckenridge and Orme, 1973). In a subject with inherited resistance to anticoagulant drugs, a chronic daily dose of 75 - 80 mg of warfarin was necessary to achieve hypoprothrombinemia and resulted in an average plasma concentration of 25 mg/L (O'Reilly, 1970).

Metabolism and Excretion. Warfarin is metabolized in man by oxidation to 6- and 7-hydroxy derivatives, which are without anticoagulant activity, and by reduction to a pair of diastereoisomeric alcohols, which are apparently active (Trager et al., 1970). The R-isomer of warfarin, which is known to be less potent than its enantiomer and to have a longer half-life in man, gives rise to significant amounts of the alcoholic metabolite. Concentrations of this metabolite in plasma have reached 2.6 mg/L by 36 hours after a 100 mg oral dose of the R-isomer, compared to a metabolite concentration of only 0.5 mg/L after the same dose of the S-isomer. No evidence was found for the presence of conjugated metabolites in plasma (Hewick and McEwen, 1973). Less than 1% of a dose is excreted unchanged in urine, and essentially no unchanged warfarin is found in the feces (O'Reilly et al., 1962). Urinary excretion accounted for 16 - 43% of a single dose of the drug over a six day period, apparently as the 7-hydroxy metabolite (O'Reilly et al., 1963).

Toxicity. Warfarin inhibits the synthesis of prothrombin and several other clotting factors by the liver, resulting in reduced blood clotting activity and leading to internal hemorrhage in overdosage.

Poisoning with warfarin is an infrequent event, since a single dose is usually insufficient to cause significant depression of prothrombin time, and continuous intentional administration of the drug over a long period of time requires a great deal of perseverance. An amount of 567 mg taken as a suicidal gesture over a six day period resulted in a state of intoxication which was successfully treated by vitamin K administration (Holmes and Love, 1952). Dermal contact with warfarin solution on multiple occasions caused hematuria, hematomas, epistaxis and bleeding of the lip in a farmer who subsequently recovered (Fristedt and Sterner, 1965). Fourteen cases of accidental poisoning were described which involved the eating of corn meal containing 0.25% warfarin for a period of 15 days, with only 2 deaths (Lange and Terveer, 1954). A death due to warfarin was reported which resulted from the ingestion of 1 g of the substance over a 13 day period, with death occurring on the 15th day (Pribilla, 1966).

Biological Monitoring. The plasma warfarin concentration is well correlated with biological effects in most subjects exposed to the chemical. The plasma concentrations which are produced during exposure to warfarin at the current TLV have not been established, but should certainly be well under 1 mg/L to prevent significant anticoagulant effects.

Analysis. Ultraviolet spectrophotometry with measurement of the absorption maximum at 308 nm has found wide application (O'Reilly et al., 1962) and has been shown to be specific for unchanged warfarin in plasma in the presence of its 7-hydroxy metabolite. A liquid chromatography technique which can distinguish both warfarin and 7-hydroxywarfarin (Bjornsson et al., 1977) is also included for its better sensitivity to low levels of the compound in plasma.

References

T. D. Bjornsson, T. F. Blaschke and P. J. Meffin. High-pressure liquid chromatographic analysis of drugs in biological fluids I: warfarin. J. Pharm. Sci. 66: 142 - 144, 1977.

A. Breckenridge and M. L'E. Orme. Measurement of plasma warfarin concentrations in clinical practice. In *Biological Effects of Drugs in Relation to Their Plasma Concentrations* (D. S. Davies and B. N. C. Prichard, eds.), University Park Press, Baltimore, 1973, pp. 145 - 154.

B. Fristedt and N. Sterner. Warfarin intoxication from percutaneous absorption. Arch. Env. Health 11: 205 - 208, 1965.

D. S. Hewick and J. McEwen. Plasma half-lives, plasma metabolites and anticoagulant efficacies of the enantiomers of warfarin in man. J. Pharm. Pharmac. 25: 458 - 465, 1973.

R. W. Holmes and J. Love. Suicide attempt with warfarin, a bishydroxycoumarin-like rodenticide. J. Am. Med. Asso. 148: 935 - 937, 1952.

P. F. Lange and J. Terveer. Warfarin poisoning. U. S. Armed Forces Med. J. 5: 872 - 877, 1954.

K. K. Midha, I. J. McGilveray and J. K. Cooper. GLC determination of plasma levels of warfarin. J. Pharm. Sci. 63: 1725 - 1729, 1974.

R. A. O'Reilly, P. M. Aggeler, M. S. Hoag and L. Leong. Studies on the coumarin anticoagulant drugs: the assay of warfarin and its biologic application. Thromb. Diath. Haem. 8: 82 - 95, 1962.

R. A. O'Reilly, P. M. Aggeler and L. S. Leong. Studies on the coumarin anticoagulant drugs: the pharmacodynamics of warfarin in man. J. Clin. Invest. 42: 1542 - 1551, 1963.

R. A. O'Reilly and P. M. Aggeler. Studies on coumarin anticoagulant drugs. Circulation 38: 169 - 177, 1968.

R. A. O'Reilly. The second reported kindred with hereditary resistance to oral anticoagulant drugs. New Eng. J. Med. 282: 1448 - 1451, 1970.

O. Pribilla. Mord durch Warfarin. Arch. Tox. 21: 235 - 249, 1966.

W. F. Trager, R. J. Lewis and W. A. Garland. Mass spectral analysis in the identification of human metabolites of warfarin. J. Med. Chem. 13: 1196 - 1204, 1970.

Plasma Warfarin by Ultraviolet Spectrophotometry

Principle:

Warfarin is extracted from acidified plasma into ethylene dichloride, and back-extracted into dilute alkali. The final extract is analyzed by ultraviolet spectrophotometry.

Reagents:

Stock solution — 1 mg/mL warfarin in methanol
Plasma standards — 1, 2, 4 and 8 mg/L
3 mol/L Hydrochloric acid
Ethylene dichloride
pH 7.25 0.5 mol/L Phosphate buffer
2.5 mol/L Sodium hydroxide

Instrumental Conditions:

Ultraviolet spectrophotometer
Record spectrum from 360 to 290 nm
Measure absorbance at 360 nm and 308 nm

Procedure:

1. Transfer 2 mL plasma to a 15 mL screw-cap tube. Add 0.5 mL 3 mol/L HCl and 10 mL ethylene dichloride and shake for 30 seconds.
2. Centrifuge and discard the upper aqueous phase. Add 3 mL pH 7.25 phosphate buffer and shake.
3. Centrifuge and discard the upper aqueous phase. Transfer 9 mL of the organic layer to a clean tube.
4. Extract with 4 mL 2.5 mol/L NaOH. Centrifuge and transfer the aqueous layer to a quartz cuvette.
5. Determine the absorbance of the solution at 308 nm against a plasma blank. Subtract the background reading at 360 nm.

Calculation:

Calculation is based on a response factor derived from a standard curve. A quality control specimen containing 3 mg/L warfarin is analyzed daily.

Evaluation:

Sensitivity: 1 mg/L
Linearity: 1 - 20 mg/L
C.V.: not established
Relative recovery: not established

Interferences:

The procedure is relatively specific for unchanged warfarin in plasma, but is inaccurate at concentrations below 1 mg/L warfarin in plasma. Other acidic drugs which absorb in the same region of the ultraviolet spectrum as warfarin, such as dicumarol, thiopental and salicylate, may interfere.

Plasma Warfarin by Liquid Chromatography

Principle:

Warfarin and an internal standard, p-chlorowarfarin, are extracted from acidified plasma into ether. The concentrated extract is analyzed by reversed-phase liquid chromatography, with detection at 308 nm.

Reagents:

Stock solution — 1 mg/mL warfarin in methanol
Plasma standards — 0.5, 1, 2 and 4 mg/L
Internal standard — 12 mg/L p-chlorowarfarin (Aldrich) in water
0.25 mol/L Sulfuric acid
Ether
Methanol
Mobile phase — methanol/0.5% acetic acid, 1:1 by volume

Instrumental Conditions:

Liquid chromatograph with 308 nm ultraviolet detector
25 cm x 2.2 mm i.d. stainless-steel column containing Micro Pak CH-10 (Varian)
Column temperature, ambient
Solvent flow rate, 1 mL/min

Procedure:

1. Transfer 1 mL plasma into a 15 mL screw-cap tube. Add 100 μL internal standard and 0.5 mL 0.25 mol/L H_2SO_4 and vortex.
2. Extract with 5 mL ether by gentle agitation for 10 min. Centrifuge and transfer ether layer to a 5 mL conical centrifuge tube.
3. Evaporate ether to dryness under a stream of nitrogen at 40° C. Dissolve the residue in 25 μL methanol and inject 15 μL into the chromatograph.

	Retention time (min)
warfarin	3.3
internal standard	6.0

Calculation:

Calculation is based on a response factor derived from a standard curve. A quality control specimen containing 2 mg/L warfarin is analyzed daily.

Evaluation:

Sensitivity: 0.1 mg/L
Linearity: 0.1 - 4.0 mg/L
C.V.: 2 - 4%
Relative recovery: not established

Interferences:

Normal plasma components do not interfere with the assay. Fifty other drugs were studied for potential interference and were found not to co-elute with warfarin or the internal standard. The known metabolites of warfarin all eluted in 2 minutes or less and did not interfere with the determination of warfarin.

XYLENE

Occurrence and Usage. The three isomers of xylene (xylol) are often found as components of the petroleum hydrocarbon solvents used in paints, lacquers, cleaning agents, pesticides and gasoline. A frequent source of laboratory exposure is in the preparation of tissue specimens for histological purposes. Commercial xylene consists of 75 - 85% of the m-isomer and only about 5% of the p-isomer. Xylene is quite similar to toluene in its spectrum of toxicity and is well-absorbed after both inhalation and dermal contact. The current industrial threshold limit value for atmospheric vapor concentrations of xylene is 100 ppm (435 mg/m^3).

Blood Concentrations. Blood xylene concentrations of 16 workers occupationally exposed to xylene-containing paint ranged up to 1.1 mg/L at the end of an 8 hour working day (Engstrom et al., 1976). Volunteers exposed daily to 100 ppm of xylene developed blood concentrations of 1.0 mg/L; during exposure to 200 ppm blood concentrations reached 2.1 mg/L (Savolainen et al., 1979).

Metabolism and Excretion. The three xylenes are rapidly metabolized in man primarily by oxidation of a methyl group to the corresponding o-, m- or p-toluic acid; an average of 72% of an absorbed dose is excreted as these metabolites in the 18 hour urine in the form of glycine conjugates, o-, m- and p-methylhippuric acid. Ring hydroxylation of the xylenes also occurs, with about 2% of a dose excreted in urine as the corresponding xylenols, probably in conjugated form. Only about 5% of a dose is excreted unchanged in the breath and less than 0.01% unchanged in urine.

The extent and rate of excretion of the major urinary metabolites have been used as indices of exposure to xylene. Unlike hippuric acid, methylhippuric acid is not a normal urinary constituent. Urine concentrations of m-methylhippuric acid in persons exposed to m-xylene at concentrations of 100 and 200 ppm for 8 hours averaged 1.9 and 4.6 g/L, respectively, in specimens representative of the whole period of exposure (Ogata et al., 1970; Sedivec and Flek, 1976). The excretion of m-methylhippuric acid in urine continues to increase during an 8 hour exposure, but declines rapidly at the termination of exposure; the half-life of xylene as estimated by urinary metabolite excretion is about 1.5 hours (Senczuk and Orlowski, 1978).

Toxicity. Xylene at concentrations of 200 ppm and above produces mucous membrane irritation, nausea, vomiting, dizziness and incoordination. Blood xylene concentrations which exceed 3 mg/L, produced by exposure of sedentary subjects to 300 - 400 ppm of xylene, cause significant impairment of equilibrium (Savolainen et al., 1979). Air concentrations of about 10,000 ppm of xylene have caused unconsciousness in workers due to central nervous system depression and at least one acute death (Morley et al., 1970). Chronic organ toxicity has not been noted in man, but xylene does cause mild hematopoietic system toxicity in experimental animals exposed to high vapor concentrations for one to two months.

A lethal dose by ingestion may be as little as 15 mL of the fluid. In three fatalities due to the ingestion of gasoline or other xylene-containing products, blood xylene concentrations averaged 21 mg/L and ranged from 3 - 40 mg/L (Bonnichsen et al., 1966).

Biological Monitoring. The measurement of xylene in breath or blood is quite feasible at the levels to which workers are exposed, but this has not been done for the purposes of biological monitoring.

A substantial amount of experience has been gained with the use of m-methylhippuric acid concentrations in urine as an index of exposure to xylene. Since at least 75% of technical xylene consists of the m-isomer, this metabolite predominates in urine and its concentration appears to be well correlated with the atmospheric xylene level and the total dose of xylene absorbed by an individual. Urine concentrations of m-methylhippuric acid in specimens collected over the entire last 4 hours of an 8 hour exposure to 100 ppm m-xylene averaged 3.14 g/L, or 2.63 g/L when corrected to a specific gravity of 1.024 (Ogata et al., 1970). Senczuk and Orlowski (1978) have found that the dose (in mg) of m-xylene absorbed by a worker over an 8 hour period could be calculated by multiplying the excretion rate of m-methylhippuric acid (in mg/hr) during the last 2 hours of an exposure by the factor 4.94.

Analysis. Xylene may be specifically determined in blood or breath by the flame-ionization gas chromatographic method described for benzene (p. 39). A gas chromatographic procedure was presented in the section on ethylbenzene (p. 138) for the determination in urine of the methylhippuric acids as their trimethylsilyl derivatives.

References

R. Bonnichsen, A. C. Maehly and M. Moeller. Poisoning by volatile compounds. I. Aromatic hydrocarbons. J. For. Sci. 11: 186 - 204, 1966.

K. Engstrom, K. Husman and J. Rantanen. Measurement of toluene and xylene metabolites by gas chromatography. Int. Arch. Occ. Env. Health 36: 153 - 160, 1976.

R. Morley, D. W. Eccleston, C. P. Douglas et al. Xylene poisoning: a report on one fatal case and two cases of recovery after prolonged unconsciousness. Brit. Med. J. 3: 442 - 443, 1970.

M. Ogata, K. Tomokuni and Y. Takatsuka. Urinary excretions of hippuric acid and m- or p-methylhippuric acid in the urine of persons exposed to vapours of toluene and m- or p-xylene as a test of exposure. Brit. J. Ind. Med. 27: 43 - 50, 1970.

K. Savolainen, V. Riihimaki and M. Linnoila. Effects of short-term xylene exposure on psychophysiological functions in man. Int. Arch. Occ. Env. Health 44: 201 - 211, 1979.

V. Sedivec and J. Flek. The absorption, metabolism, and excretion of xylenes in man. Int. Arch. Occ. Env. Health 37: 205 - 217, 1976.

W. Senczuk and J. Orlowski. Absorption of m-xylene vapours through the respiratory tract and excretion of m-methylhippuric acid in urine. Brit. J. Ind. Med. 35: 50 - 55, 1978.

ZINC

Occurrence and Usage. Zinc is extensively used as an alloying agent in brass and other alloys, in metal plating (galvanizing) and for numerous minor industrial applications. Zinc chloride in finely divided form is produced in chemical smoke generators which are used for military and other purposes. It is also a component of many soldering fluxes. Exposure to zinc or its compounds is generally by inhalation of dusts or fumes. Zinc is an essential trace metal and is supplied in the daily human diet in amounts of 10 to 15 mg. The current threshold limit values for exposure to fumes of zinc chloride and zinc oxide are 1 and 5 mg/m^3, respectively.

Blood Concentrations. Serum zinc concentrations in 17 healthy volunteers ranged from 0.66 - 1.02 mg/L, averaging 0.83 mg/L; plasma concentrations did not differ significantly from those of serum, although erythrocyte zinc concentrations averaged 12.25 mg/L in normal volunteers (Kosman and Henkin, 1979). Low plasma zinc levels have been observed in dietary zinc deficiency as well as in various other disease states (Prasad, 1979). Whole blood and plasma zinc concentrations in healthy brass foundry workers were noted to be 46% and 22% higher, respectively, than those concentrations in healthy control subjects; the investigator concluded that excess zinc which is not immediately excreted is stored in erythrocytes (Hamdi, 1969).

Metabolism and Excretion. About 20 - 30% of the zinc ingested in the diet is absorbed from the gastrointestinal tract. Of the amount absorbed, about 20% is excreted in the daily urine and up to 60% is excreted in feces (Prasad, 1979). Zinc distributes to all tissues, notably the liver, muscles and bone. Normal urine zinc concentrations are from 0.3 - 0.4 mg/24 hr, but may increase to as much as 2.1 mg/24 hr in patients with albuminuria (Vallee, 1957). Urinary zinc concentrations of 0.6 - 0.7 mg/L were observed in workers exposed to zinc oxide at levels of 3 - 5 mg/m^3 (ACGIH, 1971). Healthy brass foundry workers exposed to zinc fumes excreted zinc in the urine at an average rate of 0.4 mg/24 hr (range 0.3 - 0.6), an increase of only 14% over normal control subjects (Hamdi, 1969).

Toxicity. Poisoning from zinc compounds is primarily a result of acute exposure. Symptoms of inhalation exposure to zinc oxide dust or fume include respiratory tract irritation, chest pain and cough; after several hours, typical symptoms of metal fume fever occur, such as chills, fatigue, headache, nausea, fever, respiratory difficulty and muscle pain. The effects rarely last more than 24 hours, and no fatalities are known to have occurred (Drinker et al., 1927; Sturgis et al., 1927; Rohrs, 1957; McCord, 1960). Urinary zinc concentrations of 0.4 - 0.6 mg/24 hr were noted in workers who suffered mild gastrointestinal distress due to zinc oxide poisoning (ACGIH, 1971).

Acute exposure to zinc chloride fume, while causing similar symptoms, has produced fatal poisoning in a number of persons exposed to high concentrations of the chemical during the generation of chemical smoke. Severe respiratory inflammation was observed in these patients who developed fever and a pale cyanotic color. Death was a result of acute pulmonary edema, bronchopneumonia or interstitial pulmonary fibrosis (Evans, 1945; Milliken et al., 1963).

A case of chronic poisoning due to dermal exposure to zinc chloride was reported in which the patient suffered leg pains, fatigue, loss of appetite and loss of weight. The patient's condition improved following removal from the job (du Bray, 1937).

Biological Monitoring. Occupational exposure to zinc has been shown to produce an increase in blood and plasma zinc levels, although this increase is not always statistically significant (Hamdi, 1969).

Urine zinc concentrations are known to rise in response to exposure to the metal, and have reached 0.7 mg/L in subjects who were exposed at the level of the current TLV. Urine zinc concentrations should be evaluated on the basis of each individual's background zinc excretion, due to the fluctuations observed during certain disease processes. These concentrations are not necessarily related to the severity of symptoms after acute exposure to zinc.

Analysis. An atomic absorption spectrometric procedure is presented for the analysis of zinc in urine specimens (Allan et al., 1968).

References

ACGIH. *Documentation of the Threshold Limit Values,* American Conference of Governmental Industrial Hygienists, Cincinnati, Ohio, 1971, pp. 284 - 285.

R. E. Allan, J. O. Pierce and D. Yeager. Determination of zinc in food, urine, air, and dust by atomic absorption. Am. Ind. Hyg. Asso. J. 29: 469 - 473, 1968.

P. Drinker, R. M. Thomson and J. L. Finn. Metal fume fever: IV. Threshold doses of zinc oxide, preventive measures, and the chronic effects of repeated exposure. J. Ind. Hyg. Tox. 9: 331 - 345, 1927.

E. S. du Bray. Chronic zinc intoxication. An instance of chronic zinc poisoning from zinc chloride used in the pillow manufacturing industry. J. Am. Med. Asso. 108: 383 - 385, 1937.

E. H. Evans. Casualties following exposure to zinc chloride smoke. Lancet 2: 368 - 370, 1945.

E. A. Hamdi. Chronic exposure to zinc of furnace operators in a brass foundry. Brit. J. Ind. Med. 26: 126 - 134, 1969.

D. J. Kosman and R. I. Henkin. Plasma and serum zinc concentrations. Lancet 1: 1410, 1979.

C. P. McCord. Metal fume fever as an immunological disease. Ind. Med. Surg. 29: 101 - 107, 1960.

J. A. Milliken, D. Waugh and M. E. Kadish. Acute interstitial pulmonary fibrosis caused by smoke bomb. Can. Med. Asso. J. 88: 36 - 39, 1963.

A. S. Prasad. Clinical, biochemical, and pharmacological role of zinc. Ann. Rev. Pharm. Tox. 20: 393 - 426, 1979.

L. C. Rohrs. Metal-fume fever from inhaling zinc oxide. Arch. Ind. Health 16: 42 - 47, 1957.

C. C. Sturgis, P. Drinker and R. M. Thomson. Metal fume fever: I. Clinical observations on the effect of the experimental inhalation of zinc oxide by two apparently normal persons. J. Ind. Hyg. Tox. 9: 88-97, 1927.

B. L. Vallee. Zinc and its biological significance. Arch. Ind. Health 16: 147 - 154, 1957.

Urine Zinc by Atomic Absorption Spectrometry

Principle:

Urine is diluted with water and directly analyzed by atomic absorption spectrometry. The method of standard additions is used for determination of the zinc content of the specimen.

Reagents:

Stock solution — 1 mg/mL zinc ion (Fisher reference standard)
Aqueous standards — 0.5, 1.0 and 2.0 mg/L
Glacial acetic acid

Instrumental Conditions:

Atomic absorption spectrometer with air-acetylene oxidizing flame and Boling burner
Zinc hollow cathode lamp
Measure absorption at 213.8 nm

Procedure:

1. Immediately after collection, treat urine with 1 part of glacial acetic acid per 100 parts of urine to prevent salt precipitation. Dilute 5 mL of urine with an equal volume of water or with one of the three aqueous standards.
2. Aspirate each diluted specimen into the flame of the atomic absorption spectrometer and measure the absorption. Subtract the value of a reagent blank (0.5% acetic acid in water)

Calculation:

Plot a curve of the absorption of each specimen versus the known zinc concentration of the diluted specimen (0, 0.25, 0.5 or 1.0 mg/L). The negative intercept of a straight line drawn through these points will be equal to the original zinc concentration of the unknown specimen. A quality control specimen consisting of pooled urine is analyzed daily.

Evaluation:

Sensitivity: <0.01 mg/L
Linearity: 0.1 - 4.0 mg/L
C.V.: not established
Relative recovery: not established

Interferences:

The method is highly specific for zinc. Caution must be taken during sampling and handling of the specimen to avoid contact with zinc-containing materials. All glassware should be soaked overnight in 50% nitric acid and thoroughly rinsed in deionized water before use.

INDEX

E

F

H

I

K

L

M

N